The State of Nutrition
in the Arab Middle East

VINAYAK N. PATWARDHAN
10 January 1905–8 July 1971

(Official U.S. Navy photograph)

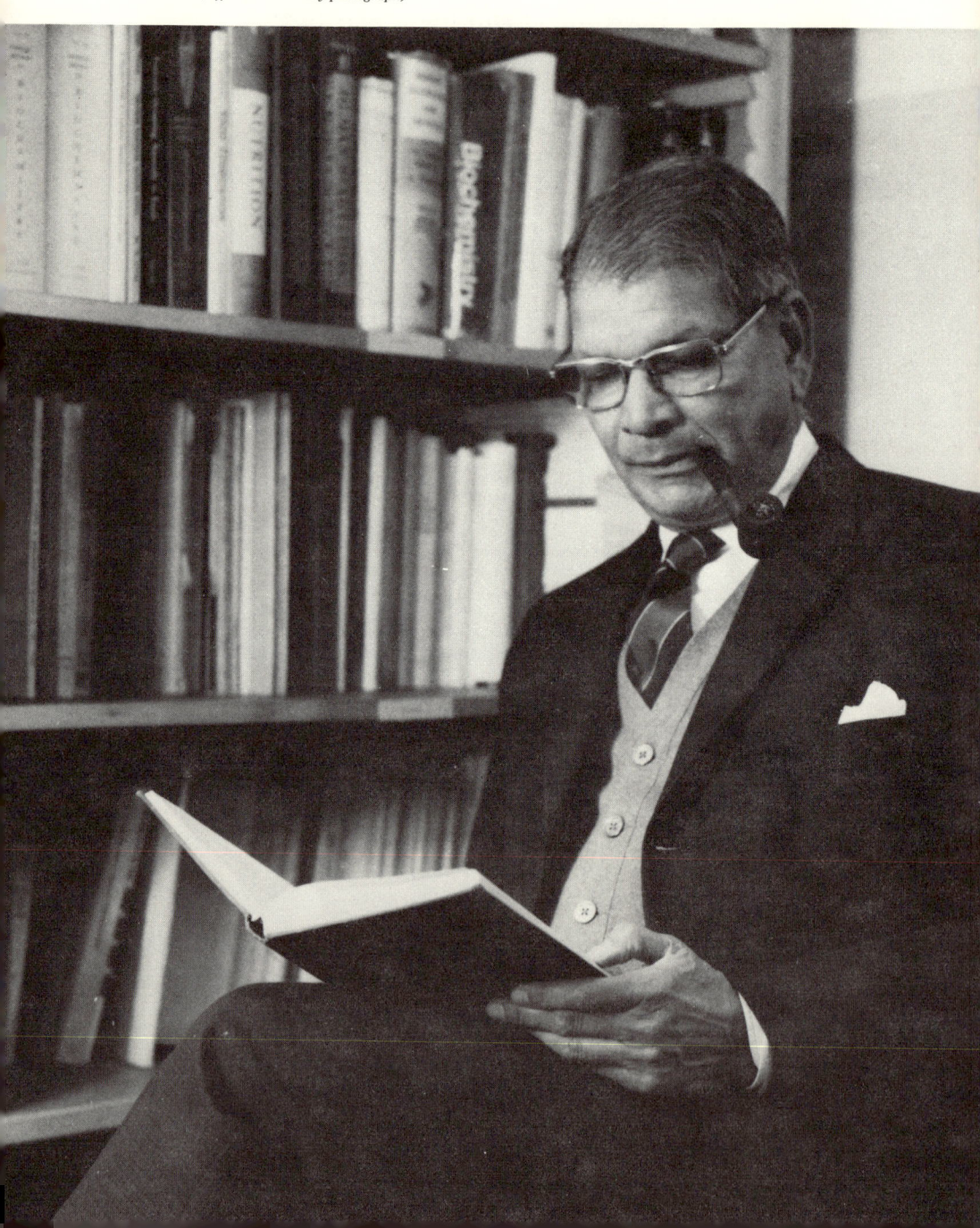

The State of Nutrition in the Arab Middle East

Vinayak N. Patwardhan, Ph.D.
and
William J. Darby, M.D., Ph.D.

VANDERBILT UNIVERSITY PRESS
Nashville • 1972

Copyright © 1972
Vanderbilt University Press

Library of Congress Cataloging in Publication Data
Patwardhan, Vinayak Narayan, 1905–1971
    The state of nutrition in the Arab Middle East.
    Includes bibliographies.
        1. Deficiency diseases. 2. Diet—Arab countries.
I. Darby, William Jefferson, 1913–joint author.
II. Title.
RC620.5.P37   616.3′9′00917671   73–123036
ISBN 0–8265–1162–7

Printed in the United States of America by
Edwards Brothers Inc., Ann Arbor, Michigan

IN APPRECIATION

It was my great privilege to be closely associated with Vinayak N. Patwardhan over a period of many years, during which he was successively Director of Nutrition of the Research Laboratories of the Indian Council of Medical Research, Coonoor, India; often an advisor to the World Health Organization and a participant in numerous joint FAO/WHO Expert Committees; a contributor to the work of the Protein Advisory Group of WHO/FAO/UNICEF; Research Officer for Nutrition, WHO; Chief of the Nutrition Unit at the Headquarters of the World Health Organization; and Professor of Nutrition, Vanderbilt University School of Medicine and Assistant Director for Biochemistry and Nutrition of the U.S. Naval Medical Research Unit No. 3, Cairo.

The impressive breadth of his knowledge, his wisdom and his tireless devotion to human betterment through improved understanding and application of nutrition were matched only by his integrity, his gentlemanly kindness and helpfulness, and his keenly critical acumen.

Through his death, international nutrition has lost a great leader, Vanderbilt University has lost a distinguished member of its faculty, and those fortunate enough to have been closely associated with him have lost a warm and wonderful friend and counselor.

William J. Darby

PREFACE

This book reviews the nutritional observations, research findings, developments, and needs as revealed by studies in several countries of the Arab Middle East. Its preparation was stimulated by the authors' increasing awareness of the wealth of material which has accumulated on nutrition in this region, much of which is not readily accessible because of the limited distribution of some of the journals, the unavailability to outsiders of many unpublished reports, and the paucity of reference by earlier reviewers to much of the material included here. There unfortunately exists a degree of scientific provincialism both in reading and credulity. Accordingly it seemed especially useful to prepare a comprehensive text on those nutritional problems and diseases which are associated with this region.

The intensive development of nutritional understanding has occurred in the Middle East in several phases. The last of these followed the WHO/FAO joint interests in pellagra and anemia in Egypt, the WHO-sponsored epidemiologic study of avitaminosis A in Jordan, the assistance from International Agencies and bilateral groups in the setting up of nutrition laboratories in several countries of the region, and the emphasis on the problems of malnutrition and broad nutritional interrelationships resulting from the ICNND Surveys in these and neighboring countries—Lebanon, Jordan, Iran, Turkey, Pakistan, Libya, Iraq, and Ethiopia. This phase has been marked by the establishment of a variety of continuing programs, examples of which are *inter alia:* The Department of Nutrition at The American University of Beirut, the National Nutrition Institute in Cairo, the Vanderbilt University–NAMRU-3 program of Nutrition Studies in the Middle East, the Ethio-Swedish Pediatric Clinic and the Children's Nutrition Unit in Addis-Ababa, and others, including nutrition interests in governmental ministries. Accordingly a rapidly growing body of information has accumulated. It seems particularly timely, therefore, to summarize critically the knowledge concerning nutrition in the region and to provide a bibliographic guide to reports in order to promote application of present knowledge, to avoid duplication of effort, and to identify needed additional information and fruitful areas for research.

The principal authors (V. N. Patwardhan and William J. Darby) have been intimately associated with a variety of nutritional developments in the Middle East and have collaborated with several of the active centers of research there. The senior author formerly served as Head of the Nutrition Section of WHO in Geneva. As faculty members of Vanderbilt University's Division of Nutrition they have been responsible for a series of intensive long-term investigations of nutrition in the Middle East, studies which have been based at NAMRU-3, Cairo, U.A.R. From this base and through other responsibilities with international agencies and bilateral programs they have a continued joint experience in the region of more than three decades.

Every effort has been made to avoid a mere recitation of regional observations. Instead, we have attempted to relate the work in the region to the development of nutritional knowledge so as to indicate its broader implication for nutritional science. Such contributions have come from the region more often than has widely been appreciated. These contributions have been made both by local scientists and by foreign investigators working in the region. The resulting nutritional and metabolic concepts have helped in clarifying the understanding of conditions and syndromes encountered in quite different milieu, including instances of conditioned malnutrition in industrialized countries.

Many opportunities exist for further elaboration of knowledge concerning ecology of malnutrition and application of such knowledge to prevention. The consciousness of governments and the existence of centers of growing activities in nutrition and related sciences augurs well for an accelerated application of such knowledge to the benefit of mankind, and especially for the betterment of the health of the population of the Middle East. If this book in any measure hastens or facilitates such application, the authors will feel more than repaid for their efforts. It is sincerely hoped, additionally, that it may contribute to a wider appreciation of the competence, resources and rich heritage of the region in the field of nutrition, as well as the vast opportunities for the future.

Finally, we would note that this might well be an example of a case study of a region which with profit could be repeated for many groups of countries with related characteristics, thereby contributing further to the international understanding through science and to the dissolution of scientific provincialism.

CONTENTS

	Preface	vii
	Acknowledgments	xi
1	The Arab Middle East	3
2	Food	19
3	Pellagra in Egypt	34
4	Anemia	57
5	Endemic Goiter	84
6	Xerophthalmia, Rickets, and Scurvy	99
7	The Zinc-Deficiency Syndrome	122
8	Protein-Calorie Deficiency Disease	141
9	Treatment of Kwashiorkor and Marasmus	175
10	Infant-Feeding Practices	182
11	Growth and Development of Children	192
12	Diets and Dietary Habits	213
13	Nutritional Status of Population Groups in Egypt, Jordan, Libya, and Lebanon	240
14	The Nutritional Situation in Iraq	267
15	Prevention	281
	Index	305

ACKNOWLEDGMENTS

We have great pleasure in placing on record our grateful acknowledgment to all those who have contributed in one form or another to the successful completion of this book. It is extremely difficult, nay, well nigh impossible, to include by name every one of those who have helped us in this task. We may, however, be forgiven if we mention a few of those to whom we owe a special debt of gratitude.

The late Professor Aly Hassan, Dr. Ismail A. Abdou, and Professor M. Rachid Barakat, experts in nutrition in Egypt, provided the sources of information, published and unpublished, without which our account would have been incomplete. Mr. Abdel Aziz Salah was extremely helpful in obtaining for us relevant information on vital statistics collected and published by the Ministry of Public Health. Miss Marguerite Aziz Farid helped with descriptions of food and food preparations in Egypt.

Miss Mona Doss, Adviser in Nutrition to the Regional Office of FAO in Cairo, and Dr. José Maria Bengoa, Chief, Nutrition Unit, WHO, Geneva, afforded us access to reports of surveys done in the Middle East under the auspices of FAO and WHO.

Dr. David Mollin, Dr. Zoheir Farid, Dr. Karim Kamel, Dr. Carol Waslien, and Mr. Louis Grivetti read and made useful comments and suggestions on several chapters of the book.

Dr. James P. Carter and Dr. Harold H. Sandstead wrote the section on treatment of kwashiorkor and the chapter on zinc nutrition.

Mr. Ahmad Sherif El-Tony prepared line drawings used as illustrative charts and Mr. Berge Sek-Zenian was responsible for photographic reproduction of these and other illustrations.

Captain Lloyd F. Miller, M.C., U.S.N., and Captain Donald C. Kent, M.C., U.S.N., successive Directors of NAMRU-3, permitted the use of facilities at NAMRU-3 and made many helpful suggestions.

National Institutes of Health, Bethesda, Maryland, furnished a grant, AM 08317 to Vanderbilt University, a grant 112501 under Public Law 840 to NAMRU-3 for investigations on nutrition which have added much to our knowledge on the nutritional situation in the Middle East. These grants also enabled us to undertake and complete the preparation of this book.

We are deeply indebted to our secretaries, Miss Alexandra Patsalidis and Miss Juanita Frazor, respectively, for their patience in typing and retyping the numerous drafts and for all the secretarial assistance uncomplainingly provided by them throughout the preparation of this book.

PERSONAL ACKNOWLEDGMENT

NAMRU-3

Captain Lloyd F. Miller	*Former Commanding Officer, NAMRU-3 (1964-1967)*
Captain Donald C. Kent	*Commanding Officer*
Mr. Abdel Aziz Salah	*Administrative Counselor*
Dr. Karim A. Kamel	*Head, Research Hematology Department*
Dr. Zoheir Farid	*Head, Tropical Medicine Department*
Dr. Carol I. Waslien	*Head, Biochemistry Department*
Miss Alexandra Patsalidis	*Secretary*
Miss Marguerite Aziz Farid	*Nurse*
Mr. Ahmad Sherif El-Tony	*Draftsman*
Mr. Berge Sek-Zenian	*Photographer*

VANDERBILT UNIVERSITY

Dr. James P. Carter	*Assistant Professor of Biochemistry in Nutrition*
Dr. Harold H. Sandstead	*Associate Professor of Biochemistry in Nutrition*
Mr. Louis Grivetti	*Anthropologist*
Miss Juanita Frazor	*Secretary*

OTHERS

Miss Mona Doss	*Adviser in Nutrition, Regional Office, FAO, Cairo, U.A.R.*
Dr. José Maria Bengoa	*Chief Medical Officer, Nutrition, WHO, Geneva.*
Dr. Ismail A. Abdou	*Director General, Food and Nutrition Institute of U.A.R., Cairo, U.A.R.*
Dr. Ali Hassan	*Adviser, Ministry of Scientific Research, Cairo, U.A.R. (Retired)*
Dr. Rachid M. Barakat	*Professor of Preventive Medicine, Cairo University, Cairo, U.A.R.*

**The State of Nutrition
in the Arab Middle East**

1 | The Arab Middle East

THE LAND AND THE PEOPLE

The terms Middle East and Near East are often used without any definite connotation of the territorial limits involved. There has never been general acceptance of their precise meaning. Historically, politically, and in military parlance, the limits of the region and the countries included in it from Libya to Afghanistan have varied from time to time. The United Nations agencies have added to the confusion, for the regions into which the world has been divided for their administrative purposes differ from one specialized U.N. agency to another. It is therefore appropriate to define at the outset the territorial limits of the region designated as the Middle and Near East for the purposes of this book.

The region covered by the account of food, nutrition, and health in this book extends from the longitude 10° East to 50° East, and the northern and southern boundaries are approximately 19° North and 40° North latitude, respectively. Within this area we have dealt with the food and nutrition situation exclusively in Arab countries, which are Libya, Egypt, Lebanon, Syria, Jordan, and Iraq. The inclusion of Saudi Arabia, the two Yemens, and the Emirates along the Persian Gulf would have covered all the Arab-speaking population in the Near and Middle East. However, so little was known about the state of nutrition in these countries that we considered it desirable to exclude them from consideration. It is to be hoped that this gap will be bridged in the near future by investigators interested in nutrition.

The purpose of this brief introductory chapter is to provide a background for the description of food, nutrition, and health of the people in these countries. It will allow only a bird's-eye view of the land, the people, their history and present conditions of life. We have kept this background description to bare essentials even at the risk of appearing to be sketchy and superficial in the treatment of the subject. However, a list of references given at the end of this chapter will indicate the sources of our information, and the publications could be consulted by those who need detailed information on any or all of the aspects dealt with in this chapter.

The Arab countries included for discussion in this book, apart from Libya, may be considered to form the fertile crescent. Egypt, with its river Nile, and Iraq, with the Euphrates-Tigris river system, form the western and eastern boundaries respectively of this crescent. Whereas the national boundaries of the other countries within the crescent are of recent origin, dating back no longer than the end of the first world war, Egypt has existed as an entity through much of its historical past. It is true that at various times in history the rulers of Egypt have held sway over territories much beyond the confines of the country, and Egypt in its turn has been subjected to foreign rules. However, in the final result its territory has undergone comparatively little alteration. Libya came into existence as a country only after World War II.

The region under consideration sits astride the lines of communication between Europe, Africa, and East Asia, and it has, as a result,

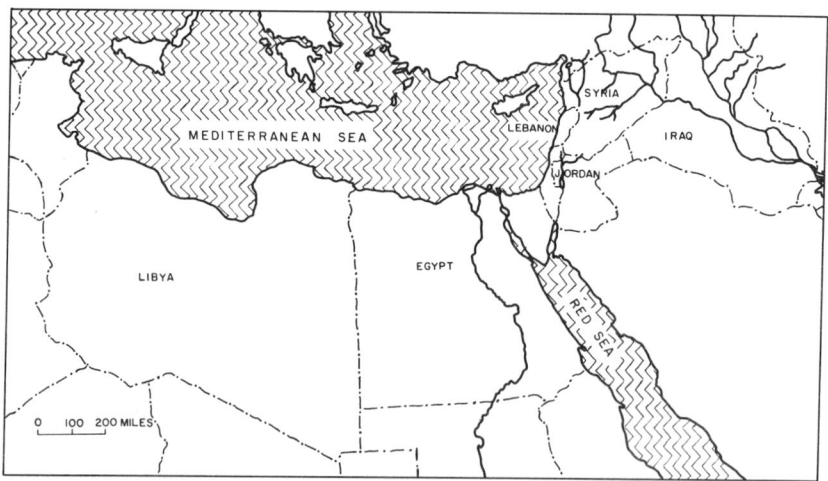

Figure 1.1. Map of the region showing the Arab countries discussed in the book.

The Arab Middle East

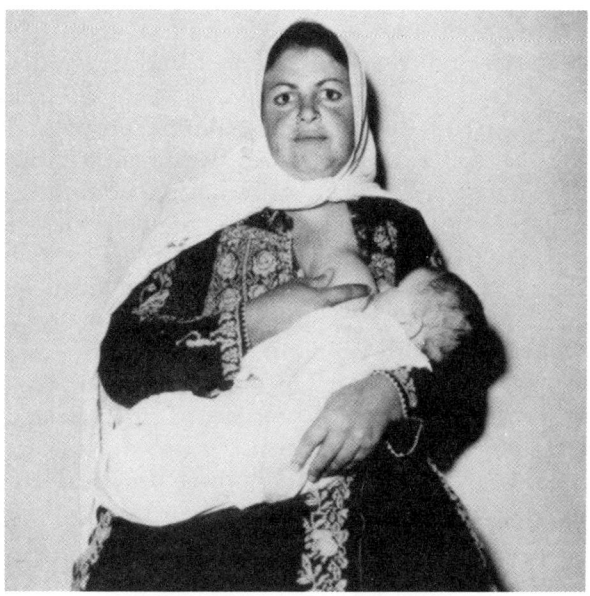

Plate 1.1. **Jordanian mother and child** (*Courtesy of ICNND*).

been subjected to influences from both the East as well as the West. In ancient times great civilizations flourished along the valleys of two great river systems, Euphrates and Tigris towards the east and Nile on the west. With the decline of these civilizations in the first millennium before Christ, Persians, Greeks, and Romans not only marched back and forth across these lands in their quest for new territories but also established themselves as rulers for varying periods of time. Of these the Romans were the last. When Rome was no longer powerful, the Orthodox Christian Byzantine Empire with its capital at Constantinople held sway over most of this region, till it succumbed in its turn to the advancing tide of Islam in a long, drawn-out process.

The followers of Muhammed the Prophet from the Arabian Peninsula, fired with the zeal to convert the world to Islam, conquered within the ten years between A.D. 632 and 642 the entire area from Iraq to Libya. They ruled over this region and even beyond for nearly eight centuries, which were punctuated by internal strife and wars with Persians, Mongols, and other invaders from Central Asia unitl the Turks conquered. The Ottoman Empire extended from Libya to Iraq and the Arabian Peninsula till the early part of this century. With the defeat of the Turks in the first world war, rivalry between the allied powers after the war and ensuing political adjustments resulted in carving out areas of influence in West Asia. From these finally emerged the countries of Lebanon, Syria, Iraq, and Jordan as we know them today.

Egypt, also a part of the Ottoman Empire, became virtually an independent state under Mohamed Ali in the early part of the last century. His successors, however, were not capable men. They had also to deal with the growing expansion and rivalry of the European powers among which Great Britain was then in the ascendant. Egypt became a British protectorate in 1882 and remained so till 1922. Thereafter, independent Egypt passed through many vicissitudes until the Revolution of 1952, which finally spelled the end of the British hegemony.

Further west, the provinces of Cyrenaica, Tripolitania, and Fezzan came under Italian influence between the two world wars. An independent state of Libya combining these three provinces was formed a few years after the defeat of the Axis powers in World War II.

The Land

The total land area covered by the six Arab countries is 1,221,600 square miles, made up as shown in Table 1. The figures for the total land area are approximate, as are those for the cultivable and cultivated land. No agreed authoritative estimates are available, as reference to any two reputable publications will show. However, for our purpose these figures serve as best possible approximations. The desert occupies 40 to 95% of the total land area in different countries. Only Lebanon has little desert area, but, as Lebanon forms less than 0.4 percent of total land area of the six Arab countries under consideration, this makes little difference to the picture.

Food production in all countries is limited to the coastal regions, the river basins, and other areas favored with adequate rainfall, such

TABLE 1
TOTAL LAND AREA IN RELATION TO ACTUAL AND
POTENTIAL FOOD PRODUCTION

Country	Total Area in Sq. Mi.	Cultivable Area %	Cultivated Area %
Libya	555,600	6	1.5
Egypt	386,000	5	4
Iraq	172,000	39	12
Syria	72,500	20	11
Jordan	37,300	9	5
Lebanon	4,000	60	44

The Arab Middle East

as plateaus and mountain valleys not far from the coast. In Libya the cultivated land lies along the coastal plains, on the rain-fed plateaus in the adjoining areas, and in the oases. An area of nearly 22 million acres is suitable for grazing camel, sheep, and goats. Of the three Libyan provinces, Fezzan, almost entirely desert, is the least suitable for agriculture. In Egypt the Nile Delta is intensively cultivated. In the region south of Cairo, also known as Upper Egypt, cultivation extends along the banks of the Nile to depths varying from a few hundred yards to well over 10 miles. The production of food is barely sufficient for its 30 million population. Lebanon is largely mountainous, with a narrow coastal belt and the fertile Beqaa valley between the Lebanon and Anti-Lebanon mountain ranges. Among the Arabs in the Middle East the Lebanese have made the best use of the cultivable land for production of fruits and vegetables. The production of cereals and grain legumes is of limited significance in Lebanon. Agriculture in Syria is also along the coastal regions, in the area fed by the rivers Orontes and Euphrates, their tributaries, and irrigation systems connected with them. In addition, bordering on the west and north of the great Arabian desert, lies a semiarid zone which with scanty rainfall forms the arable steppe and provides land for grazing. Jordan is largely an arid region, having only 9% of its area as arable land. However, the hilly region on the west bank of the Jordan is suitable for growing fruits and olives; the Jordan valley lends itself to intensive agriculture and horticulture, whereas on the Transjordan plateau seasonal rainfall and some irrigation make possible the cultivation of cereal crops. Agriculture in Iraq extends along the Tigris and Euphrates rivers with their irrigation systems. In addition, dry farming in the North is responsible for much of the wheat and barley production of the country.

The People

The inhabitants of the region from Libya to Iraq are known as Arabs. They are derived largely from the Semitic stock. However, they also provide an example of mixed ethnic derivation in which racial stock from Europe, Central Asia, and Africa have commingled to varying extent. Sumerians, Akkadians, Babylonians, Assyrians, Persians, Greeks, Romans, Arabs, Mongols, Turks, and Berbers have all contributed to the physical mixture and the resulting complexity of culture. In more recent times, slave trade in East and Central Africa, in which mainly Arabs were engaged, has introduced a negroid element into the population, but only to a minor degree. In Iraq, Kurds, who are ethnically different from the Arabs, form about 17%

of the total population. Another 8 to 9% is made up of Jews, Armenians, Lurs, and Turkomans, the last two originating in Iran and Central Asia.

The rise of Arab power initiated Arabization of the conquered people and their conversion to Islam. The process was well-nigh completed in the eight centuries of Arab rule extending from the Persian Gulf in the east to the Atlantic Ocean on the west, so that even before the Ottoman Empire became all powerful people in the Arabian Peninsula Syria (as it then was inclusive of Iraq, Jordan, and Lebanon), and in Egypt, and those living along the southern shores of the Mediterranean had all come to be accepted as being Arabs. Arabization of such a vast area was no mean feat, which in fact, should be considered unparalleled in human history. This achievement stands to the credit of the Arab civilization which flowered from the eighth to eleventh centuries, with its basis in the firm foundations of the Graeco-Roman and Persian civilizations which preceded it. Arts and sciences flourished. Chemistry has been rightfully claimed as an Arab science. Islamic medicine had its great proponents like al Rāzi and Ibn Sínā (known to the west as Rhazes and Avicenna respectively) whose learned works formed the basis of medical teaching in the Middle East and in Europe in the Middle Ages and even after the Renaissance. Islamic architecture can be seen in all its grandeur in Arab countries and in lands occupied by the Arabs in the past. The Mongol invasions in the thirteenth and fourteenth centuries, however, dealt a crushing blow to Arabs in West Asia. The rise of the Ottoman power in Asia Minor, which conquered Syria, the Arabian Peninsula, and Egypt, kept the Arabs in the Middle East under subjugation for nearly four hundred years. Conditions for the continued development of Arab culture and civilization could not have been more unfavorable.

Arab resurgence commenced in the last two decades of the nineteenth century. This gained momentum only on account of the 1914–1918 world war which saw the downfall of the Ottoman Empire. Since 1918 Arabs have gradually come into their own, a process hastened by the Second World War and the happenings during the two decades following its termination. However, it will take long years of hard work and assiduous efforts for the Arabs to overcome the degrading effect of the long Turkish subjugation, and it is difficult to predict when they will make up for lost time and take their place again among the advanced countries of the world.

Nomads and seminomads, collectively called Bedouins, form a sizable element in the Arab populations. The Bedouins lead a pastoral life, and their animals—camels, sheep, and goats—constitute their wealth. The several tribes of Bedouins lead lives independent of one another. Bedouins wander long distances in search of pasture and water for their animals. It is not unusual to find them covering hundreds of miles during their seasonal migration, usually reaching the same pastures year after year. In fact, rights to pasturage areas are jealously guarded. Life in the inhospitable desert environment has shaped the character of Bedouins, who are an independent, brave, and hospitable people. They are also suspicious and quarrelsome and have limited interests. In the past they often went on marauding expeditions, and the vast expanse of the desert made it difficult for the governments to control them. Recourse to modern means of communication and surveillance has gradually changed this, however. Some Bedouins have settled near habitations in villages on the fringes of the desert and have increasingly sought to adopt a farmer's life. These are looked down upon by the true Bedouins who consider agriculture a lowly profession and settled life a degradation. However, if the present tendency among the progressive Arab governments is any indication, serious attempts to settle the Bedouins on the newly reclaimed lands will be made with fair chances of success. U.A.R. has undertaken a large project with the help of the World Food Program, the object of which is to settle Egyptian Bedouins along the shores of the Mediterranean between Alexandria and Sollum in northwest Egypt.

It is difficult to estimate the number of Bedouins in any of the Arab countries, for census rarely reaches them and when it does they resist the counting of heads. In Lebanon their number is probably the lowest, since most of them temporarily migrate from Syria. Bedouins from the peninsula are known to go deep into Syria in search of pasture. In Libya, nomads and seminomads form nearly 30% of the total population. In other countries their population varies.

Religion

Islam is the religion of the majority of the population, and those belonging to the Sunni branch predominate. However, Muslims of the Shiya branch form nearly 50% of the Muslim population in Iraq.

Christians and Muslims are almost equal in number in Lebanon. The majority of Lebanese Christians are Maronites who are in communion with the papal church but form a distinct denomination. The original home of Maronites is Mount Lebanon, and they are in a majority in North Lebanon. Muslims predominate in the South.

Copts in Egypt form another sizable minority group of Christians who belong to one of the orthodox churches. Copts are the early native Christians of Egypt who resisted conversion to Islam and are held to be the true Egyptians. They form approximately 8 to 10% of the Egyptian population. Jews, Druses, pagans, Roman Catholics, Protestants, and Christians of other denominations form a comparatively small proportion of the total population in the six Arab countries.

In the early years of Arab conquest, the Muslim rulers showed tolerance towards Christians and Jews inhabiting the conquered regions. The process of conversion to Islam gradually gained momentum and ultimately resulted in the bulk of the population accepting Islam as their religion. Not so long ago people belonging to other religions were discriminated against and even persecuted. Although this has largely disappeared, there are undercurrents of antipathy and distrust against Christians which come to the surface at times of stress, particularly in a country where Christians and Muslims are almost equal in number. With a higher level of education and increasing understanding this state of affairs should probably improve.

Language

Arabic is the acknowledged language of the populations in these countries. The spoken Arabic may differ in different countries, and it usually does. The reasons for this difference are obvious. Many different ethnic groups have merged to constitute the present Arab-speaking people. The different vocabulary and language usage of these various ethnic groups must have influenced the spoken Arabic over the vast area which stretches from the Atlantic Ocean to the Persian Gulf. Fortunately, however, written Arabic is a common language understood by all. This has been a great unifying influence in addition to that of a common religion.

Population

Approximately 50 million people live in the six Arab countries under consideration. Egypt is the most heavily populated of these. The estimates of population as of 1965 and their respective rates of annual growth are shown in Table 2.

The over-all relative density of the population has little meaning in most Arab countries, since the bulk of the populations can be found in those areas where agriculture is possible and in large cities and towns.

The annual rate of population increase given in Table 2 is for the period 1950–1965. According to the U.N. population projections pub-

TABLE 2
POPULATION AND ANNUAL RATE OF GROWTH

Country	Population in Thousands	Annual Rate of Increase in Percent
Libya	1,580	1.5
Egypt	29,730	2.5
Lebanon	2,050	2.4
Syria	5,345	3.0
Jordan	1,972	3.0
Iraq	7,214	2.8

lished in 1964, and assuming a medium rate of growth, the population in these six Arab countries is expected to be more than doubled by A.D. 2000. This population will have to be adequately fed, housed, educated, and assured health and a reasonable standard of living. The countries concerned are fully aware of the challenge which this prospect presents and are doing their utmost to meet it.

Agricultural population in these countries is estimated to be around 55%, with the exception of Jordan, where it is 33%. The bulk of this population consists of small farmers, peasants, and landless laborers. Most of the land has belonged to town-dwellers who are primarily absentee landlords. Peasants work on the land as tenant cultivators, sharecroppers, or laborers, with only a few actually owning land. In Egypt land reforms of 1958 and 1961 broke up the large estates. A ceiling of 100 feddans (1 feddan is approximately 1 acre) per family was permitted by law, with the provision that land in excess of 100 feddans could be sold until 1970. This restriction is now to be enforced. The ceiling for individual holding has been reduced to 50 feddans. Estates of less than 100 feddans were largely untouched. By 1965 redistribution of land raised the proportion of land in small holdings of less than 10 feddans to about 75%. By and large, however, the general pattern of extremely small holdings was not altered, for the largest number of land owners (67%) still have 5 feddans or less as their family holdings.

Land reforms have also been attempted in Syria and Iraq, but their progress has been negligible as compared to the largely successful land reform in Egypt. As a result absentee landlords still own large areas of land, and the cultivation is done by tenant farmers under a share-cropping system. The landlords, being only interested in income, do little to improve the land and increase food production. The tenant farmer does not have either the resources or the incentive to do it.

The lot of the majority of the agricultural population has not been enviable. The peasant is tied to the land but is not in a position to benefit much by it. Poor to start with, faced with demands for taxes, giving a major share of the crop to the landlord, having to maintain animals necessary for plowing and to buy tools of his profession, the tenant farmer usually ends up with an income barely sufficient to maintain his family and himself at the subsistence level. Not infrequently he is in debt. Such a situation has obtained for centuries and is not unlike that which exists in many other developing countries. The absentee landlords, the economically better-placed town dwellers, and the government have thus far shown little inclination to improve the condition of the peasant, with probably a few exceptions. Informed observers agree, however, that the small tenant farmers are intelligent, hardworking, and capable of improving the yield of crops on the land they cultivate, if they had proper advice and financial resources and if the land tenure laws were such as to provide them with the incentive which they lack now. Although the land reforms enacted in Egypt after 1952 have effectively redistributed land and increased the number of small farmers, they have done little that is significant to improve his economic condition and that of the landless laborer.

It seems that in Lebanon this problem does not exist. A few large estates in the coastal belt are cultivated by tenant farmers, but in the mountain areas and the valley land is owned and cultivated mostly by small farmers. The farmer is not plagued by the obsolete land-tenure system obtaining in neighboring countries and possesses the incentive to derive fullest benefit from farming. In Lebanon modern methods of soil management and farming techniques are in use to a much greater extent than in the neighboring Arab countries. Furthermore, since the land is largely used for production of fruit and vegetables, olives and tobacco, it brings greater cash return to the farmer than would the production of staple crops. For this reason production of cereals and grain legumes forms a minor part of the total food production in Lebanon.

Education

In general the literacy rate is low, with the exception of Lebanon. Since the 1952 revolution Egypt has made great efforts to improve the situation by making primary education compulsory. In 1966-67 the number of students enrolled in primary schools had reached nearly 3.5 million. The significance of this number is in question because of appreciable proportion of absenteeism, which varies from

15 to 40%. However, there is little doubt that progress has been made. Literacy rates in Libya and Iraq were estimated to be between 10 and 15% around 1960. The situation in Syria and Jordan was probably comparable at the time. However, it is likely that during the present decade considerable progress has been made to improve the over-all literacy rate in all these countries.

Most of these countries have established an increasing number of preparatory and secondary schools and colleges of arts and sciences for higher education. Facilities for professional education in agriculture, engineering, veterinary sciences, and medicine exist and are continually expanding with national initiative and international assistance. Egypt is probably the most advanced among the Arab countries from the standpoint of educational facilities offered and the number of students benefiting from them. Considerable advances have taken place since the 1952 revolution. The number of schools and colleges has increased, and the university educational system has expanded. Recent statistics show that student enrollment at the universities in Egypt rose from 88,111 in 1959–60 to 144,981 in 1966–67, which is a 67% increase. Especially important is the increase in girl students, whose number rose from 11,600 to 30,800. This is a good augury for the future. Other countries in the region, with the possible exception of Lebanon, may not make as impressive a showing, but better things may be in the offing, given peace, stability, appropriate planning, and implementation of plans.

Economic Situation

Agriculture is the principal industry in these countries. Nearly 70 to 80% of the total working population earns its livelihood from land by engaging in direct cultivation; a further unestimated number is dependent upon the products of agriculture. A substantial, if not the major, proportion of the total national income is derived from agriculture and its products.

Among the natural resources oil is the most important. It is found in Libya, Egypt, and Iraq. Crude oil is exported and also processed for domestic use, the relative proportions being determined by the need for foreign currency, availability of capital and skilled personnel for refining operations, and the capacity for local consumption. Other mineral resources include phosphate, manganese, sulphur, chrome, etc., and further surveys may reveal fresh deposits. The existing resources are not being fully exploited because of their inaccessibility, lack of communications, and lack of skilled personnel. However, the mining industry is among those growing slowly in importance.

Considerable diversification in industrial development has been particularly noticeable in Egypt. Foods and beverages, textiles, metals and light engineering, electrical, chemical, and pharmaceutical industries employ nearly a million workers in Egypt. In other Arab countries, again with the exception of Lebanon, the tempo of industrial development has been rather slow.

In spite of the developments referred to above, the people in these countries are generally poor. Typical of most developing countries, there is great discrepancy between the incomes of a few extremely rich people and the mass of the population, which is poor. A bird's-eye view of the economic situation can be obtained by reference to the available figures for the gross national product per capita given in Table 3.

The increase in the total GNP for the developed countries is between 3 to 4% per annum. The estimate of the rate of increase for the five Arab countries for which figures are given above is 2 to 3% per annum per head. Considering the rate of the increase in the population of these countries, which almost equals the rate of increase in GNP per head, the present rate of increase in GNP apparently will make little change in the over-all picture in the near future.

With the discovery of oil in Libya and the rapid exploitation of this source of wealth in recent years, Libya must be in a much better economic situation than its neighbors, although no comparable figures for GNP can be given.

Health Situation

Only a very rough idea of the health situation in Arab countries in the Middle East can be given. Statistics are not of much help because they are often incomplete. Our main source of information in this respect is the reports compiled and published by the World Health

TABLE 3
PER CAPITA INCOME IN ARAB COUNTRIES (GROSS NATIONAL PRODUCT)

Country	GNP/Capita (1965) in U.S. $
Libya	—
Egypt	163
Lebanon	434
Syria	227
Jordan	270
Iraq	266
Average for Developed Countries	1,700

The Arab Middle East

TABLE 4
HEALTH STATISTICS FROM ARAB COUNTRIES[1]

	Iraq	Jordan	Lebanon	Syria	Egypt
Birth rate/thousand	17.8	45.5	31.6	29.3	42.8
Death rate/thousand	3.8	6.0	4.3	4.3	15.4
Infant mortality per 1000 live births	17.9	48.4		25.4	118.6
MCH Centers including prenatal and child-health centers	125	38		47	
No. of individuals who used these centers in 1963 or 1964:					
Women	17,635	82,735		18,231	517,941
Infants under 1 year	54,148	67,739		17,066	4,267,180[2]
Children 1 to 5 or 6 years	34,741	71,720		9,298	

1. Corresponding figures for Libya are not to be found in this report, and data for Lebanon, incomplete as they are, have been taken from ICNND Nutrition Survey Report, 1962.
2. Number of consultations.

Organization from time to time. Table 4, which is based on the figures contained in the Third Report of the World Health Situation, 1961–1964, published in 1967, provides some basic information which may be of interest.

The first impression one forms after scrutinizing this table is that the statistics reported from some of these countries must be incomplete and hence do not represent the actual situation. Figures for birth and death rates and infant mortality rates would obviously fall within this category. Birth rates are probably nearer to the truth, although birth registration must have been impossible to enforce and was evaded in many instances. Except for Egypt the death rates reported are half or less than half of those reported from the developed countries such as the United Kingdom, United States, and Soviet Union. Then again the reported infant mortality rates are unbelievably low for Iraq and Syria. The opening sentence in the chapter on Public Health and Welfare in Iraq by Harris (1958) mentions that 300 out of every thousand persons born in Iraq die in infancy. It is unbelievable that within a space of seven years, infant mortality has come down to the 17.9 per thousand live births found in the WHO Report. When one compares this figure with the infant mortality rates of 19 in the United Kingdom, 26.1 in the Soviet Union, and 23.7 in the United States with their highly developed health services, healthy environments, adequately nourished populations, and freedom from infections, one is driven to the conclusion that there is something wanting in the Iraqi and Syrian statistics reported to the World Health Organization. We do not wish to convey the impression that faulty statistics are being reported to WHO in order deliberately to mislead the people. WHO as well as the countries concerned know that such statistics from most developing countries are incomplete and not very useful for indicating the health situation in a country or to evaluate the progress of ameliorative projects. The defect lies in the lack of basic health services because of lack of resources and trained personnel. This becomes evident by looking at the bottom four sets of figures, which pertain to the number of maternal- and child-health centers and the number of pregnant women, infants, and children benefiting from the services offered. They must be considered totally inadequate when viewed in terms of the total population of the country. Between Syria, Jordan, and Iraq, Jordan provides a larger coverage than the other two. In contrast, Egypt is fairly well provided with basic health services, and this is reflected in the credible reporting of vital statistics from the country.

Since 1942 Egypt has undertaken plans to improve basic health services. Beginning with the year 1955 a system of combined units intended for the rural population and comprising divisions of health, education, and agricultural and social affairs has been developed, with the ultimate objective of providing such units throughout the country at the rate of one unit for every 5,000 population. Up until 1968, 315 combined units were established in different provinces known as governorates. In addition, there were 1,410 rural health centers which provided services in the fields of maternal and child health, communicable diseases control, diagnosis and treatment of diseases, and guidance in environmental health. Health statistics provided by the Egyptian government, with the help of its widespread health service, approximate the existing situation more than do those of other countries in the region.

It is to be regretted that no comparable health statistics can be found for Libya in WHO reports until 1966. Perhaps, however, it is better so in view of the unreliability of statistics from some other countries. On the other hand, Lebanon, which is known to be educationally and technologically well advanced and is also considered to be progressive, has not provided health statistics for reasons which we cannot fathom.

Communicable Diseases

Malaria is endemic in most of these countries. Malaria eradication programs sponsored and directed by WHO have made great progress in all of them. However, an appreciable number of new cases is reported every year. Bilharziasis and ankylostomiasis are endemic in Egypt and Iraq, principally, and present a major public health problem in both countires. Trachoma is another important problem in all these countries. In addition, food- and water-borne diseases occur frequently because of poor sanitary environment and unhygienic practices. Immunization programs for smallpox, diphtheria, tetanus, and whooping cough are undertaken in different countries with varying degrees of coverage and success. The total picture is not reassuring. One can only express the hope that the governments concerned are conscious of the problems in public health and are doing their best to improve the situation.

The current health situation has to be viewed in terms of the trained medical and paramedical personnel available in these countries. The number of doctors in five of these countries in 1963–64 in relation to the population is as follows: Iraq 1:4900; Jordan 1:4700; Lebanon 1:1600; Syria 1:5400; and U.A.R. 1:2500. Here again no figures are available for Libya. The existence of a large number of doctors does not necessarily mean better health services. A variable proportion of qualified personnel is engaged in private practice, mostly in towns and cities. They are of little use to the rural population. However, the large number of doctors in a country implies that a fair proportion of them can be available to the government for manning its health service. There is also great shortage of trained paramedical personnel needed to man the basic health services, special health projects, and hospitals in these countries. Considerable effort will be needed to fill this gap.

REFERENCES

Atlas of the Arab World and the Middle East. 1960. London and New York: Macmillan and Co., Ltd.
Ayrout, H. H. 1963. *The Egyptian Peasant.* London: Beacon Press.
Berger, M. 1964. *The Arab World Today.* Garden City, New York: Doubleday and Co., Inc., Anchor Books.
Fedden, H. R. 1965. *Syria and Lebanon.* London: John Murray.
Fisher, W. B. 1957. *The Middle East: A Physical, Social and Regional Geography.* London: Methuen and Co.
Harris, G. L. 1958. *Iraq Its People, Its Society, Its Culture.* New Haven, Conn.: Hraf Press.
Hitti, P. K. 1964. *History of the Arabs: From the Earliest Times to the Present.* 8th ed. New York and London: Macmillan and Co., Ltd.

Indicative World Plan for Agricultural Development 1965-85. 1966. Vols. I and II, *Near East.* Rome: Food and Agriculture Organization of the United Nations.

Lerner, D. 1958. *The Passing of Traditional Society: Modernizing the Middle East.* New York: The Free Press.

Mansfield, P. 1965. *Nasser's Egypt.* Baltimore, Maryland: Penguin Books, Penguin African Library.

May, J. M. 1961. *The Ecology of Malnutrition in the Far and Near East.* New York: Hafner Publ. Co., Inc.

May, J. M. 1967. *The Ecology of Malnutrition in Northern Africa.* New York: Hafner Publ. Co., Inc.

Rizk, F. 1968. Rural Health Services in U.A.R. *J. Egypt. Publ. Health Assoc.* 43: 3.

Sanger, R. H. 1963. *Where the Jordan Flows.* Washington, D.C.: The Middle East Institute.

World Health Organization. 1967. *Third World Report on the World Health Situation 1961-1964.* Geneva, Switzerland.

Wilcocks, C. 1962. *Aspects of Medical Investigation in Africa.* University of London, Heath Clark Lectures. London: Oxford University Press.

2 | Food

The vast land area inhabited by the Arabs, which stretches from the Atlantic Ocean to the Persian Gulf and Arabian Sea, offers extremely limited potential for food production, due to unfavorable geographic features. In the countries of the Near East and in Libya, the desert occupies from 40% to more than 95% of the land area, except in Lebanon and Syria. The cultivated area in these countries ranges from 2.5 to 12.3% of the total land area. Rainfall varies greatly, from the average annual precipitation of almost nil to more than 600 mm. The climate of the coastal regions along the Mediterranean is temperate to subtropical; in the interior it is typical of the desert with extremes of temperature and little or no rainfall. Methods of food production, storage, and marketing are still unsophisticated in most cases. Thus the limited area of cultivated and cultivable land, extremes of temperature, shortage of water, inadequate facilities for irrigation, insufficient use of fertilizers, lack of pest-control measures, and possibly inappropriate local laws of land tenure are severally and collectively responsible for the low level of food production and its inability to keep pace with the increasing population. Furthermore, food-processing industries, although they are gradually expanding in scope and production in these countries, have yet to make their full impact on food preservation and to ameliorate the situation with regard to available food supplies. Lebanon is one exception, for in this small country improved agricultural practices are current and a variety of food-processing industries has been established.

The food crops grown in the Near East comprise a variety of cereals, legumes, vegetables, and fruits. Some of these have been cultivated in these lands since ancient times. Other food crops, such as rice, sugar cane, mangoes, and bananas, have been introduced at various times from other countries in Asia. Still others, for example maize and potato, came from the New World through Europe. As elsewhere, soil, climate, rainfall, and availability of river water for irrigation must have influenced the particular types of food crops grown in different countries within the region.

FOOD PRODUCTION AND USAGE

Cereals. Wheat is the staple cereal cultivated in all countries from Libya to Iraq, although the production today is not sufficient to satisfy the needs of the population. Wheat heads the list of the cereals grown in Lebanon, Syria, and Jordan and comes second in Egypt, Libya, and Iraq. Barley is next in importance, except in Egypt. Its importance as a food crop, however, has gradually diminished; the consumption of barley is confined mainly to the desert areas. Maize has established itself as the most important cereal crop in Egypt, whereas it is a minor crop in other countries of the region. Sorghum is grown in the dry areas of Egypt and Libya, where it forms the staple for the local population. The cultivation of rice, which is dependent upon plentiful supply of water, is limited to riparian regions.

Irrespective of which cereal heads the list of those produced in any given country, wheat is the most popularly consumed cereal in all Arab states, including Egypt. The people of the Delta region of Egypt willingly would, if they could afford to do so, replace maize with wheat or at least dilute it with wheat as much as possible. The production of rice is comparatively small; it features only occasionally in the poor people's diets, even though it finds a place in many popular Arab dishes.

Balady bread (*khubz* or *aish balady*) is the most popular type of wheat bread. It is made from wheat flour, milled locally or imported, or blends of both in varying proportions. Wheat flour, water, and a little salt are well mixed with yeast or starter dough (which may be the remaining portion of the previous day's dough) and manually kneaded into a soft dough. This is then divided into balls of convenient size and allowed to stand for about one-half to one hour. At the end of this period the balls are flattened by hand or by a rolling pin into rounds about one-half inch thick and 8 to 10 inches in diameter and baked in a preheated oven for about 90 seconds. The bread rises explosively during baking, suggesting that the leavening is more due to a steam generated during baking than to the fermentative action of the starter (Dalby, 1963). The loaf collapses on removal from the oven, and the final product is a flat round loaf about an inch thick. It is separable into the hard upper crust and the spongy lower portion, with a pocket in between. This pocket serves as a space for stuffing with cheese, vegetables, meat, or pickles to make a tasty sandwich. *Aish shamy,* a Syrian type of bread, is made by brushing the once-baked bread with water and placing it in the oven again for 2 or 3 minutes. White flour is used for making *aish shamy* dough.

In towns and cities bread is almost exclusively made in bakeries. The procedures may vary slightly in detail, as Rizk *et al.* (1960) describe. In villages bread is made mostly in the homes, and neighbors usually help in the bread-making. The procedure is roughly the same as in bakeries. Enough bread is baked at a time to last the family for 8 or 9 days.

Another type of wheat bread known as *aish shamsy,* or sun bread, is made in Upper Egypt. The dough, prepared as in the making of balady bread, is flattened on a round unglazed clay tile covered with bran. It is then exposed to the sun for an hour and turned over to expose the other side for another hour. The partially sun-baked bread is then placed in the oven for final baking. This bread is stable for about a week.

Khubz balady or *khubz abyad* (white bread) is commonly consumed in Lebanon. However, a paper-thin bread, *khubz markouk,* is peculiar to the mountain regions of the country. The procedure for making the dough for this type of bread is similar to that for *khubz balady.* A ball of dough of appropriate size is manipulated deftly with hands by patting, pressing, and swinging, with the result that the dough assumes a round shape and gets thinner and larger in diameter. When it attains the desired size, it is flipped onto a concave flat iron pan heated on an open fire. It takes only a few minutes to bake. The making of this kind of bread requires great skill, which is passed on from generation to generation.

Some other preparations of wheat deserve mention. *Burghul* is parboiled wheat made either domestically or in large establishments. Wheat is soaked in water and boiled till it is soft. The grain swells and breaks open. Excess water is drained off, and the boiled wheat is dried in the sun. The dried product is coarsely ground and stored for future use. Both sweet and savory preparations can be made from *burghul* in combination with other foods. *Kishk* is *burghul* mixed with buttermilk into a soft homogeneous mass, divided into small lumps, and dried in the sun. As a mixture of wheat and buttermilk, it must be a nutritive product, although information on its nutritional assessment is not available.

Pasta made from wheat flour may substitute for bread or supplement it on occasion. It has become increasingly popular in Arab countries, and there are establishments which make it on a commercial scale.

In Lower Egypt, where most of Egypt's maize is grown, maize bread is made. Maize flour, to which is added fenugreek seed meal (about 3% by measure), is made into a loose dough and mixed with homemade starter dough. A fermentation time of about one hour is allowed. Balls of the dough are placed on a wooden board and flattened by hand at first; then the board is swung round and round till the dough spreads evenly into a thin layer. The bread is baked in the oven for 1 or 2 minutes. It is taken out and put back in the oven for a minute or two to make it drier still. The baked bread is preserved between layers of *berseem* (clover), which presumably prevents it from drying and hardening. This bread is then used for 10 to 15 days.

In Upper Egypt sorghum millet is the main cereal, and leavened bread is made from it in much the same way as bread is made from wheat or maize. It is known as *bétau*. The fermented dough is fairly loose in consistency and is not rolled into flat cakes like wheat dough. Ladlefuls of sorghum dough are dumped on a plate in a heated oven. The dough spreads a little as it bakes. Thinner *bétau* can be made from sorghum flour mixed with about 3 to 4% fenugreek seed meal. In areas where bread is made from maize and sorghum, wheat is sometimes used in combination with these grains. The proportion of wheat in the mixture depends upon its availability and the ability of the consumer to purchase the costlier wheat in preference to the locally grown sorghum or maize.

As has been mentioned before, rice is not one of the staple articles of diet in Arab countries. Its production is limited in extent and quantity. Egypt is the only country in the region, apart from Iraq, in which significant amounts of rice are grown. However for economic reasons a substantial proportion of Egyptian rice is exported, leaving limited amounts for local consumption.

Rice is milled before marketing. It is the milled and polished rice which is used as food, cooked either alone or mixed with a legume like chick-pea or with meat. Rice is first partially fried in a little oil and then cooked in water; only as much water as the rice can absorb is added, to yield a soft and discrete cooked grain. This method retains the thiamine contained in rice. In those countries of Southeast Asia where rice is the staple, it is usually cooked in excess water, which is discarded when the rice is nearly cooked. This results in losses in the nutritive value of rice. The difference in the two methods of cooking rice is worth pondering over, although one cannot find an explanation why among the people to whom rice means so much a wasteful cooking practice should prevail.

Legumes. Grain legumes are second to cereal in importance as food crops. Broad beans, haricot, lentils, chick-peas, and cowpeas are most commonly cultivated. In Egypt, however, *Vicia faba,* or the fava bean, is the most important grain legume. Fenugreek is also an important legume in Egyptian diets, for it is mixed with maize in amounts of 3 to 4% for making maize bread. Grain legumes are important sources of protein in Arab diets, containing total protein to the extent of 20% and more, as compared with about 10% protein found in most staple cereals.

Stewed beans and chick-peas and lentil soup are the commonest preparations of grain legumes. *Fool medammès,* a popular preparation in Egypt, is made by slow and gentle cooking of *Vicia faba* bean in large closed pots over a low fire for 16 to 20 hours. The excess water is drained off; oil, salt, and some spices are added. The stewed beans are either eaten alone or mixed with stewed lentils. A stew made from decorticated split chick-pea in an almost similar manner is known as *hummos. Taamiyah,* or bean cake, is another popular preparation based on beans. Broad bean (fava bean) is decorticated and soaked in water overnight. The soak water is discarded; onion, garlic, greens, fresh coriander, other spices, and salt are added to the soaked beans and the mixture ground into a thick paste. The ground mass is allowed to stand in a warm place. Amounts of 10 to 12 g are made into small, flat, round cakes and deep-fried in oil. Although the use of other legumes for making *taamiyah* has been suggested, fava bean is the only bean that is commonly used in its preparation.

Vegetables. In winter and spring vegetables are plentiful, but they are limited in quantity and variety during the dry summer months. It is noteworthy that Arabs are extremely fond of eating green vegetables raw, as salads. Lettuce, tomato, green pepper, radish, carrot, leeks or green onions, and various leafy vegetables are eaten raw. Even the poorest follow this practice and unwittingly derive the greatest benefit from the consumption of green vegetables.

Other vegetables are cooked in different ways, sometimes mixed with beans or meat, seasoned with tomato sauce and spices, and eaten with bread.

Meat, Fish, Eggs. Beef and mutton are the most common meats consumed. Camel meat is not infrequently eaten. In Egypt water buffaloes provide another source of meat. Poultry is kept in rural areas in individual homes and is sold for cash, as are the eggs. The poor people in these countries consume meat very infrequently. In some cases meat consumption may be restricted to feast days in the year, which are few.

Libya, Egypt, and Lebanon have long coast lines; yet the production of fish is meager, and its consumption is mostly restricted to the coastal areas.

Milk and Milk Products. Milk and milk products are not unimportant articles of diet in these countries. Supplies, however, are not plentiful. The FAO estimates show that in 1966 the available supplies of milk per capita per day were 61 g in Jordan; 121 g in Syria; 122 g in U.A.R.; 130 g in Libya; and 353 g in Lebanon.

The cow is not the only important milk-producing animal in these countries. Other animals contribute substantially to the total milk production. In Libya, according to the 1960 estimates, animal milks were produced in the following proportions: goat milk, 42%; sheep milk, 25%; cow milk, 20%; and camel milk, 13%. In Egypt buffalo milk constitutes 70% of the total milk produced. According to the 1958 estimates, Egypt seems to have had as many sheep, goats, and camels as Libya. The milk of these animals must be important for populations, particularly in the arid regions. Current official estimates for milk produced in Egypt by these animals were not available to the authors.

The quality of dairy husbandry varies in different countries, as is reflected in the average milk yield in kilograms per cow per year, which was as follows for the years 1964–68: Jordan, 850; Lebanon, 2120; U.A.R., 674; Libya, Tripolitania, 417; Cyrenaica, 277. There is apparently a great potential capacity for milk production which can be harnessed to improve the availability of this valuable food for human consumption.

The high environmental temperature and the lack of organized facilities for collection, refrigeration, transport, and pasteurization make it necessary that the small producer sell the milk while it is still fresh or process it domestically for conversion into products before the milk is spoiled. The major portion of the milk that is produced is converted into a variety of milk products. An estimate made in 1959 for milk used in Egypt showed that 50% of the production went for making butter and clarified butter (*samna*), 40% for making soft and hard cheese, and only 10% was available for use as fluid milk. The skimmed milk remaining after the removal of butter is made into cheese, and this adds to the available supplies of cheese made from whole milk. The skim milk cheese is popular among the poor because of its low price as compared to the whole milk soft and hard cheeses. Another important item is the fermented product known as *laban* (*zabadi* in Egypt), which is comparable to yoghurt. Milk is boiled, cooled till it is tepid, inoculated with a starter, and left in a warm place. Lactic fermentation takes place, and milk coagulates within 8 to 10 hours.

Fruits. A large variety of fruit is grown in the region. It ranges from the types found in temperate regions to those found in the tropics. Citrus fruits are among the most important in all of these countries. Apples, pears, peaches, apricots, plums, grapes, figs, olives, watermelons, and bananas are also produced in appreciable quantities. Large quantities of dates are produced and consumed both fresh and dried. Fruits in season are included in the diets, more often in those of middle-class and rich people. In times of glut the prices may be low enough to enable the poorer people to consume fruit, which would otherwise be well-nigh impossible. In Egypt mangoes rank as an important fruit crop, and they are widely consumed when in season. Another fruit popular in Egypt is the fruit of prickly pear (*Opuntia*).

In Syria, Lebanon, and Iraq considerable amounts of nuts, such as walnuts, almonds, and pistachios are produced.

Oil Seeds. Among the oil seeds from which edible oil is manufactured are the cotton seed and peanut. Sesame is also cultivated, but it is mostly used in preparations such as *tehima* and *halawa* and is one of the expensive items. Considerable quantities of edible vegetable oils are imported in the region.

Sugar. Sugar cane is cultivated in Egypt and Syria as an industrial crop for the manufacture of sugar. However, large amounts of sugar are imported to supplement the local production.

Food Imports. The major food imports in the region are wheat and wheat flour, maize (except probably in Egypt), sugar, vegetable oils, and livestock. Considerable import and export trade exists between the countries within the region. Tea and coffee required for making the most popular beverages are imported.

THE STATE OF FOOD PRODUCTION AND PROSPECTS

It might be useful to indicate the extent to which the food supplies available for human consumption meet the nutritional needs in these countries. Food Balance Sheets published every three years by the Food and Agriculture Organization (FAO) provide such information. These balance sheets are prepared principally from the statistics supplied to FAO by the respective governments. The production and processing of food within the country, including livestock and fishery, wastage of food in production and storage, needs for the seed, nonfood uses of the produce, and exports and imports are the various aspects taken into consideration by FAO before arriving at the figures for food available for human consumption.

There is an obvious limitation to the interpretation of these Food Balance Sheets. The statistics of food production in developing countries are far from satisfactory, as are also probably the estimates of wastage. The experts in FAO have to use considerable technical skill and experience to fill gaps in knowledge in preparing the final balance sheet (FAO, 1966). However, food statistics have shown gradual improvement during recent years, and the reliability of data on which Food Balance Sheets are based increases year by year.

Food Balance Sheets for the years 1957–59 to 1963–65 and the provisional estimates for 1966, taken from the FAO publication *The State of Food and Agriculture, 1968,* are given in Table 1.

The table indicates the food supplies available for human consumption per person per day. It will be wrong to conclude that every individual in a given country consumes the foodstuffs in quantities found in the table. What the table shows is that these amounts would be available to every man, woman, and child in the country, provided the food was equally distributed. This seldom happens in practice. The Food Balance Sheet indicates the capacity of a country in a given year to feed its population adequately or otherwise. Information on the actual levels of consumption can only be obtained by diet surveys in representative communities, an aspect with which we shall deal later. In the meantime some comments are necessary on the data contained in the table.

The estimated calorie supply in 1966 varied from 2,330 to 2,880 calories per capita per day. The lowest figure represents a marginal adequacy of calories for the population as judged by the FAO Calorie Requirements Report (1957) and by the norms set by the ICNND (1962, 1963) for Lebanon and Jordan. These norms should be applicable to Libya, Egypt, and Syria as well. Considered in this manner, the available calorie supplies in 1966 were adequate for the population of Syria, Lebanon, Egypt, and Jordan. In Libya they were not; however, there has been imperceptible improvement over the last ten years; for in 1959, the estimated available calorie supply was 1,870, whereas in 1966 it was estimated to be 2,340. The country has made a tremendous effort to increase food production. Since the population has also been increasing steadily, the available food supplies per capita had increased only a little by 1963–65. The preliminary estimates for 1966 present a more hopeful situation.

The situation is somewhat similar with regard to the available pro-

Food

TABLE 1
FOOD SUPPLIES AVAILABLE FOR HUMAN CONSUMPTION IN THE COUNTRIES OF THE REGION (FAO BALANCE SHEET)[1]

	Jordan				Lebanon			Syria		
	1957–59	60–62	63–65	1966	60–62	63–65	1966	60–62	63–65	1966
Cereals	348	368	386	290	303	340	365	432	438	575
Potatoes and starchy foods	34	28	35	43	40	54	64	24	25	21
Sugar and sweets	59	63	74	113	66	72	111	46	44	39
Pulses, nuts, and seeds	40	27	28	25	25	74	12	32	39	23
Vegetables	243	319	626	309	267	284	312	153	169	146
Fruit	257	315	268	236	435	486	379	435	396	257
Meat	21	33	28	28	71	87	84	38	30	32
Eggs	3	5	7	8	8	10	23	4	4	4
Fish	2	2	2	2	7	6	6	—	—	—
Milk	135	99	44	61	188	263	353	146	108	121
Fats and Oils	20	26	36	26	28	31	26	30	26	26
Estimated Calories	2180	2230	2500	2140	2320	2630	2720	2350	2330	2600
Fat g	40	45	51	40	53	63	55	48	48	49
Protein, Total g	58	61	67	55	66	78	78	69	69	78
Protein, Animal g	7.4	9.9	10.5	13.6	19.7	25.3	28.3	12.2	9.3	10.3

1. Source: FAO, *The State of Food and Agriculture*, 1968.

TABLE 1 (Cont'd.)
FOOD SUPPLIES AVAILABLE FOR HUMAN CONSUMPTION IN THE COUNTRIES OF THE REGION (FAO BALANCE SHEET)[1]

	Libya				United Arab Republic			
	1959	60–62	63–65	1966	1957–59	60–62	63–65	1966
Cereals	282	324	330	361	504	545	578	551
Potatoes and starchy foods	42	27	18	24	26	32	41	38
Sugar and sweets	70	49	46	90	44	44	48	49
Pulses, nuts, and seeds	16	9	12	24	29	29	32	35
Vegetables	116	84	92	138	214	242	282	292
Fruit	164	110	112	164	190	227	250	232
Meat	26	34	41	56	35	32	35	36
Eggs	4	3	3	3	3	3	3	4
Fish	2	5	4	5	12	14	13	9
Milk	152	111	125	130	116	125	124	122
Fats and Oils	18	20	23	26	13	16	17	19
Estimated Calories	1870	1840	1920	2340	2530	2690	2880	2810
Fat g	35	35	40	50	39	42	46	48
Protein, Total g	47	49	51	62	73	79	83	80
Protein, Animal g	10.3	10.0	11.3	14.7	11.9	12.2	12.0	11.8

1. Source: FAO, *The State of Food and Agriculture,* 1968.

tein supplies. Assuming a Net Protein Utilization (NPU) value of 65% as the estimate of the biological value of dietary protein in the Arab countries, the desirable protein intake according to the FAO/WHO Report on Protein Requirements (1965) can be placed at 54 g per capita per day as a population average. In this regard, Libya could be considered deficient in 1963-65, whereas Jordan had just a little more than was needed. In Lebanon, Syria, and Egypt the supplies were adequate. In most of these countries animal protein supplies amounted to about 10 to 11 g protein per capita per day except in Lebanon, where the animal protein was available at the level of 26 g per capita per day.

The governments in the region have been conscious of the limitations of their food supplies, and they have not been sparing in efforts to increase food production with the stimulus, advice, and assistance provided by the Food and Agriculture Organization. Information that is available with FAO indicates that considerable improvement has occurred in Libya and U.A.R. so far as the total food production is concerned.

Figure 1 illustrates the yearly estimates of total food production in Libya, Egypt, Syria, and Iraq from the estimates made by FAO for the years 1952-66. Similar estimates for Lebanon and Jordan were not available. It will appear from the figure that, whereas in Libya and Egypt there has been a steady progress in increasing food production during the fourteen years in question, the position is not as satisfactory in Syria and Iraq. There have been violent fluctuations from year to year in these two countries: the indices for food production have varied as much as 50 points from one year to the other. In general an upward trend is discernible in Iraq, but the situation in Syria remains unpredictable.

There may be several reasons for the lack of consistency in the results of efforts to increase food production in Syria and Iraq. Unfavorable climatic conditions may and do influence agricultural production. Plant and animal diseases and pests take their toll, which may vary from year to year. The wastage which may occur during inefficient storage is variable. Other reasons are inseparable from the effects attributable to the economic situation and political stability in the country. The unraveling of the relative roles of these and other factors in determining the progress in increasing food production will require specialized knowledge and an extensive study of all the factors involved. We are mainly concerned with the results which, as Figure 1 shows, are not entirely satisfactory so far as Syria is concerned and are only partially so in Iraq.

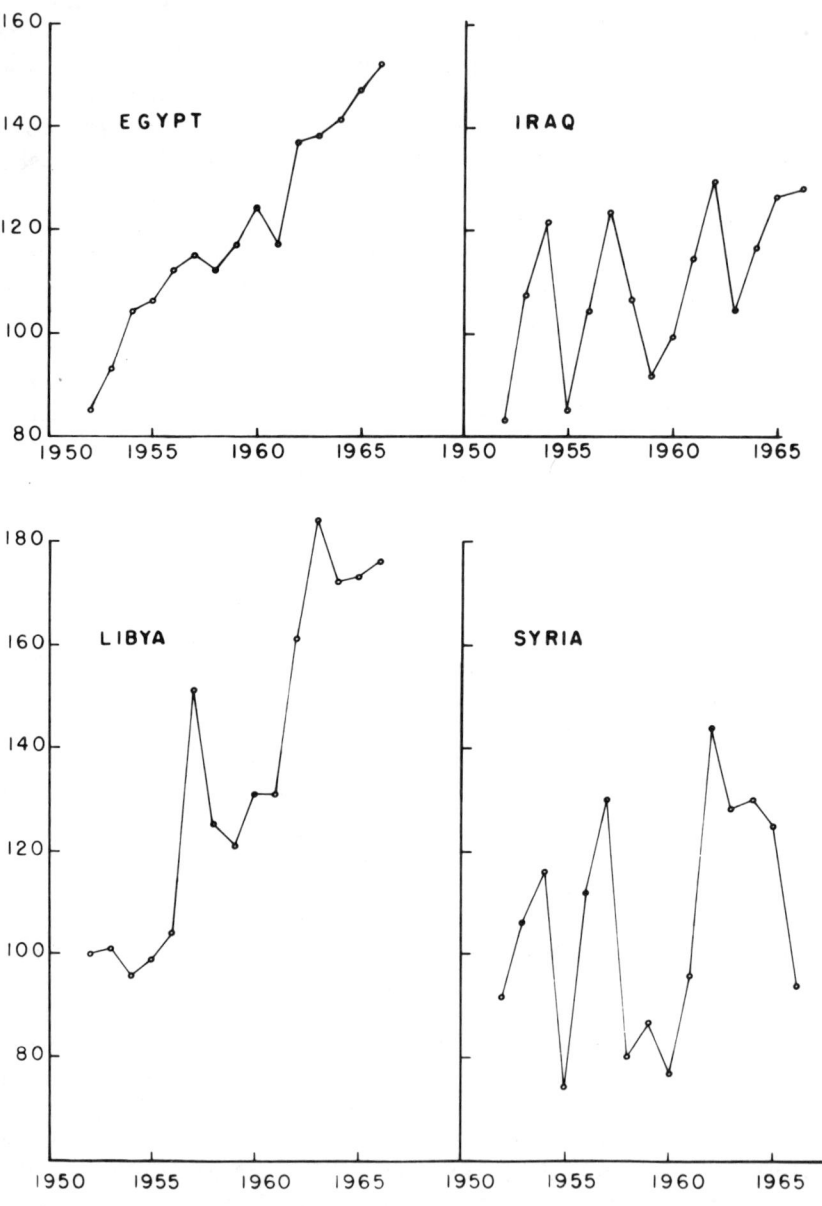

Figure 2.1. Trends of total food production from 1952 to 1966 in four Arab countries (from *State of Food and Agriculture*, FAO, 1968).

Food

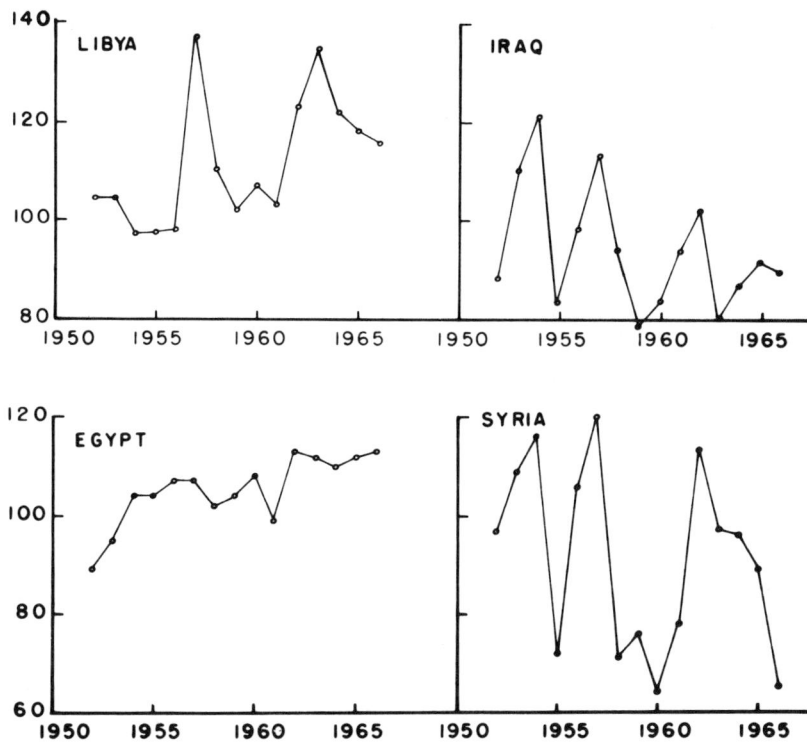

Figure 2.2. Trends in per capita food production from 1952 to 1966 in four Arab countries (from State of Food and Agriculture, FAO, 1968).

Figure 2 illustrates the achievement in food production in terms of the food produced per capita of the population, which has been increasing approximately at the rate of 3% per annum. As compared with the steady increase in population, the increase in food production has tapered off in recent years. According to the estimates made by FAO, the expansion of food production within the region was 28% between 1952–53 and 1957–58, but over the seven years which followed, the rate of increase was below 2% per annum. The levels of per capita food production illustrated in Figure 2 again indicate a steady increase for Libya and Egypt and wide fluctuations from year to year in Syria and Iraq.

The fact that food production is barely keeping pace with the population increase in some countries of the region is reflected in the continuously increasing imports of food within the region. According to an FAO estimate, the net food imports have increased between 3 and

5 times during the last fifteen years. The Indicative World Plan for Agricultural Development, 1965-85, for the Near East (FAO, 1966) envisages further stimulated efforts which should result in ensuring adequate supplies for the populations concerned, enabling them to subsist at higher levels of nutrition than prevail today.

FOOD COMPOSITION

A knowledge of the composition of foodstuffs and food is essential for the purpose of the nutritional evaluation of diets and, where necessary, for planning for their improvement. Published literature on the composition of food produced within the region and consumed by the population is comparatively small. The authors are conscious of the fact that in Egypt considerable unpublished data have been accumulated, and were assured that they were in the process of being assembled for publication.

Dr. Ismail Abdou, Director of the Food and Nutrition Institute of U.A.R. in Cairo, had made this information available to the compilers of the Food Composition Tables published in 1963 by the Division of Food Technology and Nutrition, Faculty of Agricultural Science, American University of Beirut, Lebanon. The authors of this publication, which has proved extremely valuable, have incorporated the results of food analysis then available from Egypt, Lebanon, and Iraq. These were obviously insufficient, for it is stated in the publication that the data on foods in the Middle East were limited, and there were relatively few foods on which large numbers of analyses were available so as to consider them to be representative. The results of a large number of analyses of foods in Lebanon were published later by workers from the Division of Food Technology and Nutrition of A.U.B. (Cowan et al., 1963, Simaan et al., 1964, Kuzayli et al., 1966, and Cowan et al., 1967).

A revised and enlarged edition of the Food Composition Tables for use in the Middle East has recently been published (Pellet and Shadarevian, 1970). This includes information on additional foods not found in the first edition. The other commendable features in the second edition are the inclusion of (1) data on sodium, potassium and iodine, (2) amino acid composition and (3) recipes and nutrient composition of many food preparations commonly consumed in the region. The information contained in this edition will be of great value to nutrition workers in this part of the world.

It is hoped that food and nutrition scientists in the neighboring countries will benefit by this example. An intensive effort to study the composition of common and uncommon foods consumed in different countries in the region is needed for effective nutrition programs.

REFERENCES

Ministry of Planning and Development, Kingdom of Libya. 1968. *Agriculture in Libya and a Plan for its Development.*
Cowan, J. W., A. H. Sakr, S. B. Shadarevian, and Z. I. Sabry. 1963. Composition of Edible Wild Plants of Lebanon. *J. Sci. Food Agric.* 7: 484.
———, M. Esfahani, J. P. Salji, and A. Nahapetian. 1967. Nutritive Value of Middle Eastern Foodstuffs. III-Physiological Availability of Iron in Selected Foods Common to the Middle East. *J. Sci. Food Agric.* 18: 227.
Dalby, G. 1963. The Baking Industry in Egypt. *Bakers' Digest* (Dec. 1963), p. 74.
Division of Food Technology and Nutrition, Faculty of Agricultural Sciences, American University of Beirut, Beirut, Lebanon. 1963. *Food Composition Tables for Use in the Middle East.* Publication No. 20.
Food and Agriculture Organization of the United Nations. 1964. *Regional Seminar on Applied Nutrition for the Near East.* Rome, Italy: Food and Agriculture Organization.
———. 1966a. *Indicative World Plan for Agricultural Development 1965-85.* Vols. I and II: *Near East Subregional Study.* Rome, Italy: Food and Agriculture Organization.
———. 1966b. *Joint Session of the Near East Commission on Agricultural Planning and the Near East Commission on Agricultural Statistics, Cairo, U.A.R., 26 Nov. 1966-5 Dec. 1966.* Rome, Italy: Food and Agriculture Organization.
———. 1968. *The State of Food and Agriculture 1968.* Rome, Italy: Food and Agriculture Organization.
Kuzayli, M. V., J. W. Cowan, and Z. I. Sabry. 1961. Nutritive Value of Middle Eastern Foods. II-Composition of Pulses, Seeds, Nuts and Cereal Products of Lebanon. *J. Sci. Food Agric.* 17: 82.
May, J. M. 1961. *The Ecology of Malnutrition in the Far and Near East.* New York: Hafner Publishing Co., Inc.
Pellet, P. L. and S. Shadarevian. 1970. *Food Composition: Tables for Use in the Middle East.* 2nd ed. Beirut, Lebanon: American University of Beirut.
Rizk, S. S., A. Sedky, and M. S. Mohamed. 1960. Studies on Egyptian Bread. I-Types and Methods of Baking Commercial Bread in Egypt. *Alexandria J. Agric. Res.* 8: 83.
Simaan, F. S., J. W. Cowan, and Z. I. Sabry. 1964. Nutritive Value of Middle Eastern Foodstuffs. I-Composition of Fruits and Vegetables Grown in Lebanon. *J. Sci. Food Agric.* 15: 799.

3 Pellagra in Egypt

Pellagra is a nutritional disease which occurs in many parts of the world, principally in regions where maize forms the staple article of the diet. It occurred in Spain, France, and Italy during the last two centuries and was found to occur in Rumania and Yugoslavia as late as the 1950's. Pellagra was also prevalent in the southern states of United States of America between the years 1907 and 1940, after which it diminished and has almost disappeared.

Men suffer from pellagra more often than women. The disease is uncommon in children and extremely rare in infants. The earliest manifestations of the disease seen in individuals on defective diets are usually nonspecific, such as loss of appetite, loss of weight, epigastric discomfort, indigestion, "nervousness," and a general feeling of weakness. Then appear burning sensations of the mouth, associated with the redness of the tips and margins of the tongue. The denudation of the tongue may be extensive. Cheilosis and angular lesions of the mouth may occur. These symptoms are soon followed by the skin rash which is characteristic of pellagra in its appearance and distribution. The rash starts as erythema resembling sunburn occurring with a bilateral symmetry over the exposed parts of the body (Plate 3.1). The sites are the backs of the hands and fingers, the forearms, dorsa of the feet and ankles, and the neck. In this latter location it is called "Casal's necklace" after the author who first described it (Plate 3.2). Symmetrical distribution over the malar region of the face and the bridge of the nose gives a butterfly appearance to the pigmentation. The scrotum also is involved in males, and in females there may be vaginitis. The erythematous patches soon darken,

Pellagra in Egypt

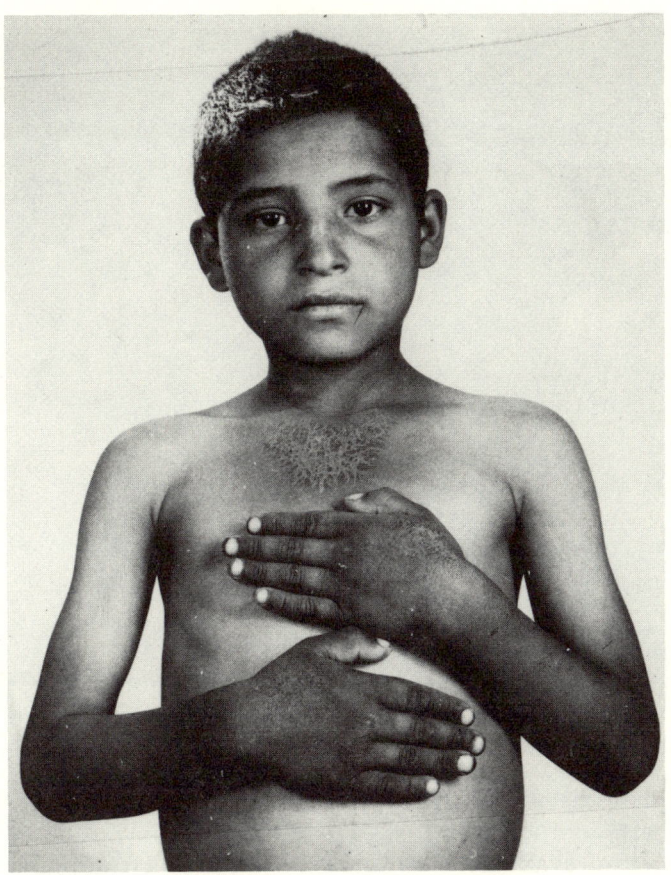

Plate 3.1. A case of pellagra showing derman lesions.

crack and peel, serosanguimous exudates may appear and the patches get encrusted. After repeated attacks the skin pigmentation becomes more general; and over elbows, knees, and knuckles the skin is darker in color, scaly, and thickened.

The other symptoms of pellagra are diarrhea and mental disturbances. Diarrhea may consist of frequent loose stools, sometimes watery with blood and mucus; it is often accompanied with proctitis.

The mental symptoms in mild cases consist of irritability, inability to concentrate, lack of interest, anxiety, and change in disposition. In acute pellagra, delirium is a common severe disturbance. In chronic cases dementia is frequently seen.

The administration of nicotinic acid or nicotinamide together with

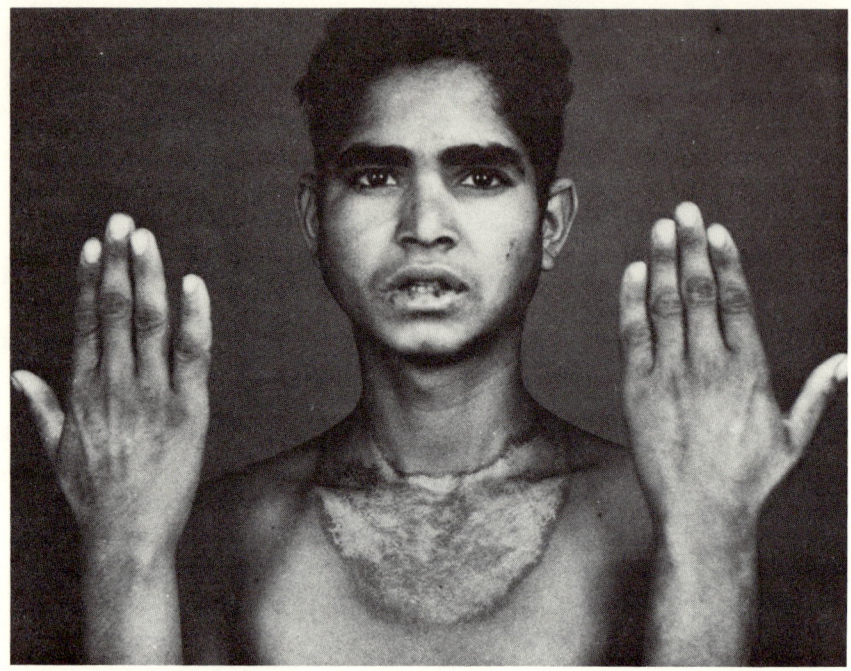

Plate 3.2. A case of pellagra showing dermal lesions (NAMRU picture).

an adequate diet brings relief from all these symptoms and a complete cure.

A search of available literature has so far failed to indicate that pellagra occurs in the Arab countries around Egypt, such as Lebanon, Syria, Jordan, Libya, and probably also Sudan. If it did occur in any or all of these, it must have done so sporadically, and the cases may have been so few as not to attract enough attention of the medical profession in these countries to warrant publication. Consequently the following account deals entirely with pellagra in Egypt.

Pellagra in Egypt was first recorded (Samborn, 1905) by Pruner in 1847 (Pruner, 1847a, 1847b). Pruner's descriptions of pellagra were as follows:

> La *pellagre* est sporadique en Egypte, et telle que nous l'avons étudiée dans le Milanais. Nous en avons vu trois cas chez des fellahs, dont l'un présente aujourd'hui, douze ans après notre première visite, la parésie des extrémités supérieures avec rétraction et atrophie des muscles (Pruner, 1847a).

> Das Pellagra. Obgleich mit den vorhergehenden Uebeln wenig oder gar nicht seinen Erscheinungen nach verwandt, glauben wir doch, dass das Pella-

gra bei ähnlichen Fehlern der Ernährung jedoch unter anderen äusseren Verhältnissen entstehe, wie die Lepra. Bekanntlich ist Oberitalien, Südfrankreich, Spanien, die Moldau u. s. f. sein eigentliches Vaterland. Wir bemerken daher nur im Vorbeigehen, dass einzelne, wenige Fälle davon auch in Aegypten von uns beobachtet wurden, mit dem Exantheme auf den Händen und im Gesichte. Wir fanden dasselbe nur im ersten Stadium von April bis August an Eigenborenen. Wir sahen ein Individuum 12 Jahre nach den ersten Anfängen der Krankheit zufällig wieder, und fanden an ihm Paresis der oberen Extremitäten mit Atrophie und Retraktion der Muskeln. Schon vor Jahren haben wir uns in Mailand überzeugt, dass die in Aegypten von uns gesehene Krankheit wirklich gleich der italienischen war. Es ist aus dem ersten Theile bekannt, das der Mais ebenfalls einen Nahrungsartikel in Aegypten bildet, jedoch nur einen sehr untergeordneten. Wir möchten fast auf diese, wenn gleich nur negative Thatsache verweisen, um der Meinung derjenigen auch von unserer Seite eine Kleine Stütze zu geben, welche das Pellagra dem fast ausschliesslichen Genusse eines noch dazu oft verdorbenen Maises oder anderer schlechter, stickstoffarmer Mehlarten zuschreiben. Gewiss ist dies die mächtigste aller inneren Ursachen, welche das Pellagra erzeugen und unterhalten (Pruner, 1847b).

Pruner's description of pellagra is inadequate per se to document its occurrence. Indeed, August Hirsch (1885) rejected Pruner's evidence as follows: "Pruner's description (as cited above) of the cases which he saw in Egypt (a brownish exanthem, paresis of the upper extremities, and muscular atrophy), does not by any means correspond to pellagra."

It is relevant to note, however, that Pruner seldom gave detailed descriptions of the conditions which he recorded in his text. His familiarity with pellagra in Italy,[1] his clear concern for the consumption of maize in relation to pellagra and the subsequent documentation by Sandwith and numerous others strongly support the validity of his report.

Nevertheless it was toward the end of the century that Sandwith confirmed its occurrence. In 1893 Sandwith (1898) noticed that a large number of his patients with ankylostomiasis showed a symmetrical eruption on exposed parts of the body which sunburn, chapping, or dirt could not explain. He concluded that these patients were suf-

---

1. Pruner wrote from Munich in the foreword of his book, *Die Krankheiten des Orient's* (1847), his qualifications as follows: "Der verfasser studirte und reiste im Jahre 1831 in Frankreich, Griechenland, Cypern, Syrien; wirkte als Professor der Anatomie 1832 an der medizinischen Schule zu Abuzabel in Aegypten, durchreiste Malta, Sicilien und Italien im Jahre 1833, und dirigirte die Centralspitäler zu Cairo und Kassr-el-ain vom Jahre 1834 bis 1839. Seine Reise nach Arabien fällt in das Jahr 1835/36. Vom Jahre 1840 bis 1846 lebte derselbe als Leibarzt S. H. Abba's-Pascha's —Enkel des Vizekönings—und praktischer Arzt in Cairo.

fering from pellagra in addition to hookworm anemia. In the following five years he saw 490 cases, the majority of them in the prime of life. According to Sandwith (1905), pellagra was common in Lower Egypt but rare in Upper Egypt. Of the 490 cases mentioned above, 437 were from Lower Egypt, including Guizeh, which is next door to Cairo. Sandwith also observed that in the villages of the Delta 20 to 50% of the poorer people suffered from pellagra. On the other hand the disease was uncommon among the well-to-do people.

Among other early accounts of pellagra in Egypt are those by Marie (1910) and White (1910) given at the National Conference on Pellagra held under the auspices of the South Carolina State Board of Health in 1909. Marie stated that in the previous ten years over a thousand cases of pellagra were admitted at the Kasr-el-Aini Hospital in Cairo and that admissions to mental asylums due to pellagrous insanity numbered 440 between 1896 and 1906. White reported that cases of pellagra admitted to mental hospitals improved after a time on a hospital diet which had no maize in it.

Numerous studies on pellagra since the days of Sandwith have dealt with different aspects of the problem, such as prevalence, the clinical and biochemical aspects of the disease, its etiology and treatment. With regard to prevalence, the more recent studies amply confirm Sandwith's original observations that pellagra is far more common in Lower than in Upper Egypt.

PREVALENCE

Wilson in 1932 carefully examined the evidence on the incidence of pellagra in Egypt and its etiology. He was of the opinion that the estimate of Sandwith with regard to the prevalence of pellagra in villages was probably too high. This, according to him, was due to the fact that Sandwith regarded as indicators of pellagra certain skin lesions and alimentary symptoms which today are considered as nonspecific. In 1915, Stiven who surveyed the villages of Sharkia in the Delta and around Assiout in Upper Egypt, considered that only about 4% of the rural population was affected with pellagra. This is in general agreement with the range of 1 to 7% prevalence in the villages in the Delta region as mentioned in *Global Epidemiology* by Simmons *et al.* as late as 1951.

Wilson's conclusion on incidence reported in 1932 was based on three different sources of figures: (1) admissions to government hospitals; (2) pellagra cases in prisons; and (3) admissions of pellagra cases to mental hospitals. In the main, Wilson confirms the distribution of pellagra in Egypt as previously indicated by Sandwith.

A review of pellagra cases admitted to hospitals between 1919 to 1928 gave a prevalence figure as 4.7 per 100,000 population for Lower Egypt and 1.4 per 100,000 population for Upper Egypt. The Suez Canal Zone had very high prevalence at 22.7 per 100,000 of population.

Vilter, Darby, and Glazer (1954), who as consultants of WHO surveyed the pellagra problem in Egypt in the year 1954, give figures for the number of pellagrins who attended the endemic diseases hospitals in different provinces of Egypt between the years 1938 and 1943 and then again for the years 1948 to 1953. We have obtained through the courtesy of the Ministry of Health the more recent figures for the attendance of pellagra patients at the endemic diseases hospitals for the years 1958–66. The annual averages based on the period 1958–63 can be compared with those given by Vilter *et al.* These figures are given in Table 1 together with the annual average attendance for a three-year period, which represents the latest available information. Using the 1937, 1947, and 1960 census figures for the Egyptian population (exclusive of the population of 5 large cities—Cairo, Alexandria, Port-Said, Ismailia, and Suez) one gets the figures for prevalence of pellagra in the predominantly rural areas of the country. These prevalence figures are very much higher than those given by Wilson in 1932 (see Table 1).

It will be wrong to argue that the prevalence of pellagra increased

TABLE 1
PREVALENCE OF PELLAGRA IN EGYPT

	Upper Egypt	Lower Egypt
	Annual averages for pellagra cases	
1919–1928[1]	79	199
1938–1943[2]	840	11,177
1948–1953[2]	2921	8,523
1958–1963[2]	4220	12,511
1964–1966[2]	1454	10,138
	Pellagra prevalence per 100,000 population	
1919–1928[1]	1.6	3.5
1938–1943[2]	13.1	156.5
1948–1953[2]	40.4	95.9
1958–1963[2]	45.7	114.4
1964–1966[2]	10.3	83.2

1. Hospital admissions.
2. Attendance at endemic diseases hospitals.

considerably during the years between 1928 and 1938 and subsequently. It is more probable that the difference in the prevalence rate may lie in the basic figures used by Wilson on the one hand and by Vilter *et al.* and by us on the other. Wilson calculated the prevalence from the annual average hospital admissions only, whereas the prevalence figures calculated from the data of Vilter *et al.* and those obtained recently from the Ministry of Health are based on the total average annual attendance at the endemic diseases hospitals. This includes ambulatory patients seen at outpatient departments as well as those admitted as inpatients. It was the practice to provide free meals to the patients attending the endemic disease hospital outpatient departments. This offered an incentive for the sick people from the surrounding areas to go there for treatment. Whether this practice helped to exaggerate the figure for prevalence is a question which is difficult to answer. However, the difference between the prevalence rates given by Wilson and those calculated from the attendance figures at the endemic diseases hospitals is much too large to be attributed to the single factor of free meals provided at these hospitals. On the other hand the prevalence rates based on the observations of Vilter *et al.* and confirmed by still later figures are more likely to be indicative of the true situation than those arrived at by Wilson.

It will be seen from Table 1 that the difference in the prevalence rates between Upper and Lower Egypt continues; the latter region can be considered as truly endemic for pellagra. However, there have been fluctuations within each region. The prevalence of pellagra showed an almost threefold increase in Upper Egypt between 1948 and 1953. It was even slightly higher in the period 1958–63, reaching 45.7 per 100,000. In the following triennium the prevalence dropped to a low figure of 10.3 per 100,000. Fluctuations in prevalence were also seen in Lower Egypt; in general, however, a declining trend is apparent.

There is a feeling among nutrition scientists in Egypt that pellagra in Egypt has been on the decrease (Barakat, 1958). This also becomes evident from Table 1. On the other hand a report of Abdou (1965) on a recent survey in different provinces of Egypt mentions that about 0.2% of the population suffers from pellagra, thus giving a prevalence rate of 200 per 100,000 population. This is even higher than the estimates for earlier years. Bearing in mind the limitations of methods used in arriving at prevalence rates, one may reasonably conclude, therefore, that although there may be local changes in prevalence in different provinces of Egypt and a general decline apparent from the health statistics, the prevalence of pellagra still remains high. In the light of this information we feel that pellagra is still a public health problem in Egypt.

Considerable emphasis has been laid by various workers on the incidence of pellagra among the mental patients in Egypt. This has been largely based on the diagnosis of pellagra in patients at the time of admission and the development of pellagra during the stay in the mental hospital. According to Wilson (1932), an average of 163 patients with pellagra was admitted per year to the Egyptian mental hospitals between 1916 and 1931. Ismail (1932) reported on 978 mental cases of pellagra admitted to the Khanka Mental Hospital alone between January 1920 and December 1931. Of these, 301 cases were reported to have died from pellagra and concomitant disease. The occurrence of pellagra in mental patients seems to have continued. Barakat (1958) stated that 2.6% of new admissions to the Khanka Mental Hospital in 1953–54 were diagnosed as pellagra. Vilter, Darby, and Glazer reported that 26% of all deaths of the patients in the same hospital between 1946 and 1950 were attributed to pellagra and that 20% of the discharged patients were pellagrins. Abdou (1965) considered that 0.4% of all new admissions to mental hospitals were pellagra cases. What is more significant probably is that 2.7% of all inmates of mental hospitals suffered from pellagra. It is noteworthy that a certain proportion of patients of mental hospitals developed pellagra during their stay in the hospitals, an aspect which is discussed later in this chapter.

On the other hand there is some doubt about the accuracy of diagnosis of pellagra in the mental cases. Vilter, Darby, and Glazer were of the opinion that the diagnosis was too lightly made on the presence of anemia (which almost always accompanies pellagra in Egypt also because of parasitism), on papillary atrophy of the tongue associated with it, and on some symptoms of mental aberrations which are not specific. Vilter *et al.* found that niacin alone seldom reversed the papillary atrophy which, however, subsequently responded to therapy with iron. Thus it is possible that the occurrence of pellagra among mental patients may have been an overestimate.

ETIOLOGY IN EGYPT

Maize in Diets. The etiology of pellagra in Egypt is of considerable interest. To a large extent the disease is associated with maize. According to Abdou (1965), maize was reported to have been introduced into Egypt from Syria in about 1840; only seven years later

Pruner recorded the appearance of pellagra. The time interval between the introduction of maize and the appearance of pellagra in such countries as Spain, Italy, Rumania, etc., has been over a hundred years in each country. The reasons for this lapse of time before the disease appears are simple. After its introduction, maize must be accepted by the people and cultivated extensively before it can form the staple article of their diets. This requires time, and hence a decade, or even less, elapsing between the introduction of maize in Egypt and the appearance of pellagra as suggested by Abdou seems incredibly short. In fact there is incontrovertible evidence that maize was introduced into Egypt much earlier, for Clot Bey,[2] who was the Inspector General of Civil and Military Medical Services in Egypt in the early years of the nineteenth century, makes a mention of maize in his book *Aperçu Général sur l'Egypte* (1840), as follows:

Mais (Zea mais Linn). Dourah Chamy.
Le nom de Chamy a été donné au mais parce qu'il a été apporté de Syrie (Châm en Arabe). Son grain est jaunâtre et plus gros que celui du dourah du pays. On en fait deux récoltes par an, l'une en été, l'autre en automn. Les Fellahs coupent les épis à demi mûrs, les font rôtir et s'en nourrissent. La farine du mais donne un pain meilleur que le dourah.

Maize must have established itself in Egypt long before the publication of this book. In fact Clot Bey, in another part of his *Aperçus,* gives the production of maize estimated in 1833 as 294,000 Hectolivres (equivalent to 13,382 metric tons), having the fifth most important place as a food crop, following wheat, dourah (sorghum), fava beans, and barley in that order. This information should place in proper perspective Pruner's observations on pellagra, which were first published in 1847.

The association of pellagra in Egypt with maize becomes clear by the observation of Sandwith (1898), who noted that in his cases there was a history of a fairly exclusive diet of maize with little else, against a background of general poverty and peasant life.

---

2. Antoine Bertelemy Clot Bey, Grenoble, France, undertook in 1824 under contract with Mohammed Aly's government the reorganization of the Egyptian Medical Service; he subsequently established a school of medicine in the village of Abou Zaabal. In 1837 the school was transferred to Kasr-el-Aini. He left Egypt in April 1849, to return for two additional years, 1856-58. It was he who modernized medicine in Egypt. His *Aperçu Général sur l'Egypte,* published in 1840 contains a wealth of information on all aspects of Egypt. It was during Clot Bey's directorship that Pruner joined the medical faculty.

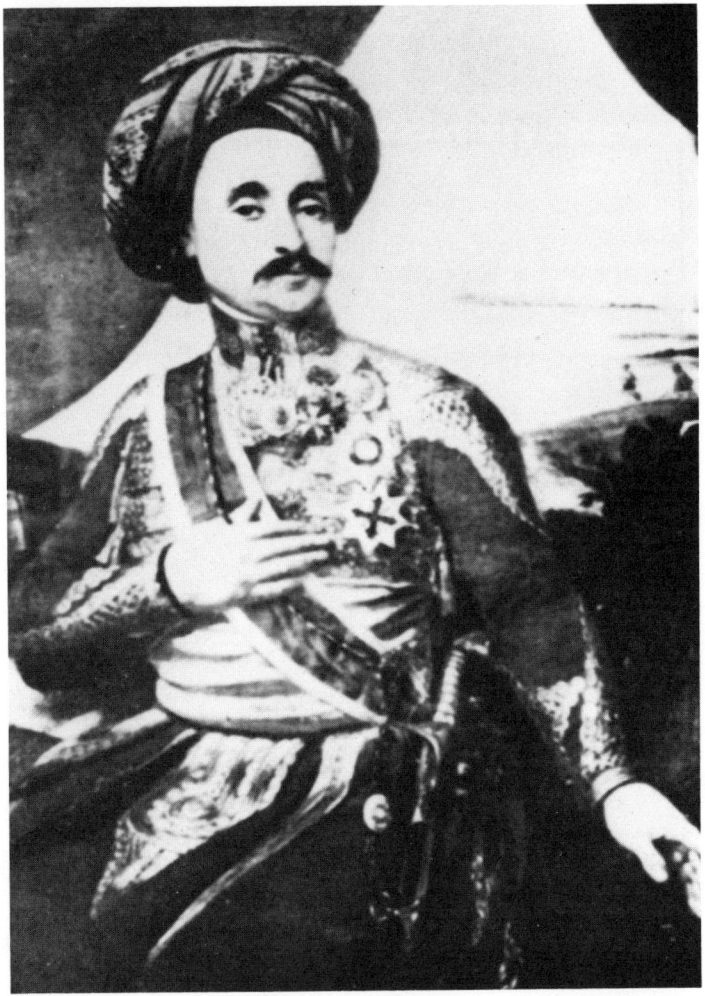

Plate 3.3. Clot Bey

The first extensive and well-considered study in Egypt on the relation between diet and pellagra is that of Wilson, which he published in detail in 1921 and later described in a lecture in Cairo in 1932. As has happened in the history of a few nutritional diseases, pellagra and its association with maize were explained as being due to the consumption of microbially infected maize. The early background of this historical association between pellagra and maize is admirably summarized by Hirsch (1885). Sandwith, who had considerable

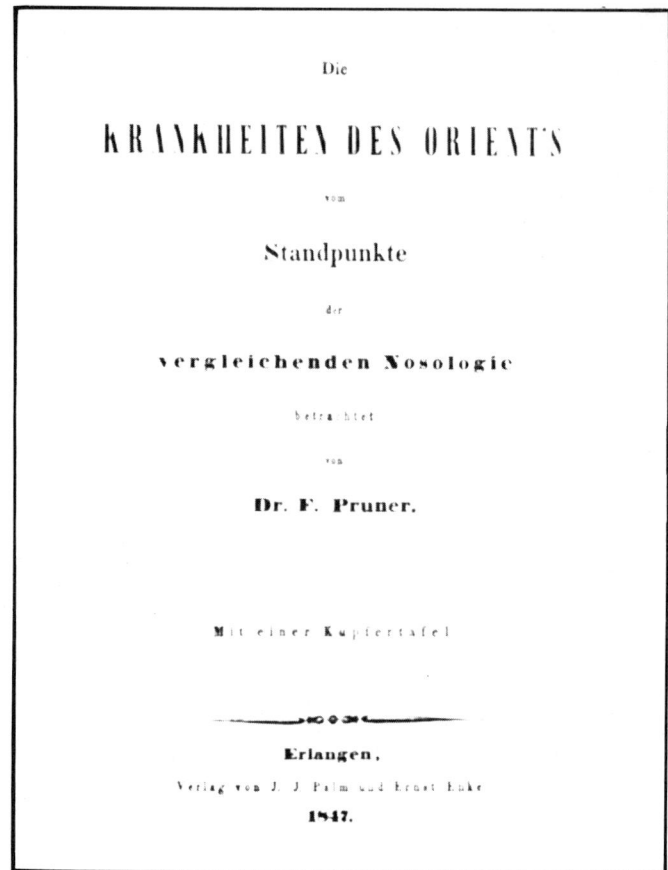

Plate 3.4. **Title page of Pruner's Krankheiten des Orients**

experience with pellagra in Egypt, was strongly of this view in the early days of his acquaintance with the disease. Apparently influenced by Wilson, however, he was convinced in later years that the consumption of bacterially infected or moldy maize was not the cause of pellagra but that it was the defective quality of maize protein which was responsible. Indeed, Sandwith (1913) was the first to advance the view that the absence of amino acid tryptophane from the chief protein component of maize, i.e., zein, was probably responsible for pellagra.

Nutritive Value of Dietary Protein and Pellagra. Wilson's interest in pellagra was considerably stimulated by his observations on the outbreak of pellagra in the Armenian refugees at Port-Said in Egypt in 1916 during the First World War. Furthermore, the occurrence of pellagra in a large number of Turkish prisoners of war interned in Kantara in Lower Egypt in 1916-17 and in German prisoners of war in Egypt in 1919 (Enright, 1920) provided Wilson fresh opportunities for study. The British Military Authority in Egypt appointed a Committee of Enquiry on Pellagra in Turkish Prisoners of War to investigate whether: (a) the disease in question was true pellagra; (b) it was spreading or existed before capture; (c) it was spreading from case to case; and (d) a defect in diet and other environmental conditions were responsible.

The Committee of Enquiry of which Wilson was a member concluded that: (a) most prisoners (Turkish) were already suffering from pellagra before capture; (b) it was not spreading; (c) there was no infective element concerned in the occurrence of pellagra; and (d) evidence pointed to a defect in nutritional quality of protein as the probable causative factor (Editorial; *Lancet,* 1919). Boyd (1919) reported these findings at a meeting of the Royal Society of Medicine in London, stating that deficiency of certain essential amino acids as reflected in the low biological value of protein played an essential role in the causation of pellagra. This view was probably based on Wilson's study of biological value of a variety of dietary proteins. The results of this study were reported by Wilson in 1921.

A study of Wilson's paper reveals the astonishing fact that the rations prescribed for the Armenian refugees, the Turkish prisoners of war, convicts at Tura, or inmates of Abbassia Mental Asylum in Cairo did not contain maize in any appreciable amounts, except that bread made for the Armenian refugees was from a mixture containing wheat flour, 75% and maize flour, 25%. The diets on which pellagra developed in all these locations are given in Table 2.

The diet of the Armenian refugees was the poorest, with a low dietary protein (57 g), having the lowest biological value (21%), and with little variety. In 1916 pellagra broke out among the refugees, and at one time 20% of them suffered from the disease. Wilson advocated certain modifications in the diet involving the addition of rice (31.2 g), edible oil (18.7 g), and fresh vegetables (100 g) and increasing the lentils and beans to 125 g per day. The total protein content increased to 99 g per day, as did its biological value (59.7%). Pellagra gradually disappeared. The high level of lentils and beans was not acceptable to the refugees, so further modifications, which made the diet more balanced than before, were suggested.

Wilson compared the protein content of the variety of reputedly

TABLE 2
DIETS ON WHICH PELLAGRA IS BELIEVED TO HAVE DEVELOPED
IN CAMPS OR INSTITUTIONS[1]

Daily Rations in grams

Foodstuffs	Armenian Refugees	Turkish P.O.W.	Tura Prison	Abbassia Asylum
Bread	750[2]	906[3]	936[4]	562[5]
Meat	8.6	114[6]	118.5[7]	150[6]
Lentils &/or beans	18.1	65	131.2	100
Rice	8.6	85	37.4	50
Burghoul	5.5			
Fresh vegetables	53.4	114	100	250
Onions	2.5	14.2	12.5	50
Dates		56.7		
Oil	5.3	14.2	25	20
Sugar & treacle	18.8	28.4		50
Salt		14.2	12.5	18
Flour & wheat				38
Milk				50
Margarine				25
Cheese	17			
Olives	14.3			
Total Protein g	57	89.7	123.5	99
Biological Value acc. Thomas	21%	38.6%	48.3%	49.4%
Net Calories		2629	2920	2720

1. Source: Wilson, 1921.
2. Made from wheat flour containing 25% maize flour.
3. Flour made from wheat 90% and millet 10%.
4. Made from millet flour.
5. Made from wheat flour.
6. Meat with bone.
7. Meat without bone.

pellagragenic and pellagra-preventive diets and also the biological value of protein contained in them. He also tried to relate the "vitamin B_2" content of these diets to their pellagragenic effect. Wilson came to the conclusion that diets which contained protein of biological value less than 40 were pellagragenic.

He observed that the biological value of dietary protein in general ran parallel to its vitamin B_2 content. However, he pointed out that there was "no consistent relation between this value and the incidence of pellagra." These conclusions are illustrated in Fig. 1, reproduced from Wilson's paper published in 1932. As will appear from the figure, Wilson's conclusions in general were in line with his obser-

Pellagra in Egypt   47

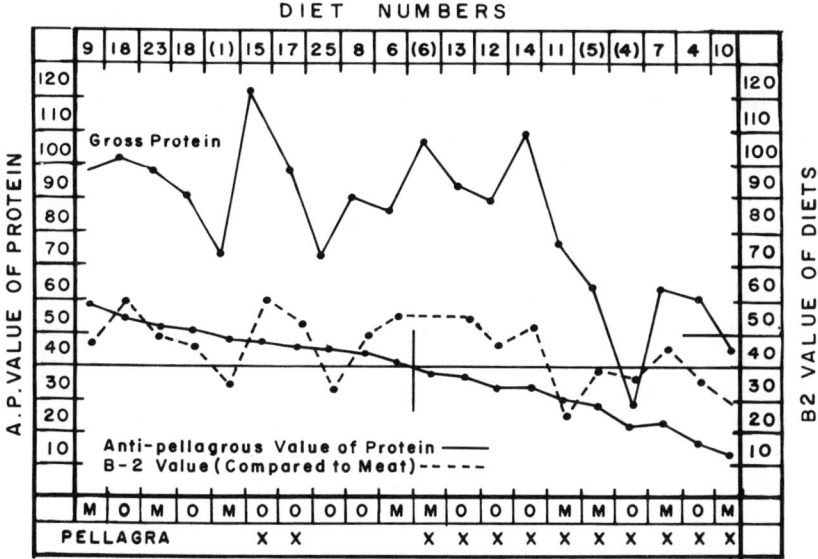

Figure 3.1. Relation of pellagra to (a) total protein in diet; (b) biological value of protein as animal protein (A.P.) value; and (c) vitamin B_2 value of diet. For explanation see text. The presence or absence of maize in diet is shown by letters M and O. Occurrence of pellagra on diet indicated by X. (From Wilson, H., 1932; *J. Egyptian Med. Assoc.* **15**: 415. By courtesy of the *Journal*).

vations. However there were two exceptions: diet 15 for Egyptian convicts at Tura prison, total protein 123 g, B.V. 48%; and diet 17, ordinary diet Abbassia Asylum, total protein 99 g, B.V. 46%. Pellagra occurred in the prison and asylum inmates on these diets, which were apparently high in total protein and had a high biological value of protein and a relatively high vitamin B_2 content.

Assuming the validity of Wilson's argument for the moment, it becomes difficult to understand why the inmates of the prison at Tura and the asylum at Abbassia should develop pellagra. There is, however, some revealing information in Wilson's paper regarding the Abbassia situation. Wilson states that the asylum diet was not pellagragenic. In fact some cases of pellagra admitted for mental disorder rapidly recovered, an observation which had already been recorded by White in 1910. Sometime in 1917 the making of bread in the asylum kitchen was discontinued, and bread was bought from a contractor from outside who could, as Wilson admits, easily have mixed with wheat flour the cheaper maize flour in large proportion or could have made bread from maize flour alone. Cases of pellagra started appearing after the substitution of contract bread for hospital-baked bread, and those who already suffered from pellagra did not improve.

The possibility of admixture of maize in diets of prisons and in prisoner-of-war camps cannot altogether be excluded, knowing what human nature is; the temptation to adulterate wheat or millet flour with cheaper maize flour must have been irresistible where contractors for the bread supply were concerned. The Egyptian villager is accustomed to eating maize bread or bread prepared from mixtures in varying proportions of maize, wheat, and millet. Hence, there were probably no complaints about the quality of bread.

There was another objection to the hypothesis of low biological value as the sole causative factor in pellagra. Proteins vary in their amino acid composition, and the deficiency of one or more essential amino acids limits the biological value of a protein. In the diets examined by Wilson, the dietary protein was derived from a variety of foods, and the amino acid composition of these diets may have been different although the estimated low biological values were comparable. Goldberger was conscious of this aspect of the question: although he was in agreement with Wilson about the deficiency of an amino acid being a causative factor in pellagra (Goldberger and Tanner, 1922), he felt, however, that a low biological value of protein by itself was not indicative of a pellagra-producing defect. Furthermore, in determining the biological value of dietary protein, Wilson merely added the biological values of proteins of foods individually determined in proportion to the protein contributed by each article of diet. This must have given him an unduly low value, for we know now that proteins, when present in mixtures as they are in most diets, have a supplementary effect so that the resultant biological value is not merely additive.

Thus, although the diets found pellagragenic by Wilson were not based principally on maize, one cannot escape the thought, for reasons given above, that apart from the low biological value of dietary protein, maize must have played a role in the outbreak of pellagra in Egypt among refugees, prisoners of war, convicts, and inmates of a mental asylum. According to Wilson the causative factor in pellagra was the deficiency of tryptophan and not the deficiency of any vitamin. Darby and Hassan (1967) have quite recently traced the development and maturation of this concept, which emerged from Wilson's investigations in Egypt undertaken independently but simultaneously with those of Goldberger in the southern United States.

The other possible contributory factor may have been the reduction of food intake over a prolonged period. Commenting on the outbreak of pellagra in German prisoners of war on an apparently good diet, Goldberger (1920) pointed out that none of the 65 patients suffering from pellagra could be considered to have been normal, for all of them had suffered repeatedly from malaria, dysentery, and chronic diarrhea. These illnesses must have resulted in low food consumption, for there was no evidence that the prisoners consumed all that was believed to have been provided. So far as the inmates of the mental asylum were concerned, Wilson also mentioned the possibility of low food consumption mainly due to the apathy of the patients. Thus it appears that more than one factor must have contributed to the outbreaks of pellagra in camps and institutions at that time, namely low nutritive value of protein in the diet most probably largely based on maize, low food consumption, and presence of parasitic infection.

The observations of Goldberger on the antipellagra activity of yeast and yeast extracts led him to the conclusion that in some foods there was present a pellagra preventive (P-P) factor other than protein. In subsequent years the isolation and identification of niacin as the P-P factor and the discovery by Elvehjem and coworkers of the conversion of tryptophan to nicotinic acid within the body not only showed that pellagra is due to niacin deficiency but also explained the role of tryptophan in relation to the disease. Sandwith, Wilson, and subsequently Goldberger had in fact drawn attention to this finding much earlier.

The successful treatment of pellagra cases in Egypt by Alport, Ghalioungui, and Hanna (1938) and Ayad (1940) added to the already mounting evidence regarding the role of nicotinic acid in the causation of pellagra. The maize diets, because of the relatively low amounts of tryptophan in maize protein and the unavailability of niacin contained in it, are pellagragenic. This, however, is not the whole story. It is well known that in Central America, where people treat maize with lime water before making tortillas, pellagra is rare, in spite of the high consumption of maize and the inadequacy of the diet in other respects. It is also possible that the consumption of food made from whole maize may have a protection effect not found in the degermed maize meal consumed in the southern United States during the 1920's and 1930's when pellagra was widespread.

Pellagra in Egypt occurs principally in villages. Its association with poverty has been documented (Sandwith, 1898; Wilson, 1921). Apart from a high consumption of maize, the diet of the poor fellaheen rarely contains enough foodstuffs or even other cereals, such as rice or wheat. The situation seems to have changed but little since Clot Bey in 1840 made the statement that "Les paysans son très sobres. Le pain de Dourah forme leur principale, quelquefois même leur unique nourriture."

Slightly over a hundred years later H. H. Ayrout (1963) wrote "the ordinary diet of the fellah, then, consists of bread, which he makes from maize of his own growing; vegetables from the edge of the field, or others of poor quality bought by his wife from the market; cheese from the buffalo, where it has not been necessary to sell the milk; and occasionally eggs, meat and fish. Briefly, he eats the cheapest products he can obtain."

The high prevalence of parasitism, such as ankylostomiasis and schistosomiasis, is another contributory factor. It is noteworthy that in cases observed by Sandwith in 1893–98 pellagra was associated with hookworm disease. Even now it is the common experience that a pellagrous patient is found to be infected with ankylostome or schistosome or both. Indeed, the frequent association of anemia and pellagra has as stated, led to diagnostic confusion. This association of pellagra, iron deficiency, and hookworm likewise occurred in the southern United States of America and at one time Bliss (1930) even hypothesized that pellagra was due to iron deficiency.

In towns and large cities of Egypt pellagra rarely occurs, for there the government-subsidized wheat bread is the staple even among the poor, and the prevalence of parasitism is low because of better sanitary environment.

Pellagra is admittedly less common in Upper Egypt. However, according to the hospital attendance reports compiled by Vilter *et al.*, its estimated prevalence had increased in the fifties. Maize is not grown and consumed in Upper Egypt to any great extent. The staple cereal in that region is sorghum millet (*Sorghum vulgare*) known in vernacular as *durra awega* as distinct from *durra chami*, which is maize. However, we have already discussed the outbreaks of pellagra in Egypt on diets which presumably did not contain maize. The evidence on the occurrence of pellagra in India on sorghum diets has been reviewed by Patwardhan (1961), and amino acid imbalance has been suggested as one of the causes (Gopalan and Srikantia, 1960). In commenting on pellagra in Upper Egypt, Vilter, Darby, and Glazer (1954) state that the disease was often found among the poorest villagers, where poverty forced the people to rely on maize flour, imported into the region, for their principal dietary cereal. This may be true to a large extent. However, it cannot be denied that pellagra can occur on sorghum-based diets, whatever may be the reason. It is also possible that in Upper Egypt, as more land is brought under perennial irrigation, agriculture is often restricted to the cultivation of a cash crop such as sugar cane. This may necessitate the transport of food supplies for the labor population—chiefly maize flour, which is the cheapest foodstuff—from areas further north.

Vilter, Darby, and Glazer (1954) give in their report other examples of the appearance of pellagra when the economic situation deteriorated. In upper Nubia where fertile land had been inundated by successive elevations in the height of the Aswan High Dam, the villagers deprived of cultivable land had become poorer and had to subsist on maize as the chief article of diet. In Edfu the draining of the lake which yielded income from fishing had affected the earning capacity of the people with the same result. Pellagra made its appearance in 1954 in these areas, where before it was rare. It is possible that this situation may have changed because of the resettlement policy of the government.

Other Observations. Reference has already been made to the role of parasitic infections in pellagra. The effect of hookworm and schistosome infections in causing gastrointestinal disturbances, anemia, and general debility may be considered as potentiating the effects of the inadequacies of maize diets in causing pellagra and other nutritional disorders.

Seasonal variation in the incidence of pellagra in Egypt has been commented upon by several investigators. The incidence is high between the months of February and May, the peak being reached usually in March or April, followed by a sharp fall. There is a second and much smaller peak in September or October. Barrada (1932) found a parallelism between the seasonal incidence of pellagra and the rate of admissions to two mental hospitals in different months of the year, suggesting that the mental aspects of pellagra contributed substantially to the population of these mental institutions.

Clark (1937) analyzed the figures for admissions in 1936–37 to the "General Hospital" (this must be the Kasr-el-Aini Hospital) in Cairo. He found that the incidence of pellagra admissions began to rise in January, reached a peak in April, and then gradually declined to reach the lowest level in August–September.

The influence of the season of the year on the incidence of pellagra has been observed in other parts of the world. Sambon (1905) commented upon it while describing pellagra in Italy. The report of the Pellagra Commission of the State of Illinois (1912) noted that peak incidence in the years 1909 and 1910 occurred in June of each year, with a smaller peak in August–September. Goldberger in his extensive studies noticed that the skin lesions started appearing early in the year. These and subsequent observations by other workers pointed to an association between the exposure to solar radiation and the incidence of pellagra. This aspect was investigated in detail by Smith and Ruffin (1937). They showed that over a period of five years, the peak of incidence of pellagra in 11 southern states of U.S.A. occurred in June–July and that the seasonal variation in the incidence of pellagra ran parallel with the incidence of solar radiation, expressed as calories per square centimeter per day on a surface at normal incidence at sea level. They further demonstrated the effect of direct sunrays on the occurrence of pellagra. Some patients who had been maintained on pellagragenic diets developed the characteristic rash and other symptoms of pellagra only after being exposed to sunrays. Following therapy these same patients did not so respond to repeated exposure to sunrays.

In villages spring and summer are the seasons for agricultural operations. This necessitates greater exposure by the farm worker to direct solar radiation than at other seasons, and this probably explains in large part the high incidence of pellagra in these seasons in Egypt as well as in other countries where pellagra occurs.

Clark (1937) does not agree with the concept of a relationship between the solar radiation and seasonal variations in pellagra. He was probably unaware of the work of Smith and Ruffin referred to above. However he had a very plausible explanation for the seasonal variation of incidence of pellagra in Egypt. Clark related this largely to the difference in staple food at different times of the year, depending upon the time of the respective harvests. Thus, Clark states that *durra* (it could be maize or sorghum) ripens in January and wheat and barley crops in April. The peasant and his family therefore presumably subsist on *durra* from January to April, which coincides with the period of the rising incidence of pellagra. From April onwards, when pellagra declines, the wheat and barley become the staple foods. Fellaheens consume dates between August and December, which, in the opinion of Clark, afford protection against pellagra.

According to Clark (1937) the relation between solar radiation and pellagra should not hold in Egypt because November to April are months characterized by cold winds and often cloudy skies. Also, the heaviest agricultural labor, which would necessarily involve direct exposure to sun, are the months of May and June, November and December.

The observations of Clark are not inherently in contradiction of the solar-radiation hypothesis. An exposure to solar radiation alone will not cause pellagrous rash, as the experiments of Smith and Ruffin show. It is only when a person has been subsisting on a pellagragenic diet for some appreciable time, probably a little over two months, that the solar effect manifests itself. The harvesting of the *durra* crop in December–January and operations connected with it result in exposure to sun, for these operations are done in the open. Furthermore, as *durra* is the cheapest grain, it probably forms the staple food of the fellaheens through a major portion of the year. Much of the wheat harvest is probably sold for cash, only a fraction being retained for home consumption. There are few other things which enter the dietary of the poor peasant. Thus reliance on *durra chami* (maize) for a large part of the year, leading to subnutrition or malnutrition, followed by continued exposure to sun from November–December, in spite of the often cloudy skies and cold winds, triggers the onset of dermal rash and with it the other symptoms of pellagra in the spring.

The mental involvement of pellagra in Egypt is probably not as uncommon as Vilter, Darby, and Glazer indicated. It is possible that an imbalance between different members of the vitamin B complex and their relative deficiencies associated with pellagra may influence the development of mental changes seen in this disease. Barrada (1932) suggests that chronic cases of pellagra with one or more annual relapses show advanced mental changes and qualify for admission to the mental hospitals.

Ismail (1932) estimated that 4 to 15% of pellagrins showed some kind of mental symptoms. As has already been stated, Barakat (1958) estimated that 2.6% of new admissions to institutions were pellagrins; the later estimate of Abdou (1965) is much lower at 0.4% of all admissions to the mental hospitals in Egypt as pellagrins. Nabi and Okasha (1964) have studied 124 cases of pellagra admitted to the Abbassia State Mental Hospital and Nile Sanatorium during ten years. They are of the view that there is no specific psychosis in pellagra. The commonest presentation in their cases was acute or subacute delirious state and affective disorders. Of the 124 cases treated with niacin and vitamin B complex, 59 were cured and 19 improved. The mental symptoms in 29 remained unchanged in spite of full recovery from pellagra. The observations of these authors indicate that patients suffering from schizophrenia or depressive states may develop pellagra through "self neglect and disinterest in their food." This was indeed suggested by Wilson almost fifty years ago.

It may reasonably be assumed that the mental condition of pellagra cases admitted to mental hospitals is not always due to pellagra. It may also well be, as already mentioned, that in some cases the diagnosis of pellagra itself is not correct. El Ridi and Ismail (1960), while examining the vitamin B_{12} status of six cases of pellagra with neurological symptoms, found that three of them had histamine-fast achlorhydria and these same cases had also lesions of the posterior and lateral columns of the spinal chord.

Of the other studies on pellagra, those on gastrointestinal absorptive function are of interest. Alport, Ghalioungui, and El Ghariny (1939) found an abnormal oral-glucose-tolerance response in pellagrins; the peak of the blood sugar was much lower than in the controls. Furthermore, after an oral dose of 300 mg ascorbic acid, pellagrins excreted in urine much less ascorbic acid in a four-hour period than the controls similarly treated. The authors concluded that the absorptive function in pellagra was impaired. They also felt that this adverse effect on absorption was probably due to intestinal parasites which were present in all the patients. On the other hand, the lower urinary excretion of ascorbic acid after a loading dose could be interpreted as a reflection of depleted body store of the vitamin and may have little to do with a defect in absorption, which later studies have been unable to confirm. Abdallah *et al.* (1963) investigated D-xylose excretion and fecal fat excretion in 20 pellagrins. Impairment was found only in one patient, who also suffered from giardiasis. The authors feel that this infestation may have been responsible for the defect in absorption in this case. Halsted and coworkers (1969) tested absorption in 11 pellagra cases with the help of D-xylose excretion, stool fat analysis, and tritiated folic acid absorption tests; they also examined jejunal biopsies obtained from these patients, comparing them with those taken from apparently healthy Egyptian controls.

Halsted and coworkers (1969) found that in Egyptian normal subjects the villous pattern was characterized by thin leaves and rarely by fingerlike villi such as are described in Europe and U.S.A. The villous pattern found in Egyptian pellagra patients was similar to that observed in normal Egyptians so far studied, and the tests for absorptive function in pellagra patients failed to reveal any abnormality. The available over-all evidence thus points to the fact that pellagra as seen in Egypt does not cause significant alterations in intestinal structure nor in its absorptive function.

REFERENCES

Abdalla, A., N. Gad-el-Mawia, A. El Rooby, M. Shaker, and N. Galil. 1963. Studies on the Malabsorption Syndrome among Egyptians. *J. Egypt. Med. Assoc.* 46: 544.

Abdou, I. A. 1965. A Study of Pellagra in the Egyptian Region, UAR. *Bull. Nutr. Inst., UAR* 1: 61.

Alport, A. C., P. Ghalioungui, and G. Hanna. 1938. Pellagra and Its Treatment with Nicotinic Acid and Nicotinamide with a Review of the Literature. *J. Egypt. Med. Assoc.* 21: 750.

Alport, A. C., P. Ghalioungui, and A. El Ghariny. 1939. Defective Gastrointestinal Absorption in Pellagra. *J. Egypt. Med. Assoc.* 22: 191.

Ayad, N. 1940. Treatment of Pellagra by Combined Nicotinic Acid and Eggs. *J. Egypt. Med. Assoc.* 23: 379.

Ayrout, H. H. 1963. *The Egyptian Peasant.* Translated from the French by John Alden Williams. Boston: Beacon Press.

Barakat, M. R. 1958. Pellagra in Egypt. *J. Egypt. Publ. Health Assoc.* 33: 267.

Barrada, Y. 1932. Clinical Aspects of Pellagra. *J. Egypt. Med. Assoc.* 15: 609.

Bliss, S. 1930. Considerations Leading to the View that Pellagra is an Iron-Deficiency Disease. *Science* 72: 577.

Boyd, F. D. 1919. Pellagra in Turkish Prisoners in Egypt. *Lancet* ii: 979.

Clark, A. 1937. Notes on Pellagra in Egypt 1936–1937. *J. Trop. Med. Hyg.* 40: 221.

Clot-Bey, A. B. 1840. *Apercu General sur l'Egypte.* Paris: Fortin, Masson et Cie.

———. 1949. *Memoires de A. B. Clot-Bey.* Publiees et annotees par Jacques Tagher. Cairo: L'Institut Francais d'Archeologie Orientale.

Darby, W. J., and A. Hassan. 1967. William Hawkins Wilson—A Biographical Sketch (1868–1956). *J. Nutr.* 92: 3.

El Ridi, M. S., and A. A. Ismail. 1960. Cyanocobalamine in Pellagra. *J. Egypt. Med. Assoc.* 43: 836.

Enright, J. I. 1920. The Pellagra Outbreak in Egypt. II-Pellagra Amongst German Prisoners of War: Observations upon the Food Factor in the Disease. *Lancet* i: 998.

Goldberger, J. 1920. The Pellagra Outbreak in Egypt. *Lancet* ii: 41.

———, and W. F. Tanner. 1922. Amino Acid Deficiency Probably the Primary Etiological Factor in Pellagra. *U.S. Publ. Health Rep.* 37: 462.

Gopalan, C., and S. G. Srikantia. 1960. Leucine and Pellagra. *Lancet* i: 954.

Halsted, C. H., S. Sheir, N. Sourial, and V. N. Patwardhan. 1969. Small Intestinal Structure and Absorption in Egypt. *Amer. J. Clin. Nutr.* 22: 744.

Hirsch, A. 1885. *Handbook of Geographical and Historical Pathology.* Vol. II, *Chronic Infective, Toxic, Parasitic, Septic and Constitutional Diseases.* Translated from the second German edition by Charles Creighton, M.D. London: The New Sydenham Society.

Ismail, A. S. 1932. The Mental Aspect of Pellagra. *J. Egypt. Med. Assoc.* 15: 504.

Marie, A. 1910. *Trans. National Conference on Pellagra: Held under the Auspices of South Carolina State Board of Health Nov. 3–4, 1909.* Columbia S.C.: The State Company.

Nabi, S. A., and A. Okasha. 1964. Psychosis in Egyptian Pellagrins. *Med. J. Cairo Univ.* 32: 325.
Patwardhan, V. N. 1961. *Nutrition in India.* Bombay: Indian J. Med. Sci. Publ.
———. 1919. Pellagra Among Turkish Prisoners of War in Egypt. *Lancet* ii: 490.
Pruner, F. 1847a. *Topographie Medical du Caire avec le Plan de la Ville et des environs.* Munich.
———. 1847b. *Die Krankheiten des Orient's vom Standpunkte der vergleichenden Nosologie.* Erlangen: J. J. Palm und Ernst Enke.
Report of the Pellagra Commission of the State of Illinois. 1912. Springfield, Illinois: Illinois State Journal Company.
Samborn, L. W. 1905. The Geographical Distribution and Etiology of Pellagra. *J. Trop. Med.* 8: 250.
Sandwith, F. M. 1898. Pellagra in Egypt. (Abstract). *Brit. Med. J.* ii: 881.
———. 1905. *The Medical Diseases of Egypt.* Part I. London: Henry Kimpton.
———. 1913. Is Pellagra a Disease Due to Deficiency of Nutrition? *Trans. Roy. Soc. Trop. Med. Hyg.* 6: 143–148.
Simmons, J. S., T. F. Whayne, G. W. Anderson, H. M. Horack, and R. A. Thomas. *Global Epidemiology.* Vol. II. New York: J. B. Lippincott Company.
Smith, D. T., and J. M. Ruffin. 1937. Effect of Sunlight on Clinical Manifestations of Pellagra. *Arch. Int. Med.* 59: 631.
Vilter, R. D., W. J. Darby, and H. S. Glazer. 1954. A Survey of Pellagra and Nutritional Anemia in Egypt. Geneva: World Health Organization.
White, R. C. 1910. *Trans. National Conference on Pellagra: Held under the Auspices of South Carolina State Board of Health Nov. 3–4, 1909.* Columbia, S.C.: The State Company.
Wilson, W. H. 1921. The Diet Factor in Pellagra. *J. Hyg.* 20: 1.
———. 1932. Pellagra in Egypt. Part I-Incidence of Pellagra in Egypt. Part II-Aetiology of Pellagra. *J. Egypt. Med. Assoc.* 15: 405, 421, 490.

4 | Anemia

EGYPT

In 1950, Dr. W. R. Aykroyd of FAO and Dr. F. W. Clements of WHO examined the nutritional situation in Egypt at the invitation of the Ministry of Public Health and recommended in outline a program of nutrition for the country. They recognized the health and economic significance of the widely prevalent anemia in Egypt, for it led to the serious impairment of health and capacity for physical effort and hence of productivity. According to them, anemia in Egypt was due to the interaction of malnutrition and parasitic infection, the latter being the predominant factor. They said "Nutrition workers in Egypt have strongly emphasized the importance of parasitic diseases—notably bilharziasis and ankylostomiasis—in accentuating the ill effects of malnutrition." However, until 1950, when the above-mentioned report was made, there were no systematic observations—at least so far as we are aware—correlating the prevalence of anemia with either one or the other or both of these incriminated factors, malnutrition and parasitism.

In 1954, WHO sent a team of consultants to survey pellagra and nutritional anemia in Egypt. The report made by Vilter, Darby, and Glazer (1954) on this survey deals in great detail with the problem of pellagra. However, it is clear even from the comparatively brief reference made in the report that anemia must be a serious problem in the Egyptian population and that it affected men, women, and children. Abdou (1960) lists anemia as one of the problems of malnutrition in Egypt. According to him, surveys among the population groups of different socioeconomic segments of the communities in villages revealed that 40% of those examined had hemoglobin levels below 11 g per 100 ml blood. It is principally through such surveys and through the results of hematological studies carried out in association with surveys on parasitism that one obtains an idea of the magnitude of the problem and of its multiple etiology.

No attempt seems to have been made to establish normal hemoglobin values for the Egyptian population. Abdou (1965) has arbitrarily selected 14 g per 100 ml as the normal hemoglobin value for adult males and females as well as children from 7 years onwards, thus making no allowance for age or for sex difference, factors that are known to influence hemoglobin levels.

The reported values in the world literature indicate a difference of about 1 to 2 g per 100 ml between the accepted mean values for adult males and females. Wintrobe (1967) gives the average value as 16.0 ± 2.0 for males and 14.0 ± 2.0 for females. Whitby and Britton (1963) consider the normal range for adult males from 14 to 17 g hemoglobin per 100 ml of blood with an average of 15.6 g; the corresponding values for adult females were 12–15.5 g with an average of 13.7 g. Admittedly the average hemoglobin levels in children are lower than in adults. Here too, however, differences in the published normal values are evident; for example, the values given by Nelson (1959) and Wintrobe (1967) do not necessarily agree for the different age groups during childhood and adolescence. These considerations should indicate the difficulty inherent in assuming any single figure as the normal value in order to express the observed values in terms of percentages. Another difficulty arises because various Egyptian authors have expressed hemoglobin values as the percentage of the standard, whose hemoglobin content is not given. However, although no adequate studies have been made on healthy Egyptians or other Arab populations, this may not be of serious consequence. The WHO Study Group on Iron-Deficiency Anemia reviewed in 1958 the large body of hematological data derived from studies of apparently normal persons throughout the world and expressed the view "that optimum hematological values in tropical and temperature zones are the same." It is therefore reasonable to conclude that the normal values would not be any different in Egyptians and other Arab populations.

In 1967 at a WHO meeting on iron deficiency and megaloblastic anemias, it was recommended that anemia should be considered to exist if hemoglobin values at sea level were below the following: 6 months to 6 years, 11 g; 6 to 14 years, 12 g; adult males, 13 g; adult females, 12 g; and pregnant women, 11 g. At all these ages the mean corpuscular hemoglobin concentration should be 34 percent. More than 95% of normal individuals are believed to be above these levels.

Anemia

The above values have been used as criteria in the discussion on anemia in the following pages.

Hemoglobin Levels in Infants, Children, and Adolescents

Abdou, Ali, and Lebshtein (1965), in a survey on 1,143 infants up to 24 months of age examined at Maternal and Child Health (M.C.H.) Centers in Cairo, found the average hemoglobin level in the neighborhood of 8.5 g per 100 ml. Hemoglobin at birth ranged from 15.5 to 18.5 g per 100 ml. The levels fell gradually till the lowest aver-

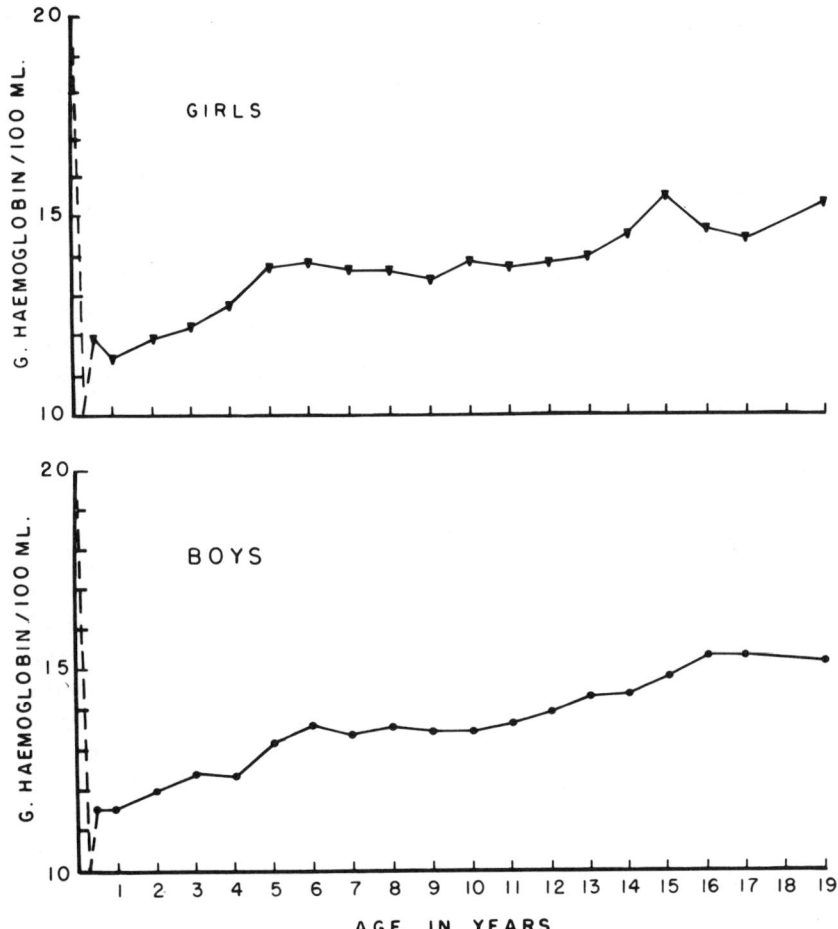

Figure 4.1. Average hemoglobin levels in British Children. Survey by Medical Research Council (1945).

age level of 8.0 g per 100 ml was reached between 9 and 12 months. There was a slight increase between 12 and 24 months. In the first year of life, between 43 and 68% of infants had hemoglobin levels between 5.6 and 8.5 g per 100 ml. These values compare unfavorably with those recorded for British children of comparable ages as observed in a survey made during World War II (Whitby and Britton, 1953) and illustrated in Figure 1. Thus infants from the community served by the M.C.H. Centers in Cairo included in the survey of Abdou *et al.* suffered from varying degrees of anemia. However, the situation may not be so bad in comparatively well-nourished Egyptian children, as the observations of Abdou *et al.* would indicate. For example, Taha and Shaker (1957) reported findings on 79 normal full-term infants whom they observed at birth and some of whom they followed for 30 months. At one day after birth the average hemoglobin was 18.9 g per 100 ml, at one month 11 g, and at six months 9.7 g per 100 ml. At this period the values are suggestive of moderate anemia. The hemoglobin level showed a rise in subsequent periods, giving an average of 13.2 g per 100 ml at 30 months. The findings of Taha and Shaker have to be interpreted with caution, for, although they started with 79 infants, the number examined at subsequent follow-up observations was not sufficient to allow a statistical interpretation of the findings. However, they should be considered suggestive of what hemoglobin levels one could expect in Egyptian infants, given proper nutrition among other things, even though the average values at six months were low. On the other hand the report of Abdou *et al.* probably indicates the state of affairs among the majority of the Egyptian infant population.

The gap in our knowledge regarding the hemoglobin levels of Egyptian children of 3 to 6 years is regrettable. Sherbini (1961) examined 210 children of 6 to 13 years from primary schools of Alexandria. He arrived at this number by a system of multi-stage sampling, and he considers the sample as representative of 116,909 primary school children in Alexandria. Sherbini found that mean hemoglobin values varied between 11.3 and 12.1 g per 100 ml. The differences between different yearly age groups were not statistically significant. The grand mean for the total sample was 11.76 g per 100 ml with a standard deviation of 1.38.

Abdou *et al.* (1967), in a survey among Cairo school children, examined hemoglobin levels in 1,637 boys and 1,219 girls of 6 to 19 years of age. His findings are given in Table 1.

In the absence of relevant information, it is difficult to determine if the small difference in the mean values between the sexes in the age group 14 to 19 was significant. The results of a survey in British chil-

Anemia

TABLE 1
HEMOGLOBIN LEVELS IN CAIRO SCHOOL CHILDREN

Age Groups Years	Average Hemoglobin g/100 ml			
	Cairo Children		MRC Averages for British Children	
	Boys	Girls	Boys	Girls
6–10	11.8	11.9	13.5	13.6
10–14	12.5	12.3	14.0	14.0
14–19	13.1	12.8	15.1	14.9

dren by the British Medical Research Council (1945) are given in the last two columns of the table. The British survey was done in wartime when the food situation in U.K. was precarious, requiring rigid control on food distribution. However, as the food distribution was carefully controlled with special attention to meeting the needs of the vulnerable groups of the population, the average hemoglobin levels of the British children were far more satisfactory than those found in U.K. before the war and can therefore be considered as the average normal values for healthy children.

In a sample of 90 growth-retarded boys of 11 to 17 years in a village school about 20 miles north of Cairo, Carter et al. (1969) found the average hemoglobin value of 12.6 g per 100 ml. The average underwent very minor variations for a year during which these boys were under observation and supplementation therapy with zinc and iron preparations. The latter had no significant effect on hemoglobin levels. The boys (30) from the school who were not retarded in growth gave an average value of 13.2 g per 100 ml. The difference was not significant.

As has already been mentioned, the reasons for such low average values for hemoglobin in Egyptian children may be partly dietary and partly parasitic infections, which are usually common in the Delta region of Egypt. Salah in 1935 had pointed out that parasitic infection was an important cause of anemia in the hospital patients seen by him. It is necessary to appreciate the importance of the widespread parasitism in Egypt and the role that it plays as a contributory factor in influencing the hemoglobin levels in the general population.

Role of Parasitism in Anemia

Prevalence of Parasitic Infections. Rifaat and Nagaty (1958) examined a single fecal sample in 948 residents of Cairo and 70 inhabitants of the Delta region from among the cases attending the skin outpatient department of the Ain Shams group of hospitals. They found that 50% of the patients from Cairo and 76% from the country were carrying protozoal or helminthic infection. Among the protozoa, *Entamoeba histolytica, Entamoeba coli, Entamoeba nana,* and *Giardia intestinales* were the common infective agents. The helminths commonly met with were *Ascaris, Ankylostoma, Hymenolepis nana,* and Enterobius. *Schistosoma mansoni* was rare. Mixed protozoal and helminth infections were common.

Nagaty, Gindy, and Rifaat (1961) examined urine and feces of school children (136 boys and 64 girls) of 6 to 15 years in Kerdasa village of Giza governorate. They found 64% of boys and 42% of girls infected with *Schistosoma hematobium* and 28% boys and 22% girls infected with *Ankylostoma duodenale*. These were the predominant parasites among other helminths and protozoa that were found. The same authors (1961b) found in Barnasht area of Giza Province an infection rate of 84% in 1,000 individuals of all ages after a single examination of urine and feces. In this population sample, too, *Schistosoma hematobium* and *Ankylostoma duodenal* were the most common infecting agents; the prevalence of schistosomiasis and ankylostomiasis was considered to have increased since 1955 when the last survey was done in this area. The high incidence of infection, from 76 to 85%, in the 1-to-9-year age group was a noteworthy feature of their findings. Almost similar observations were reported by Nagaty and Khalil (1960) at a health center in Damietta Province in the Delta bordering on the Mediterranean. Seventy-four percent of 273 persons examined were infected with one or more parasites. *Ascaris lumbricoides, Schistosoma hematobium, Schistosoma mansoni,* and *Ankylostoma duodenale* were again the most common helminths. The peak incidence of *Schistosoma hematobium* was in the 10-to-19-year age group and that of *Schistosoma mansoni* in the 20-to-29-year age group. Ankylostome infection showed no such definite trend. In Alexandria, at the northwest end of the Delta, Sherif (1961) found 64.9% of the primary school children and 20.3% of the 200 adults from the families of school children infected with Ascaris. He also found 26 out of 30 soil specimens from the small streets of Alexandria positive for *Ascaris* eggs. In a more detailed investigation on 1,150 urine and stool samples collected from school children in Alexandria, Sherif, Abdou, and Sawi (1961) found the following predominant infections among others not mentioned here: *Entamoeba histolytica,* 14.9%; *Entamoeba coli,* 2.2%; *Ascaris lumbicoides,* 65.0%; *Trichuris trichiura,* 14.6%; *Hymenolepis nana,* 7.9%; and *Enterobius vermicularis,* 10.5%. It was noteworthy that schistosome infection was found only in 1.1% of the children examined.

The association of parasitic infection with lowered hemoglobin levels becomes clear from the observations of Saif (1959), who deter-

TABLE 2
PARASITIC INFECTION AND AVERAGE HEMOGLOBIN CONCENTRATION
IN BLOOD OF EGYPTIANS[1]

	No.	% Hb.	S.D.
No parasites	972	91.25	9.62
Ankylostoma	373	75.28	17.29
Ascaris	530	84.42	10.81
Trichostrongylus	111	85.94	13.74
Oxyuris	202	88.56	8.17
Hymenolepis nana	119	81.98	11.54
Intestinal bilharziasis	67	78.23	18.52
Urinary bilharziasis	667	84.65	11.6
Urinary + Intestinal bilharziasis	43	81.94	14.48
Urinary bilharziasis + Ankylostoma	284	74.96	15.18

1. Source: Saif, 1959.

mined hemoglobin in the blood of 4,214 individuals by the acid hematin method. Saif also examined urine and feces for evidence of parasitism and found 77% of the total sample infected with one or more parasites. Taking 14.2 g hemoglobin per 100 ml blood as the normal level and expressing his results in percentage of this value, he demonstrated an association between the hemoglobin levels and parasitism. His results are given in Table 2.

Although the association of anemia with parasitism has been accepted for a long time, it is only recently that sufficient scientific evidence has been assembled which establishes beyond doubt the direct role of some of the parasites such as hookworm and bilharzia in the causation of anemia.

Hookworm. Roche and Layrisse (1966) have reviewed the world literature on the relationship between hookworm infection and anemia. In Venezuela, they found a significant negative correlation between the worm load (as determined by egg count) and hemoglobin concentration in blood in the population. According to them counts beyond 2,000 eggs/g feces cause a significant decrease in hemoglobin levels in relation to the severity of infection. The principal cause for the lowering of hemoglobin level in hookworm infection is bleeding in the intestine, with the resultant drain of iron from the body. This gives rise to a state of iron deficiency leading to anemia of iron-deficiency type.

Investigators have determined the relation between the worm load and the amount of blood loss (Roche and Layrisse, 1966). The observations of Roche, Pérez-Giménez, Layrisse, and Di Prisco (1957) in pure *Necator americanus* infections indicate that on an average, 0.031 ± 0.017 ml blood per worm is lost per day. In a single case of

TABLE 3
BLOOD AND IRON LOSS IN INFECTION WITH
ANKYLOSTOMA DUODENALE IN EGYPTIANS[1]

	Series I 12		Series II 12	
Number of Patients	Range	Average	Range	Average
Age in years	10–49		12–45	
Ova per g feces	4,133–10,933	5940	33–16,000	5636
Worms collected				
Male	21–77	39	3–217	65
Female	37–101	62	3–202	71
Hemoglobin g per 100 ml	2.8–11.2	7.5	3.2–12.5	6.4
Serum Fe μg/100 ml	12–43	21	20–42	28
TIBC μg/100 ml	381–763	563	308–615	443
Blood loss				
total in ml per day	13.6–45.0	26.4	2.3–120.3	31.4
in ml per day per worm	0.16–0.34	0.26	0.11–0.29	0.20
Iron loss mg per day	3.56–9.94	6.06	0.33–13.00	5.69

1. Source: Farid et al., 1965 and 1966.

mixed (71% ankylostoma and 29% necator) infection and allowing for the blood loss due to necator, these authors estimated the blood loss per *A. duodenale* at 0.205 ml per day. Working in Egypt with pure *A. duodenale* infections and also using the technique of Cr^{51} tagging of erythrocytes to estimate blood loss, Farid et al. (1965, 1966) studied two series of 12 infected subjects each. Their data from the two series of observations are reproduced in Table 3 in a modified form.

The slight difference between the average blood loss per worm in the two series of Farid et al. was due to the fact that in the first series no correction was made for the normal blood loss in the intestines, which may be as much as 2 ml per day (Roche et al., 1957). The difference, however, is immaterial in so far as the over-all magnitude of iron loss in ankylostome infection is concerned. It will appear from Table 3 that with the average worm loads of 100 and 136 worms, the total iron lost through bleeding could approach 6 mg a day. This is a gross estimate. The net iron loss may be smaller; by tagging erythrocytes with Cr^{51} and Fe^{59} in infected patients, Roche and Pérez-Giménez (1959) and also Layrisse and Roche (1962) found that some of the iron lost through bleeding was reabsorbed. The observed range was wide, but the average reabsorption in 40 subjects was found to be 39.2%. Farid and coworkers are now engaged in examining the reabsorption of the hemoglobin iron in *A. duodenale* infection. Preliminary results seem to confirm the findings of Roche and his group of workers in necator infection.

At the average level of gross iron loss observed by Farid *et al.* the net iron loss would still be substantial and possibly could not be compensated through dietary iron. This would partly account for the observations of Farid and Miale (1962) on the association between the intensity of ankylostome worm load and severity of anemia in 35 of their patients.

Bilharzia. The other common parasitic infection in Egypt is with schistosomes. As the earlier discussion must have shown, urinary (*Schistosoma hematobium*) and intestinal (*Schistosoma mansoni*) infection with the two species of the parasite are common particularly in the rural populations of the Delta region of Egypt. Not uncommonly, the same individual may harbor both types of infections. In chronic infection with *Schistosoma hematobium,* blood loss occurs through sporadic or continuous hematuria. Chronic infection with *Schistosoma mansoni,* on the other hand, gives rise to multiple polyipi in the colon and rectum, through which bleeding occurs. In double infections bleeding may occur through both the channels. Bleeding through one or both routes, when continued over prolonged periods as it is in chronic infections with these parasites, leads to a depletion of body iron stores and eventually to iron-deficiency anemia. Farid *et al.* (1967, 1968) have studied the contribution of schistosomiasis to iron depletion in both types of infections, and their findings are summarized in Table 4.

Recently Layrisse *et al.* (1967) have demonstrated that blood loss also occurs in infection with *Trichuris trichiura,* and this may be one of the causes of iron-deficiency anemia in children.

TABLE 4
BLOOD LOSS IN CHRONIC SCHISTOSOME INFECTION[1]

	Schistosoma Mansoni		Schistosoma Hematobium	
	Range	Average	Range	Average
Number of subjects	7		9	
Age in years	13–52	25	10–40	18
Hemoglobin g per 100 ml	2.8–13.2	8.2	5.0–13.2	8.8
Serum Fe μg/100 ml	6–56	31.5	15–45[2]	28
TIBC μg/100 ml	246–615	409	246–553[2]	407
Blood loss per day ml	7.5–25.9	12.5	2.6–126.0	22.7
Iron loss per day mg	0.6–6.7	3.5	0.6–37.3	6.9

1. Source: Farid *et al.*, 1967, 1968.
2. 6 patients only.

In Egypt, therefore, parasitic infections should be considered as a very important cause of the wide prevalence of anemia of varying degrees of severity. It will appear from the information contained in the preceding pages that no age group is exempt. However, the chronicity of infection, the existence of multiple infections, and the frequency of reinfection of treated cases will ultimately determine the state of iron deficiency and hence anemia in the Egyptian population, particularly in the Delta region. In urban areas where the prevalence and severity of infection are low, anemia does not occur with such frequency and with such severity as is found in the rural populations; nevertheless a mild degree of deficiency anemia does exist which might depend upon dietary inadequacy. When physiological stress supervenes, as happens during pregnancy, the deficiency state, and hence anemia, may be aggravated.

Hemoglobin Levels of Populations in the Oases

Abdou's (1965) observations in the Kharga and Dakhla oases indicate that mild degrees of anemia prevail in Egypt, even in the relative absence of parasitism. Out of the 429 urine samples examined in these oases, only 6 turned out to be positive for *Schistosoma hematobium*. In 132 stool specimens, the findings were as follows: Ascaris, 2; Hymenolepis, 2; Oxyuris, 6 and Ankylostoma, 2. Among the hospital patients 72 out of 458 in Dakhla and 13 out of 547 in Kharga had bilharziasis, and 6 patients in all from Kharga and Dakhla had ankylostomiasis. The hospital figures, and more so the results of the survey of the inhabitants, indicate a low prevalence of parasitic infections in these oases. In spite of this the average hemoglobin levels were lower than normal in these locations. This will become clear from Figure 2, which shows the frequency distribution of hemoglobin levels in children examined in Kharga and Dakhla oases as compared with children of comparable ages (7 to 13 years) from Namoul village in the Delta region. Most of the children in all the three locations had low hemoglobin values. However the percentage of children of both sexes having hemoglobin less than 11.3 g per 100 ml was far greater in Namoul than in Kharga and Dakhla, demonstrating once again the added effect of parasitism in Namoul against the general background of malnutrition in the three locations.

Hemoglobin Levels in Adult Population

The average hemoglobin levels in adults of the Kharga and Dakhla oases and Namoul village were found as follows:

| | Average Hemoglobin g/100 ml | |
	Males	Females
Dakhla	12.7	12.4
Kharga	11.3	11.0
Namoul	11.6	11.0

The frequency distribution of hemoglobin values in adults, also illustrated in Figure 2, shows a picture not dissimilar to that observed in children from these areas.

At the northern end of the Delta, in Alexandria, Khalifa and Salah (1951) had found higher average hemoglobin levels in 234 Egyptian male adults from the army, navy, and the Alexandria University Faculty of Medicine. The average for the whole group was 13.10 g per 100 ml. Of the total 234 subjects studied, 52 were free from parasites, and their average hemoglobin was 14.23 g per 100 ml. In the remaining 182 subjects with ankylostome and/or bilharzia infections, the average hemoglobin was 12.76 g per 100 ml. The higher average hemoglobin values for the Alexandria subjects were probably due to the fact that those subjects may have been better nourished than the population groups studied by Abdou in the oases and at Namoul.

Anemia Associated with Pregnancy

The low hemoglobin values found in women assume particular significance because of effects of pregnancy and lactation during their reproductive period. In a survey of 1,143 mothers of infants attending the Maternal and Child Health Centers in Cairo and 763 pregnant women, Abdou, Ali, and Lebshtein (1965) found that over 80% of nursing women and 90% of pregnant women had hemoglobin levels less than 10 g per 100 ml. Only 11% of nursing women had hemoglobin levels lower than 8.4 per 100 ml as against 54% of pregnant women. This really presents a grim picture of the status of health of possibly a majority of Egyptian women. It is possible that the situation may not be as bad even in Cairo as seems to be from the report of Abdou *et al*. Fathalla and Kamal (1964) reported on the findings in 300 pregnant women admitted for delivery in the Department of Gynecology and Obstetrics of the Medical Faculty of Cairo University. It is noteworthy that at the terminal period of pregnancy they found the average hemoglobin value of 11.02 g per 100 ml; about 34% of the cases had hemoglobin above 12 g per 100 ml and an equal number below 10 g per 100 ml.

Fathalla and Kamal found that increasing parity had an adverse

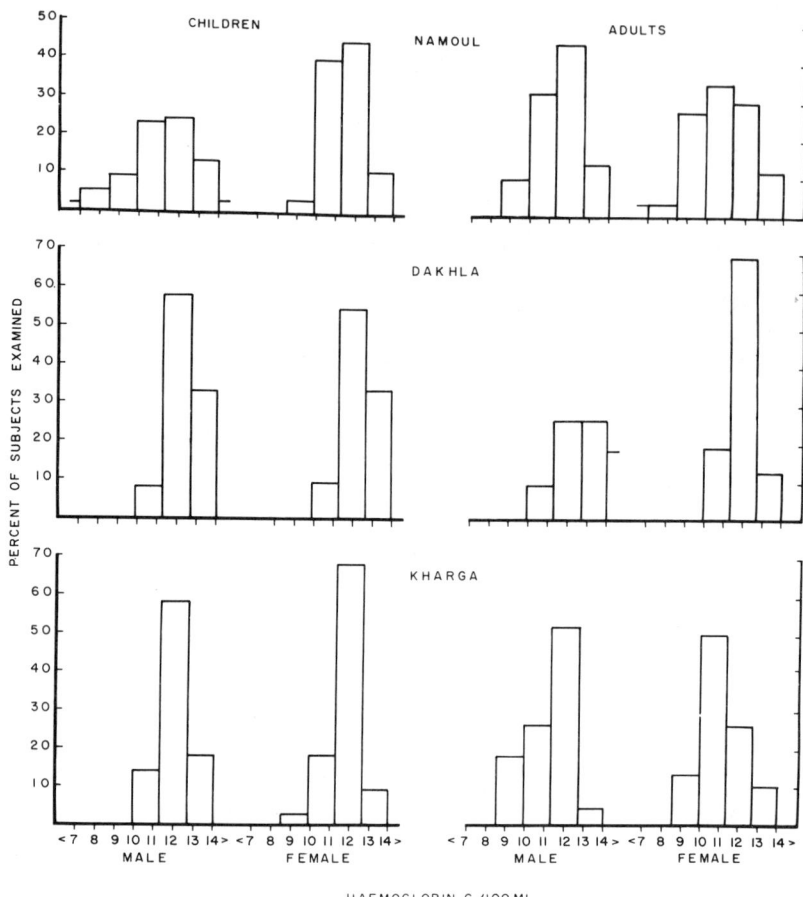

Figure 4.2. Hemoglobin levels in Egyptian adults and children of 7 to 13 years of age from the oases of Kharga and Dakhla and Namul village in the Delta.

effect of hemoglobin levels in their subjects. This will become clear from Table 5.

The table thus shows that hemoglobin decreased progressively as parity increased, indicating that during the intervals between successive pregnancies women in most cases were unable to regain the prepregnancy levels of hemoglobin. The cause may be nutrition, parasitic infection, or both.

Fathalla and Kamal also observed that six days after delivery the average hemoglobin level fell to 9.75 g per 100 ml. They ascribe this to blood loss at delivery. Based on the difference between hemoglobin

TABLE 5
HEMOGLOBIN LEVELS IN BLOOD AND PARITY IN 300 PREGNANT WOMEN AT TERM[1]

Parity	P	M_1	M_2	M_3	M_4 and Over
Percentage of cases	20.5	14.5	19	31	15
Average Hgb g/100 ml	12.4	11.9	12.1	10.2	8.5

1. Source: Fathalla and Kamal, 1964.

levels before and after delivery, their estimate of the average total blood loss in relation to delivery was 588 ml. The average is much higher than the reported figures elsewhere. The authors mentioned that blood loss depended on the ease of delivery and demonstrated that the fall in average hemoglobin after delivery was twice as high in difficult labor as in easy labor and four times higher in Caesarean section. The average blood loss, if it had been corrected for the cases undergoing Caesarean section, would have been much smaller.

Anemia associated with pregnancy in Egypt is largely of the iron deficiency type. Youssef, Ali, and El Mahdi (1954) investigated 50 unselected pregnant women between 28 weeks and term. Only three women had normal hematological values (values not stated), whereas 28 of them had hemoglobin levels below 10 g per 100 ml. Of these anemic cases 12 belonged to hypochromic microcytic type, 2 were orthochromic macrocytic, and 14 belonged to the hypochromic macrocytic or mixed type of anemia. The greatest number of these anemic pregnant women were iron deficient. Bone marrow aspirations were not done, and the factors responsible for macrocytosis were not investigated.

Mohi el Din (1954) studied 200 normal pregnant women. Of these 44 had hemoglobin levels above 10 g per 100 ml, with an average of 10.6 g per 100 ml, which was lower than the average value of 12.4 g per 100 ml for 20 nonpregnant women belonging to the comparable socioeconomic groups. Of the remainder who had hemoglobin levels below 10 g per 100 ml, the distribution of the types of anemia was as follows:

Microcytic hypochromic	100	MCHC	28.9%
Normocytic hypochromic	24	MCHC	29.5%
Macrocytic normochromic	4	MCHC	31.8%
Macrocytic hypochromic	28	MCHC	25.3%

If one considers 32 to 38% as the range for normal MCHC values and interprets the MCHC values given by the author accordingly, not only all the above-mentioned cases, but also those who had hemoglobin above 10 g per 100 ml, as well as the 24 controls, suffered from iron deficiency, the degree of deficiency being the only difference. Bone marrow aspirations were not done. Mohi el Din has described the results of treatment of some cases in each group. The majority of the microcytic hypochromic group responded to treatment with iron. The macrocytic anemia cases improved on a high protein diet, consisting of half a chicken, 3 eggs, and 750 g milk per day. The cases of mixed deficiency (macrocytic hypochromic) improved on high protein diet and additional iron. The other articles of diet are not mentioned. It is possible that a certain proportion of the anemia of pregnancy may be due to folate and/or vitamin B_{12} deficiencies, but we do not have enough evidence to appreciate its extent.

It would thus appear that irrespective of considerations of its prevalence, anemia associated with pregnancy presents a problem of public health importance in Egypt.

Anemia Associated with Protein-Calorie Deficiency

Anemia of varying degrees of severity almost always accompanies protein-calorie-deficiency disease (PCDD), and the Near East is no exception. The problem has recently been studied in some detail in Egypt, Lebanon, and Jordan in particular. Nabawy (1959) stated that hemoglobin levels of kwashiorkor cases in his experience ranged between 8 and 10 g per 100 ml and that the anemia was normocytic in a majority and macrocytic in a small number of cases. Gholmy et al. (1962) investigated 27 cases and concluded that anemia in most of them was due to iron deficiency. This conclusion was based on the examination of peripheral blood picture and determinations of serum iron and iron-binding capacity. A more detailed study with bone marrow findings in 17 cases has been published by Sandstead et al. (1965b). They confirmed that iron deficiency was frequently seen in their cases, but they also found megaloblastic changes in the bone marrow of 12 of the 17 cases examined. Serum vitamin B_{12} levels varied widely, but in most cases they were within the normal range or elevated. The authors did not determine folate in serum. Sandstead et al. concluded that anemia in PCDD must be due to a multiplicity of factors and that it would be unwise to attribute it to a single cause.

Weiler et al. (unpublished) studied in detail 77 cases of anemia associated with full-blown kwashiorkor. The anemia was moderate to severe, hypochromia being a common feature (MCHC 30.1% average); the MCV showed great variation from 49 to 179 $c\mu$ with an average of 93 $c\mu$. Bone marrow aspiration biopsies were examined in 61 cases. Megaloblastic changes were found in 16 of them with an elevated MCV (102 cμ average). Nine cases had also iron deficiency as judged by the absence of stainable iron in the bone marrow. Serum vitamin B_{12} levels were elevated in the whole group as well as in megaloblastic anemia cases. The mean serum folate level for the whole group was 4.1 ± 2.2 ng/ml and for 16 megaloblastic cases 4.0 ± 1.4 ng/ml. The tocopherol levels in serum were in general much higher than those observed by Sandstead et al. in their cases. It appears from the average serum folate values given by Weiler et al. that several of their patients had marginal folate levels and a few were within the range of clinical deficiency (values below 3 ng/ml). Out of 16 cases of megaloblastic anemia, Weiler et al. treated 10 cases with folic acid, vitamin B_{12}, and vitamin E. Three patients fully responded to folic acid, and two more gave an equivocal response. Five other cases which were complicated by iron deficiency and severe infection failed to respond to folic acid, vitamin E, or vitamin B_{12}. These investigations thus point to the possible role of the deficiency of other nutrients, not as yet known, in megaloblastic anemia associated with kwashiorkor.

More recently Halsted et al. (unpublished) have investigated in detail 24 more cases with complete hematological and bone marrow examinations, determinations of iron, folate, vitamin B_{12}, and vitamin E levels in serum. They were cases exhibiting signs and symptoms of kwashiorkor with a mean serum albumin level of 2.1 g and mean hemoglobin level of 8.5 g (range 3.7 to 12.2 g) per 100 ml on admission. The mean corpuscular volume ranged between 75 and 130 cμ with an average value of 89.5 cμ. The mean corpuscular hemoglobin concentration was 30.3%, with a range of 19 to 36%. Various degrees of bone marrow maturation abnormality were found in 17 out of 24 cases and marrow hemosiderin absent or minimum in 18 cases. Serum vitamin B_{12} levels were either normal or elevated (range 214–1390 pg/ml); serum folate levels ranged from 1.5 to 8.8 ng/ml and serum vitamin E from 0.15 to 0.78 mg per 100 ml. Thus the majority of cases in this group had iron and folate deficiencies contributing to the development of anemia in addition to protein deficiency. A significant number showed a reticulocyte response to realimentation with protein-rich diet without the administration of any hematinic. In these patients, as well as others of the series on whom observations could be completed (4 died and 3 left the hospital prematurely), therapy with iron and folic acid evoked further reticulocyte responses and brought about the restoration of normal hematological values.

Basic hematologic and related data from the investigations referred to above are summarized in Table 6.

TABLE 6
HEMATOLOGIC AND RELEVANT DATA ON ANEMIA IN KWASHIORKOR IN EGYPT

	Gholmy et al.		Sandstead et al.		Weiler et al.	Halsted et al.
	M^1 (12)[3]	K^2 (15)	K (39)		K (77)	K (24)
Hemoglobin g/100 ml	7.79	7.39	(31)	8.3 ± 2.2		8.5 ± 2.14
Hct %			(31)	26.5 ± 5.9	26.5 ± 4.3	28.2 ± 6.36
R.B.C. mill/cmm			(31)	2.82 ± 0.77		3.27 ± 0.95
MCV cuμ			(31)	96.7 ± 16.3	92.9 ± 22.0	89.5 ± 14.8
MCHC %			(31)	31.1 ± 3.1	30.1 ± 3.3	30.3 ± 3.45
Retics %			(17)	2.4 ± 4.2		
Serum Fe μg/100 ml	50.8 ± 15	28 ± 0.93	(33)	44 ± 20.5		62.9 ± 28.2
T.I.B.C. μg/100 ml	351 ± 38	144 ± 5.4	(21)	88 ± 61.0		257 ± 133
Serum Cu μg/100 ml		133	(34)	94 ± 53.0		
Serum folate ng/ml					4.1 ± 2.2	4.4 ± 2.97
Serum vitamin B_{12} pg/ml			(26)	367 ± 321	924 ± 791	592 ± 276
Serum tocopherol mg/100 ml			(9)	0.15	0.64 ± 0.61	0.42 ± 0.21
Serum protein						
Total g/100 ml	5.47 ± 0.55	3.61 ± 0.16	(39)	4.12 ± 0.86	4.1 ± 0.8	4.4 ± 0.99
Albumin g/100 ml	2.18 ± 0.32	1.06 ± 0.08	(39)	1.17 ± 0.67	1.1 ± 0.6	2.1 ± 0.68

1. M = Marasmus
2. K = Kwashiorkor
3. Figures in parentheses indicate number of cases.

Anemia

LIBYA, LEBANON, JORDAN

Anemia in General Population

That anemia, probably of the iron-deficiency type, prevails in these countries is to be concluded from the reports of ICNND Surveys done in these countries between 1957 and 1963. The mean levels of hemoglobin in the population groups examined in these surveys have been given in the chapter on nutritional status. However a distribution of values for hemoglobin and the mean corpuscular hemoglobin concentration together should give a better idea of the prevalence of anemia in these populations and the probable underlying deficiency than the mean values for hemoglobin levels alone. Such an attempt is made here and summarized in Tables 7, 8, and 9.

It has been stated earlier in this chapter that the normal range for MCHC values is 32 to 38%, although according to WHO Report (1968) it should not be less than 34%. Assuming that the range of 32 to 38% represents the normal distribution of values, those below 32 should be indicative of iron deficiency. In the ICNND Survey in Libya, the intervals for MCHC distribution as given in the report are somewhat awkward from the standpoint of interpretation. Individuals are grouped according to their MCHC (1) < 28.0; (2) 28.0–29.9; (3) 30–33.9; and (4) above 34 percent. Whereas there is no doubt about iron deficiency in the first two groups, there must be a certain number of individuals in the third higher group whose MCHC was between 30 and 31.9%, values which would be indicative of iron deficiency. In the Libyan sample the proportion of those individuals cannot be estimated. However, the percentages of individuals below 30% MCHC and between 30 and 33.9% have been shown separately.

TABLE 7
HEMOGLOBIN AND MCHC VALUES AS INDICATED OF ANEMIA
IN POPULATION GROUPS IN LIBYA[1]

	Number	Hemoglobin < 12 g/100 ml	MCHC 30%	MCHC 30–33.9%
		%	%	%
Army	67	3.0	14.9	76.1
Defense & Police Forces	77	3.9	23.2	66.2
Civilians				
Men	97	3.1	15.6	69.8
Nonpregnant women	37	24.3	21.6	67.6
Pregnant women	35	64.6	26.5	61.8

1. Source: Adapted from ICNND *Report on Nutrition Survey in Libya*, 1957.

TABLE 8
HEMOGLOBIN AND MCHC VALUES AS INDICATORS OF ANEMIA IN POPULATION GROUPS IN LEBANON AND JORDAN[1]

| | | Number | | Hgb < 12 g/100 ml | | MCHC | | | |
| | | | | | | Nonrefugees | | Refugees | |
	Age	Nonrefugees	Refugees	Nonrefugees	Refugees	< 29.9%	30–31.9%	< 29.9%	30–31.9%
				%	%	%	%	%	%
Civilian				*Lebanon*					
Males & Females	5–9	47	53	60.5	57.5	39.5	37.2	42.5	25.0
Males	10–14	22	15	22.7	25.0	22.7	50.0	0	66.7
	15–44	44	12	0	0	35.6	57.8	50.0	33.3
	45+	28		3.7		51.8	37.0		
Females	10–14	32	12	38.7	50.0	45.2	29.0	40.0	40.0
	15+	33	7	43.8	42.8	53.1	40.6	71.4	0
Pregn. & Lactat.		12	48	66.7	85.7	66.7	25.0	71.4	24.5
				Jordan					
Males	5–9	29	32	27.6	40.6	17.2	48.3	24.9	28.6
	10–14	26	25	7.7	28.0	34.6	42.5	24.0	40.0
	15–44	41	17	7.3	5.9	17.0	24.4	5.9	52.9
	45+	29	24	6.9	4.2	13.7	27.6	29.2	33.3
Females	5–9	24	32	25.0	25.0	27.2	54.5	12.5	21.9
	10–14	35	24	31.4	20.8	32.4	41.2	13.0	43.5
	15–44	41	28	29.3	17.8	29.3	36.6	25.0	35.7
	45+	28	4	17.8	25.0	7.1	57.1	—	—
Pregn. & Lactat.		46	30	39.1	43.3	19.6	45.6	31.0	41.4

1. Source: Adapted from ICNND *Reports on Nutrition Surveys in Lebanon* (1962) *and Jordan* (1963).

Bearing in mind the above limitations, one does find that a small percentage of men examined had hemoglobin lower than 12 g per 100 ml, but a much greater proportion gave an indication of iron deficiency. Among women there was a greater proportion of anemic subjects. One can also see that a larger proportion of pregnant women was anemic than the women who were not pregnant. The number of subjects whose blood was examined was small. However, this was a subsample of a total of 3,592 individuals of different categories coming from different parts of the country. One could justifiably conclude, therefore, that anemia of iron-deficiency type is not uncommon in Libya and that women are affected more than men.

The situation with regard to anemia prevalence in Lebanon and Jordan as revealed by surveys carried out in 1961 and 1962 respectively was not much different (Table 8). Trends similar to those found in Libya were also observed in these two countries. The interpretation of findings is rendered easier by the inclusion of a new group of MCHC values, i.e., 30–31.9%. The prevalence of anemia was higher in women than in men, and pregnancy and lactation were associated with still higher prevalence. The cutoff point taken by ICNND for hemoglobin for children 5 to 9 years of age was probably higher than it ought to be. However the MCHC values should indicate a high prevalence of iron deficiency in this age group. Comparative figures for the refugee population and the other civilians are to be found in Table 8. In Lebanon as well as in Jordan there does not appear to be much difference between these two groups.

In Table 9 are summarized the hemoglobin and MCHC values

TABLE 9
HEMOGLOBIN AND MCHC VALUES AS INDICATORS OF ANEMIA
IN JORDANIAN INFANTS AND YOUNG CHILDREN[1]

Age Group	Number	Hemoglobin g/100 ml		MCHC	
		Mean	Less than 10g	< 29.9%	30–31.9%
			%	%	%
< 1 yr.	29	10.12	44.8	44.8	27.6
1 yr.	66	10.12	41.0	47.6	17.5
2 yr.	79	10.36	31.7	44.0	24.0
3 yr.	88	11.23	15.9	16.3	32.6
4 yr.	84	11.23	20.3	21.0	32.1
5 yr.	86	11.94	5.9	9.6	20.5
0–5 yr.	432				
Nonrefugees	336	11.06	21.5	26.1	24.2
Refugees	96	10.66	30.2	33.0	31.9

1. Source: Adapted from ICNND-ICNJ *Report on Jordan Pediatric Study* (1964).

taken from the report of a pediatric study done in 1963 jointly by ICNND and ICNJ (Interdepartmental Committee on Nutrition for Jordan). This study covered infants and children up to 5 years of age from all the areas of the Hashemite Kingdom of Jordan. The cutoff point for hemoglobin has been arbitrarily selected as 10 g per 100 ml, and the mean values for hemoglobin are included for each year's age group.

A comparison of the hemoglobin levels with Figure 1 will show that the average values in Jordanian infants and children were much below the MRC average values for British children of comparable age. A similar finding has been recorded by Patwardhan and Kamel (1967) for 845 children of 0-6 years belonging to randomly selected families from the east and west banks of the Jordan. It will be clear from Table 9 that moderate to severe anemia was more common during the first two years of life. The low values of hemoglobin became progressively less frequent after this period. The values for MCHC indicate that iron deficiency probably was the important contributory factor. As in adults, there was not much difference between the refugee and other children of comparable age, although the figures in Table 9 would indicate a slightly higher prevalence among the refugee children. The difference, however, is probably not significant.

Anemia Associated with Protein-Calorie Malnutrition

The report of the Jordan Pediatric Study includes reference to some special investigations in protein-calorie malnutrition. In 30 malnourished children (1 marasmus, 9 kwashiorkor, and 20 pre-kwashiorkor), the average hemoglobin was 9.00 g per 100 ml, and the average hematocrit value was 31.7%. The resulting MCHC value of 28.2 indicates a degree of iron deficiency greater than that in the total group of children, as shown in Table 9. Other factors may also have been responsible for anemia associated with protein-calorie malnutrition. Pharaon (1960) mentioned that out of 216 cases studied by him in Amman, anemia was clinically diagnosed in 163. Of these 25 suffered from severe anemia requiring blood transfusion; 33 others had moderately severe anemia as determined by the blood counts. All cases were treated with iron and multivitamins together with a protein-rich diet. The results of treatment so far as anemia was concerned were not described.

Majaj (1960), working at the Augusta Victoria Hospital in Jerusalem, has reported on 183 cases of protein-calorie malnutrition. He studied anemia in some detail in 65 cases of kwashiorkor and 32 cases of what appears to have been marasmus. Although the average and the range of values are not given, the distribution of cases according to red blood cell count and hemoglobin values indicates that Majaj was dealing with a severe degree of anemia associated with protein-calorie malnutrition more so than had Pharaon in his report from Amman. In infants under one year of age, anemia was more severe in those with kwashiorkor than in patients with no edema. This was not so clear in the older children, mainly because the number in one group (marasmus) was very small. It is noteworthy that 70% of 97 cases had an MCV over 100 cμ and an almost equal percentage had a MCHC below 28%, indicating that these were cases mostly of macrocytic hypochromic anemia. Pharaon in Amman had found macrocytosis in only 10 of the 25 cases of severe anemia on whom MCV was determined. The reasons for this difference were not quite clear. Pharaon and Majaj were dealing with two different population groups within the country. Whereas Pharaon's patients were drawn from the civilian population, those of Majaj were almost wholly if not entirely from the Palestine Arab refugees living in Jordan. This in itself is not a sufficient explanation. Neither Pharaon nor Majaj examined the bone marrows, thus leaving the characterization of anemia incomplete. Majaj observed that intramuscular administration of B_{12} was necessary to lower the MCV. If so, vitamin B_{12} deficiency was probably involved in addition to that of iron in the pathogenesis of anemias associated with protein-calorie malnutrition in a majority of cases seen by him. The experience in other parts of the world and even in Cairo has been that serum vitamin B_{12} levels in kwashiorkor are either within the normal range or are elevated, and it seems that vitamin B_{12} deficiency is rare in this condition. Unfortunately Majaj at that time did no determinations of serum vitamin B_{12}. In a later paper, Majaj, Dinning, Azzam, and Darby (1963) give more detailed investigation of 12 cases of anemia, all of which proved to be megaloblastic on bone marrow examination with characteristic changes in the red and white cell precursors. In 9 cases in which serum vitamin B_{12} was determined, two had values of 46 and 64 pg/ml whereas in 7 others they were between 170 and 948 pg/ml. The patients were maintained for two to four weeks on a skim milk-casein-enriched diet before starting any specific therapy. During this period a transitory reticulocytosis was seen without significant hemopoiesis. Plasma vitamin E levels were low, with an average of 0.43 mg/100 ml, and the urinary creatine:creatinine ratios were higher than the normal range of 0.4 to 0.6. Thus there was evidence of vitamin E deficiency in these patients. Serum folate levels were not determined. Based on the biochemical evidence of vitamin E deficiency and on the occurrence of binucleated megaloblasts in bone marrow similar to those described by Porter, Finch, and Dining (1962) in vitamin E deficient monkeys the authors instituted treatment with vitamin E. This consisted of 100 mg α-tocopherol phosphate intramuscularly and 280 mg α-tocopherol acetate orally per day for 5 days. A reticulocyte response followed this treatment, accompanied by a rise in r.b.c., hemoglobin, and plasma vitamin E and a reduction in urinary creatine:creatinine ratios. The megaloblastic marrow became normoblastic; the MCV was reduced from 112 ± 5 before treatment to 91 ± 5 after treatment. The final hemoglobin values for all patients are not given, but in the two cases graphically illustrated in the paper hemoglobin had risen to about 8 g per 100 ml from the initial values of about 2 and 4 respectively. Since the MCHC had remained unchanged after treatment (mean 28%) with vitamin E, iron deficiency may probably have limited the rise in hemoglobin.

In commenting on their results, Majaj *et al.* pointed out that the hematologic response to vitamin E was similar to that obtained with vitamin B_{12} or folic acid, and they suggested that vitamin E should be considered as one of the hemopoietic factors of importance in man. They further expressed the opinion that similar cases may be found elsewhere. Indeed this hope was partially fulfilled, for a year later Marvin and Audu (1964) published a note describing the results of vitamin E therapy in anemia of kwashiorkor in Nigeria. They found extremely low levels of vitamin E (0 to 0.09 mg/100 ml) in 14 children with kwashiorkor. They administered tocopherol, 100 mg orally and 100 mg by injection, for 5 days and elicited a reticulocyte response. Further information on the rise of hemoglobin is not given in the paper. Recently Whitaker, Fort, Vimokesant, and Dinning (1967) demonstrated in an empirical trial in Thailand the hemopoietic effect of vitamin E in anemia associated with protein-calorie malnutrition. The trial included 41 cases which were maintained on a high protein diet alone and 19 cases which received in addition a supplement of 250 mg α-tocopherol acetate for 5 days. The children in both the groups were followed for 17 to 37 days. Out of 19 children receiving tocopherol, 18 showed a rise in hemoglobin ranging between 1.2 to 6.1 g per 100 ml, whereas the hemoglobin level actually showed a fall in the unsupplemented group. Between 25 to 28 days after tocopherol administration the vitamin E-supplemented group had an average hemoglobin value higher by 2.7 g per 100 ml than the average in the control group. These reports therefore confirm the observations of Majaj *et al.* (1963). Dinning *et al.* (1963) found 4 cases of megaloblastic anemia in Jordanian kwashiorkor children, with kwashiorkor responding to a dosage of 6-chromanol of hexahydrocoenzyme Q4 at the level of 300 mg per day given orally for 7 days. The response was similar to that previously obtained with tocopherol phosphate and acetate. The authors, however, felt no reason to assume a deficiency of coenzyme Q10 in these children. In a recent publication, Majaj (1966) reported that the administration of vitamin E to six infants with megaloblastic anemia associated with kwashiorkor and marasmus brought about an increase in serum levels of folate and ascorbic acid, although these nutrients had not been given. These findings point to a possible interrelationship between vitamin E, folate, and ascorbic acid metabolism.

In Lebanon, Asfour and Firzli (1965) tried the effect of vitamin E in malnourished anemic infants 12 to 24 months in age. All these infants had very low serum vitamin E (0 to 0.16 mg/100 ml). The average hemoglobin level was 8 g per 100 ml and the average MCHC 26.6%. These were cases of iron-deficiency anemia, for bone marrow examination did not show any abnormality in maturation. However, Asfour and Firzli found that vitamin E administration did not evoke a reticulocyte or hematologic response, whereas iron administration did as was to be expected. They conclude that vitamin E deficiency did not contribute to the state of anemia of iron-deficiency type. It must be stated here that these findings do not contradict those of Majaj *et al.* in Jordan, for the type of anemia studied in the two locations was different.

In Cairo, Egypt, a series of investigations (Sandstead *et al.*, 1965, Weiler *et al.*, unpublished, and Halsted *et al.*, 1969) show that the search for anemia associated with protein-calorie malnutrition which would respond to vitamin E has not been very encouraging. The object of the two latter studies was to identify vitamin E responsive anemia as an entity apart from those types which respond to the already known hematinics such as iron, folate, and vitamin B_{12}. All these investigators in Cairo have found low serum vitamin E levels in a majority of their anemia cases. A certain proportion of these anemias were megaloblastic. The serum levels of folate were also low. In addition to the megaloblastic change in the bone marrow, the complete absence of hemosiderin, or a considerable decrease in stainable iron in the bone marrow, indicated that deficiencies of folic acid and iron were the causative factors in anemia of kwashiorkor in Egypt. This conclusion was confirmed on therapy with these two hematinics as described by Halsted and coworkers. Thus the megaloblastic anemias studied in Cairo resembled those investigated by Majaj in Jerusalem in their pathology and biochemical features. Whether they could have responded to vitamin E instead of folic acid is an open question. To our knowledge, nowhere has Majaj claimed that his cases failed to respond to folic acid, nor is there a record of his having tried folic acid.

Darby (1968) has reviewed most recently the evidence of the hemopoietic role of vitamin E in man and animals. Vitamin E is essential for hemopoiesis in the monkey, pig, trout, and rat. Anemia of prematurity in the human infant responds to vitamin E. In infants fed diets rich in polyunsaturated fatty acids but low in vitamin E, there is an increase in reticulocytosis, poikilocytosis, and anisocytosis and increased sensitivity to peroxide hemolysis of erythrocytes. These changes respond to treatment with vitamin E. These facts, taken together with the observations in malnourished infants of Majaj *et al.* (1963), Marvin and Audu (1964), and Whitaker *et al.* (1967), provide reasonably convincing evidence that vitamin E has a role in hemopoiesis in man as well. The later finding of Majaj (1966) of the effect of vitamin E on the serum levels of folate and ascorbic acid, already referred to, point to a possible interrelationship between these nutrients. Whereas at the present moment there is no satisfactory explanation for the mechanism of vitamin E action in hemopoiesis, Darby's suggestion that a study of the interrelationship between vitamin E and the known hematinics might provide the answer appears to be the possible approach to the problem.

Summarizing the situation with regard to anemias in the Middle Eastern Arab countries, one cannot escape the conclusion that anemia is an important public health problem and one of the causes of ill health among the population. In Egypt, malnutrition and parasitic infection together are responsible for moderate to severe degrees of anemia among the majority of the adult population. In the other countries of the region, it is probably the inadequacy of dietary intake of iron or, in cases where it is adequate, interference in its absorption, exerted by other dietary constituents such as phytate, that may be responsible for the prevalence of anemia, which in general is mild to moderate. The prevalence and severity of anemia is greater in women of child-bearing age, and pregnancy and lactation seem to aggravate the severity. Anemia also commonly accompanies protein-calorie malnutrition in infants and young children in all these countries.

The prevailing anemia is mostly of the iron-deficiency type, as the description of findings so far would indicate. In malnourished children, however, since they suffer from panhypoalimentation, there may be more than one nutritional deficiency involved in the causation of anemia.

REFERENCES

Abdou, I. A. 1960. Nutrition Problems in the Egyptian Region. *J. Egypt. Publ. Hlth. Assoc.* 35: 137.

Abdou, I. A., H. E. Ali, A. K. Said, W. A. Moussa, H. G. Demian, A. M. Soliman, and L. H. Hawary. 1967. Incidence of Nutritional Deficiencies, Goiter, and Dental Caries among School Children in Cairo. *J. Egypt. Publ. Hlth. Assoc.* 42: 175.

Asfour, R. Y., and S. Firzli. 1965. Hematologic Studies in Undernourished Children with Low Serum Vitamin E Levels. *Amer. J. Clin. Nutr.* 17: 158.

Aykroyd, W. R., and F. W. Clements. 1950. *A Nutrition Program for Egypt.* Report to FAO and WHO. Document FAO/54/3/1813. Rome, Italy: Food and Agriculture Organization.

Darby, W. J. 1968. Tocopherol Responsive Anemias in Man. *Vitamins and Hormones* 26: 685.

Dinning, J. S., A. S. Majaj, S. A. Azzam, W. J. Darby, C. H. Shunk, and K. Folkers. 1963. Response of Macrocytic Anemia in Children to the Coenzyme Q_4-Chromanol. *Amer. J. Clin. Nutr.* 13: 169.

Farid, Z., and A. Miale. 1962. Treatment of Hookworm Infection in Egypt with Bephenium Hydroxynaphthoate and the Relationship between Iron Deficiency Anemia and Intensity of Infection. *Amer. J. Trop. Med. Hyg.* 11: 497.

Farid, Z., J. H. Nichols, S. Bassily, and A. R. Schulert. 1965. Blood Loss in Pure *Ancylostoma duodenale* Infection in Egyptian Farmers. *Amer. J. Trop. Med. Hyg.* 14: 375.

Farid, Z., S. Bassily, A. R. Schulert, J. H. Nichols, and S. Guindy. 1966. Blood Loss in Egyptian Farmers Infected with *Ancylostoma duodenale*. *Trans. Roy. Soc. Trop. Med. Hyg.* 60: 486.

Farid, Z., S. Bassily, A. R. Schulert, F. Raasch, A. S. Zeind, A. S. Rooby, and M. Sherif. 1967. Blood Loss in Chronic *Schistosoma mansoni* Infection in Egyptian Farmers. *Trans. Roy. Soc. Trop. Med. Hyg.* 61: 621.

Farid, Z., S. Bassily, A. R. Schulert, A. S. Zeind, E. McConnell, and M. F. Abdel Wahab. 1968. Urinary Blood Loss in *Schistosoma hematobium* Infection in Egyptian Farmers. *Trans. Roy. Soc. Trop. Med. Hyg.* 62: 496.

Fathalla, M. F., and I. Kamal. 1964. Hemoglobin Levels Before and After Parturition. *J. Egypt. Med. Assoc.* 47: 373.

Halsted, C. H., N. Sourial, S. Guindi, K. A. H. Mourad, A. K. Khattab, J. P. Carter, V. N. Patwardhan. 1969. Anemia of Kwashiorkor in Cairo: Deficiencies of Protein, Iron, and Folic Acid. *Amer. J. Clin. Nutr.* 22: 1371.

Interdepartmental Committee on Nutrition for National Defense. *Reports of Nutrition Surveys in Libya, 1957; Lebanon, 1962; Jordan, 1963.* Bethesda, Md.: National Institutes of Health.

Interdepartmental Committee on Nutrition for National Defense (USA) and Interdepartmental Committee on Nutrition for Jordan. 1964. *Nutrition Survey on Infants and Preschool Children in Jordan.* Bethesda, Md.: National Institutes of Health.

Khalifa, A. A., and M. K. Salah. 1951. A Survey of the Hemoglobin Content of Blood of Egyptians. *J. Egypt. Med. Assoc.* 34: 647.

Layrisse, M., and M. Roche. 1962. Reabsorption of Hemoglobin Iron Lost into the Intestine in Hookworm-Infected Patients: Conference on Malabsorption and Allied Hematological Problems. *Amer. J. Digest. Dis.* 7: 976.

Majaj, A. S. 1960. Protein Malnutrition and Macrocytic Anemia among Palestine Refugees in Jordan. *Gaz. Egypt. Pediat. Assoc.* 8: 611.

Majaj, A. S. 1966. Vitamin E Responsive Macrocytic Anemia in Protein-Calorie Malnutrition: Measurements of Vitamin E, Folic Acid, Vitamin C, Vitamin B_{12}, and Iron. *Amer. J. Clin. Nutr.* 18: 362.

Majaj, A. S., J. S. Dinning, S. A. Azzam, and W. J. Darby. 1963. Vitamin E Responsive Megaloblastic Anemia in Infants with Protein-Calorie Malnutrition. *Amer. J. Clin. Nutr.* 12: 374.

Marvin, H. N., and I. S. Audu. 1964. A Preliminary Study of Vitamin E and the Anemia of Kwashiorkor. *West. Afr. Med. J.* 13:3.

Medical Research Council U.K. 1943. Special Report Series No. 252. London: H.M.S.O.

Mohi-el-din, O. 1954. Studies on Anemias of Pregnancy. *J. Egypt. Med. Assoc.* 37: 613.

Nagaty, H. F., M. S. Gindy, and M. A. Rifaat. 1961. A Helminthological Survey of the School Children of Kerdasa Village, Giza Governorate, Egypt, U.A.R., in 1960. *J. Egypt. Med. Assoc.* 44: 516.

———. 1961b. A Parasitological Survey of the Inhabitants of the Barnasht Area, Giza Province, Egypt, U.A.R., in 1959. *J. Egypt. Med. Assoc.* 44: 68.

Nelson, W. E. 1959. Textbook of Pediatrics. Seventh Edition. Philadelphia and London: W. B. Saunders Company.

Pharaon, H. M. 1960. Nutritional Deficiency Syndrome in Jordan. *Gaz. Egypt. Pediat. Assoc.* 8: 469.

Porter, F. S., C. D. Fitch, and J. S. Dinning. 1962. Vitamin E Deficiency in the Monkey. IV—Further Studies of the Anemia with Emphasis on Bone Marrow Morphology. *Blood* 20: 471.

Rifaat, M. A., and H. F. Nagaty. 1958. The Incidence of Intestinal Parasitic Infections among the Inhabitants of Cairo. *J. Egypt. Med. Assoc.* 41: 164.

Roche, M., and M. Layrisse. 1966. The Nature and Causes of "Hookworm Anemia." *Amer. J. Trop. Med. Hyg.* 15: 1032.

Roche, M., and M. E. Perez-Gimenez. 1959. Intestinal Loss and Reabsorption of Iron in Hookworm Infection. *J. Lab. Clin. Med.* 54: 49.

Roche, M., M. E. Perez-Gimenez., M. Layrisse, and E. Di Prisco. 1957. A study of Urinary and Fecal Excretion of Radioactive Chromium Cr^{51} in Man: Its Use in the Measurement of Intestinal Blood Loss Associated with Hookworm Infection. *J. Clin. Invest.* 36: 1183.

Sherbini, A. F. 1961a. The Blood Picture of the Alexandria Primary School Children. *Alexandria Med. J.* 7: 137.

———. 1961b. Ascaris Infection in Alexandria. *Alexandria Med. J.* 7: 427.

Sherif, A. F., A. H. Abdou, and F. Sawi. 1961. Incidence of Parasitic Infections among School Children in Alexandria. *Alexandria Med. J.* 7: 483.

Taha, M. M. and Y. K. H. Shaker. 1957. A Study of Serum Iron in Infancy. Part I-In Health. *Alexandria Med. J.* 3: 423.

Vilter, R. W., W. J. Darby, and H. S. Glazer. 1954. A Survey of Pellagra and Nutritional Anemia in Egypt. Geneva, Switzerland: World Health Organization.

Weiler, R. J., M. K. Gabr, S. Shukry, A. Hifney, K. Anderson, and W. J. Darby. Anemia of Kwashiorkor in Egypt: Studies on Folic Acid, Vitamin E and Vitamin B_{12}. Forthcoming.

Whitaker, J. A., E. G. Fort, S. Vimokesant, and J. S. Dinning. 1967. Hematologic Response to Vitamin E in the Anemia Associated with Protein-Calorie Malnutrition. *Amer. J. Clin. Nutr.* 20: 783.

Whitby, L. E. H., and C. J. C. Britton. 1963. *Disorders of the Blood.* 9th ed. London: J. and A. Churchill Ltd.

Wintrobe, M. M. 1967. *Clinical Hematology.* 6th ed. Philadelphia, Pa.: Lea and Febiger.

World Health Organization. 1968. *Nutritional Anemias-Report of a WHO Scientific Group.* Wld. Hlth. Org. Techn. Rep. Ser. 405.

Youssef, A. F., A. M. Ali, and M. A. H. Mahdi. 1954. Anemia in Pregnancy in Egypt: A Problem of National Importance. *J. Egypt. Med. Assoc.* 37: 319.

5 Endemic Goiter

The thyroid gland is one of the endocrine organs of the body. It is situated at the base of the neck in front of the trachea and consists of two lobes joined by a narrow band of thyroid tissue. Ordinarily the gland is not visible and not even palpable.

The average weight of the thyroid gland in an adult varies between 20 and 30 g. At birth it weighs less than 2 g. It gradually increases in size and weight with an accelerated growth at puberty and assumes its normal weight after adolescence.

The function of the thyroid gland is to control the general metabolic activity of the body. It does this through a hormone, thyroxine, which it synthesizes. The thyroid gland has the capacity to concentrate iodine from the circulating blood and to use this iodine for the synthesis of thyroxine, which is then secreted back into the blood circulation in combination with a protein. The amount of iodine needed per day to keep an individual in health and his thyroid gland functioning normally is extremely small; nevertheless it is an essential nutrient. Stanbury (1960) believes that the average daily consumption of iodine in nongoitrous areas is above 75 μg/day. The estimates of daily iodine requirement vary between 150 and 200 μg/day. All of it must be derived through food, both of plant and animal origin. Iodine occurs in soil and water, and through these it is incorporated in plant food grown and in animals that thrive on such food.

There are situations where the iodine content of soil and water is low. Man in these regions subsists on iodine-deficient food and suffers from iodine deficiency. Under these conditions the thyroid gland enlarges, and the resulting condition is known as simple goiter. This enlargement is considered a compensatory mechanism for counteracting the effects of the deficiency in the supply of iodine to the gland. When the proportion of individuals with visibly enlarged thyroid exceeds 5% in a population, the area is considered endemic for iodine deficiency and the condition termed endemic goiter.

The endemicity of goiter can be ascertained by examining the thyroid gland as a part of the nutrition survey program. The actual techniques of examination and recording of the enlargement of thyroid in such surveys have varied in the past. In recent years, however, the investigators have generally followed the lead given by a WHO Study Group in 1952, recording the results of surveys on endemic goiter in 4 categories as follows:

Grade 0—Persons without goiter. By definition these are persons whose thyroid glands are less than 4 to 5 times enlarged.

Grade I—Persons with palpable goiter. The thyroid is considered to be more than 4 to 5 times enlarged, although not visible with the head in normal position. Most of these will be readily visible with the head thrown back and neck fully extended.

Grade II—Persons with visible goiter. Persons with goiters which are easily visible with the head in normal position but which are smaller than in Grade III. Palpation may be helpful in determining the mass of the gland but is not needed for diagnosis.

Grade III—Persons with very large goiters. The goiters of persons in this category can be recognized at a considerable distance. They are grossly disfiguring and may be of such size as to cause mechanical difficulties with respiration.

The above descriptions given by Perez, Scrimshaw, and Munoz (1960) in the WHO monograph on endemic goiter has been acceptable also to the Interdepartmental Committee on Nutrition for National Defense (See the ICNND *Manual for Nutrition Surveys,* 1963). In the earlier surveys the ICNND teams recorded only one category of thyroid enlargement, for according to the first edition of the ICNND *Nutrition Survey Manual* (1957) the recording of enlarged thyroids was to follow the criterion "must be definitely palpable with or without swallowing and at least slightly perceptible to visual inspection." The revised classification of goiter in the 2nd Edition of the ICNND *Manual* is more meaningful, for it not only indicates prevalence but also the severity of the condition. A prevalence of 5% denotes that the area is endemic, and that of over 10% means that endemic goiter is a public health problem.

Goiter in Egypt

It is highly probable that simple goiter must have existed in Egypt for a long time. However, one cannot trace with a certainty references to it in ancient Egyptian history. Ghalioungui (1965) questions the validity of the interpretation of carvings on ancient tombs showing what was considered to be goitrous individuals, cretins, or those suffering from myxedema. Even as late as the nineteenth century one fails to find specific reference to goiter in the writings on diseases in Egypt such as those contained in *Description de l'Egypte* and the accounts of Pruner.

Attention to the occurrence of goiter in Egypt in recent times was first drawn by Dolby and Omar in 1924. They described 198 cases of colloid adenomatous goiter and 3 of cretinism admitted to the Kasr-el-Aini Hospital between 1919 and 1923. These were all fellaheens or the poor people from villages—landless laborers, peasants, and small farmers. The authors expressed the opinion, without giving figures to support it, that the incidence was higher in Copts, Jews, and the Saiyeds, i.e., the minorities with considerable degree of inbreeding. According to them, villages along the Nile had no goiter, whereas goiter was frequently encountered in villages remote from the river where people used well or canal water. They stated that the canal water was highly polluted and by implication considered water pollution as an important factor in the occurrence of goiter.

A few years later Ibrahim (1932) described goiter in the oases of Kharga and Dakhla. Only men were available for examination in both the oases. In Kharga oasis 5 out of 195 men examined had goiters. In Dakhla oasis the prevalence was greater, but the number examined was small. Ibrahim reported the following figures for three different villages in Dakhla oasis: In Kalamoun 18 out of 100, in Moot 3 out of 53, and in Gedida 3 out of 33 had goiters. Water supply in this oasis was from artesian wells often 200–300 meters deep with only traces of iodine and a high degree of permanent hardness. For example, the water of Kalamoun had 420–750 degrees of hardness. Although women were not available for examination, Ibrahim saw four women with enlarged thyroid gland.

Our knowledge of the occurrence and distribution of goiter in Egypt is almost entirely due to the researches of the indefatigable investigator Ghalioungui, who has summarized his findings in a publication, "Thyroid Enlargement in Africa with Reference to the Nile Basin" (1965). We have drawn extensively on this publication for the following account, which is necessarily brief.

Ghalioungui has studied goiter in different locations in Egypt along the Nile from Nubia to the Mediterranean and in the oasis in the Western Desert. He reported the prevalence varying between 10 and 50%. His findings are summarized in Table 1.

There are some difficulties in interpreting these figures which need some explanation. Ghalioungui accepted the WHO (1953) classification of goiter; however, in recording the thyroid enlargement of Grade I, he has indiscriminately used a variety of terms such as Grade I, palpable, slight enlargement, and enlarged. One is not certain whether all these terms are interchangeable and are meant to convey approximately the same degree of enlargement. Furthermore, on some occasions Ghalioungui includes among those affected with goiter only the individuals with visible and nodular goiters. Entries made in the various columns of Table 1 are as Ghalioungui has described them, and it is left to the reader to interpret those in the third column.

If one takes into account only the categories "Diffuse X4 and over" and "Nodular," about which there can be no dispute, the following comments would be justified.

The prevalence of goiter along the Nile and in the oases varied between 1.3 and 22.0%. The prevalence figure of 22.0% for Alexandria is based on the examination on one day of 186 individuals attending the out-patients clinic at the University Hospital. This can hardly be considered as indicative of the true prevalence in the town or the region. Apart from this instance the prevalence of simple goiter in the Nile Valley was the highest in Nubia (20%) and lowest (1.3%) in Cairo.

The prevalence of 26% goiter in Dakhla oasis reported by Ghalioungui is difficult to interpret for lack of details about the degree of enlargement. However, in an examination of a smaller number of children of school age in Kharga and Dakhla oases, Ghalioungui (1955) found visible goiter in 5 and 20% respectively of those examined.

In a nutrition survey done in the oases of Kharga and Dakhla, Abdou (1965) classified goiters as: "A"—those in which the thyroid gland was enlarged 4 times the normal size and was visible with the head retracted; and "B"—those in which the thyroid gland was enlarged to more than 4 times its normal size and was visible with head in the normal position, the enlargement being soft and diffuse or hard and nodular. These observations are summarized in Table 2.

According to Abdou, the total prevalence of goiter in Dakhla was no different from that in Kharga. The visible goiters of diffuse and nodular varieties were found with only slightly less frequency (7.7% in

TABLE 1
DISTRIBUTION OF ENDEMIC GOITER IN EGYPT[1]

	Number Examined	Grade 1 Goiters × 4 Diffuse %	Grade 2 Goiters Diffuse × 4 & Over %	Nodular %	Total of Grade 2 and Nodular %	Remarks
Nubia (9 villages)	1387	29±	2.9	17.1	20.0	± Grade 1
Luxor—Komo Ombo	1092	15.2±	7.4	0.01	7.4	± Palpable
Assiyut—Beni Mur	1547	39.5±	3.2	3.1	6.3	± Slight enlargement
Kharga—(higher values in three villages of Kharga not included)	512	36.6±	9.0	4.4	13.3	± Slight enlargement
Dakhla	543				26.0	
Cairo	1000	17.1±		1.3	1.3	± Enlarged
Alexandria	186	25.0	7.0	15.0	22.0	
Ras Hekma	116	10.6				

1. Source: Ghalioungui, 1965.

Goiter

TABLE 2
PREVALENCE OF GOITER IN KHARGA AND DAKHLA OASES[1]

	Males		Females	
	No.	%	No.	%
Kharga				
Total examined	1353		918	
Thyroid normal size	855	63.1	481	52.2
Thyroid palpable A	370	27.4	331	36.2
Thyroid visible B	128	9.5	106	11.6
Dakhla				
Total examined	419		281	
Thyroid normal size	267	64.6	157	55.6
Thyroid palpable A	120	28.7	97	34.5
Thyroid visible B	32	7.1	27	9.6

1. Source: Abdou, 1965.

males and 9.6% in females) in Dakhla than in Kharga (9.5% in males and 11.6% in females). These estimates agree with those of Ghalioungui so far as the Kharga oasis is concerned. In other respects there are marked differences which are difficult to explain.

In general the prevalence of goiter was higher among females than in males. The age distribution was such that peak incidence was found between 10 and 19 years, which include the ages of puberty and adolescence.

The information summarized in Tables 1 and 2 indicates that goiter is a health problem in Egypt, and in certain areas, such as Nubia, it can be a major problem.

Ghalioungui has examined the causes of the prevalence of goiter in Egypt, among which are iodine deficiency, dietary goitrogens, and genetic factors.

There is not much information on the iodine content of Egyptian soils. However a great deal is known about iodine in water (Table 3). The water of the river Nile in Cairo has an average iodine content of about 6 μg per liter. The level varies during the year and reaches a peak value between 10 and 12 μg per liter in August. This rise has been traced to the waters of the Atbara, one of the Nile tributaries which is in flood in August and whose water is richer in iodine than that of the Blue or the White Nile. Processing and purification of the river water to make it safe and potable results in a decrease in iodine content, for tap waters at different sites in Cairo have been found to contain between 1 and 7 μg per liter with the mean values between 3 and 4 μg per liter. In Lower Egypt the canal waters approximate Nile water in their iodine content, whereas well waters are variable. Wells in the Nile Valley receive their water from the Nile after seepage and percolation through the soil. The iodine content of these well waters fluctuates according to seasonal changes in the iodine content of the Nile water, partly modified by the nature and composition of the soil and rocky formations through which water seepage occurs. Ghalioungui has found in well waters of Upper Egypt a tendency for iodine concentration to diminish as one proceeds south: for example, in Beni Suef the average of 4 samples gave a value 37 µg per liter, whereas in Aswan the average of 3 samples yielded a figure of 10.8 µg per liter. Wells in the desert and in the Nubian region possess waters whose iodine content depends upon the composition of the strata of the rock through which the water flows, unmodified by contribution from the Nile water.

Ghalioungui believes that an association exists between iodine content of water and prevalence of goiter in Egypt. However owing to uncertainties regarding the interpretation of his data, this association cannot be convincingly demonstrated.

TABLE 3
IODINE CONTENT OF WATERS IN EGYPT[1]

	Iodine µg/liter	
Cairo	Nile Water	Tap Water
Giza	6.37	3.54
Rod el Farag	7.06	3.97
Alexandria	Mahmoudia Canal	
	10.1	8.5
Suez		5.57
Lower Egypt	Well Waters	
Gharbia	14–43	
Menufia	12–29	
Sharkiya	15–29	
Kaliubieh	11–26	
Upper Egypt		
Beni Suef	28–45	
Minya	11–42	
Assiyut	6–14	
Quena	10–21	
Aswan	10–11	
Oases		
Kharga	4–13	
Dakhla	5–11	
Siwa	14–50	

1. Source: Ghaliounghi, 1965.

Goiter 91

The iodine content of soil and water are indications of the iodine status of the environment. However, the presence of iodine in soil and water does not necessarily mean that crops grown in such soil will contain iodine in amounts reflecting those of the soil and water. Ghalioungui mentions a few examples of foodstuffs from Egypt which on analysis showed no iodine at all or much less than the values reported elsewhere. Furthermore, the crude sea salt and rock salt used in different parts of Egypt were poor in iodine. Thus it would appear that in spite of comparative richness of the river and most well waters in iodine, the iodine needs of Egyptians in certain locations are not met. Such a situation exists in Nubia and in the two major oases, Kharga and Dakhla in the Western Desert.

Evidence on the role of other factors in the causation of goiter in Egypt is not conclusive. Ghalioungui considers that the high uptake of I^{131} in goitrous subjects and low urinary excretion of iodine argue against the role of dietary goitrogens. The occurrence of familial sporadic goiter with evidence of defective iodine utilization by the thyroid gland has been described in the endemic goiter areas of Egypt. However, it seems certain that iodine deficiency must be the principal reason for the endemicity of goiter in Egypt.

Goiter in Libya, Lebanon, and Jordan

Libya. The ICNND survey in Libya revealed a low prevalence of simple goiter. A prevalence between 0 and 0.2% was recorded in more than 2,700 individuals comprising the army, police, civilians, and boys of 5 to 15 years. Slightly higher prevalence figures of 3.6% and 4.9% were found in women. Goiter was not associated with any specific geographical areas in the country, as it occurred in coastal as well as inland regions.

Lebanon. Goiter is endemic in Lebanon. Matovinovic (1961), a WHO consultant, examined over 3,400 school children from 20 different locations widely separated on the coast, high mountains, and in the valley. He found an over-all prevalence of 49%, with the highest prevalence in the mountain villages.

A year later ICNND (1962) reported the results of a nutrition survey in different areas of Lebanon. The report indicated that goiter occurred at all ages and in both sexes. The prevalence was the lowest in infants and children up to 4 years and increased sharply thereafter. According to the data extracted from the ICNND Nutrition Survey Report and presented in Table 4, the peak prevalence occurred between 10 and 14 years. The females were affected to a

TABLE 4
GOITER IN LIBYA AND LEBANON[1]

	Number Examined	Thyroid Enlarged %	Number	Thyroid Enlarged %
		Libya		
Men				
Police	808	0.1		
Army	941	0		
Civilian	865	0.2		
Boys 5–15 years	120	0		
Women				
Nonpregnant	303	3.6		
Pregnant	61	4.9		
		Lebanon		
Military	1938	49.1		
		Nonrefugee Civilians	Refugee Civilians	
Children M & F				
0–4 years	98	4.0	138	7.2
5–9 years	492	46.1	546	31.9
Males				
10–14 years	238	41.6	184	48.9
15–44 years	263	44.9	103[2]	27.2
> 45 years	121	14.0		
Females				
10–14 years	303	67.7	163	49.7
15–45 years	171	67.8	44[2]	86.4
> 45 years	127	27.6		
Pregnant	16	43.8	78	79.5
Lactating	42	69.0	30	86.7

1. Source: ICNND Surveys, 1962.
2. 15 to > 45 years.

greater extent than the males. It is noteworthy that differences in goiter prevalence among the refugee and nonrefugee civilians were most marked in women. A prevalence of 80% and over was found in 152 refugee nonpregnant, pregnant, and lactating women as compared to a prevalence of 44 to 69% in a corresponding group of 229 nonrefugee women.

The belief that goiter occurs less frequently in the coastal region of Lebanon than in the mountains and the valley lying between the Lebanon and Anti-Lebanon mountain ranges is not borne out by later observations. Najjar and Woodruff (1963) examined 1,548 school children from 5 to 18 years of age in Beirut and found 31% had enlarged thyroids of Grade I and over. They also observed that chil-

Goiter

dren of comparable age in orphanages showed a higher prevalence of goiter than the children of the higher socioeconomic classes attending private educational institutions (Table 5).

Cowan et al. (1965) examined 424 boys and girls of school age in a village 1,500 meters high in the mountains and found an over-all prevalence of 25.4%. The results of the studies conducted by Najjar and Woodruff and Cowan et al. are summarized in Table 5.

The differences in prevalence between the different regions of Lebanon are not marked, as Table 5 shows. Similarly the over-all sex difference in the prevalence of goiter in school age children is noticeable in only two sets of observations. All these studies show beyond doubt, however, that goiter is a public health problem for the whole of Lebanon, irrespective of the geographical differences in this small country.

Supporting studies on radioiodine uptake by the thyroid, urinary iodine excretion, and the effect of iodine supplementation have also been reported by Najjar and Woodruff and Cowan et al. The mean iodine uptake was elevated but not to as great an extent in non-goitrous as in goitrous children. Both the reports mention a drop in iodine uptake after iodate administration; Cowan et al. observed a decrease from 83.3% to 14.3% when measured nine months after the start of the consumption of iodized salt. On the other hand, Najjar

TABLE 5
GOITER IN SCHOOL-AGE CHILDREN IN LEBANON

	WHO Survey[1]		ICNND Survey		Najjar and Woodruff		Cowan et al.	
	No.	Goiter %	No.	Goiter %	No.	Goiter %	No.	Goiter %
Coastal								
Boys	2134[2]	44.5	337	24.0	550	11.8		
Girls			317	24.6	408	24.0		
Orphan Boys					359	51.1		
Orphan Girls					231	60.5		
Mountain								
Boys	1051[2]	53.3	201	38.8			226	23.4
Girls			444	31.4			198	27.8
Valley								
Boys	236[2]	72.5	448	19.4				
Girls			264	36.8				

1. J. Matovinovic, Goiter Survey in Lebanon: Report to World Health Organization, Geneva, 1960.
2. Boys and girls together.

and Woodruff administered 8.5 mg potassium iodate daily for 11 days and registered only a reduction from 88.2% to 62% after two months. In children receiving the placebo the corresponding values before and after therapy were 88.3% and 78%. The average urinary excretion of iodine (I-127) in the series of Najjar and Woodruff was 11.75, 17.33, and 23.25 µg per 24 hours in goitrous orphans, non-goitrous orphans, and control subjects respectively.

Cowan et al. (1965) found in 67 subjects from a mountain village an average urinary iodine excretion of 20.9 µg/g creatinine. The normal value for urinary iodine excretion per day is 50 µg and over per g creatinine (Follis et al., 1962). In 13 families consuming iodized salt (1 part iodine in 50,000 parts salt), the urinary iodine excretion in 3 months rose to 341 µg/g creatine, whereas it was only 27 µg/g creatinine in families not receiving the fortified salt.

In a later study extending over the coastal, high-mountain, and valley regions of Lebanon, Cowan et al. (1966) found higher urinary excretion of iodine per g of creatinine in the coastal area as compared with the mountainous and valley regions (Table 6). In the latter two locations, urinary excretion of iodine was in the low and deficient ranges.

Thus there is little doubt that iodine deficiency is the principal cause of goiter in Lebanon. This conclusion is further strengthened by some other studies of Cowan and coworkers.

Cowan, Silahian, and Djibelian (1968) have determined the iodine content in 47 different foods in common use in Lebanon. They collected the samples, 443 in all, from different areas of Lebanon with

TABLE 6
AVERAGE URINARY EXCRETION OF IODINE IN LEBANON
(µg I/g CREATININE)

	ICNND Data		Cowan et al.	
	No.	µg I / g Creat.	No.	µg I / g Creat.
Coastal			44	62.7
Nonrefugees	16	30.2		
Refugees	46	49.8		
Mountain			47	33.5
Nonrefugees	56	30.9		
Refugees	9	30.2		
Valley			40	21.2
Nonrefugees	13	28.8		
Refugees	7	29.3		

TABLE 7
AVERAGE DAILY IODINE INTAKE IN LEBANON[1]

Location	No. Samples Analyzed	μg I Intake Per Capita Per Day	
		Mean	Range
Kalamoun (Sea coast)	39	54.6	0 to > 70
Faraya (High mountain)	40	41.7	0 to > 70
Ain Zalta (Valley)	39	22.0	0 to 60

1. Source: Cowan et al., 1966.

different goiter endemicity. They found a large variation in iodine content from sample to sample: for example, in 22 samples of white bread, iodine varied from 0 to 185 μg/kg, in green beans the range was < 5 to 32, in mature onions 0 to 368, and in white cheese from 33 to 245 μg/kg. Cowan et al. (1968) also determined the iodine content in the soil and water and found that the average values of iodine in soil and water diminished as one progressed from an area of low to an area of high endemicity. Their experience with the iodine content of parsley collected from these same regions indicated that much of the variation in iodine content of food found by them must be due to the varying concentrations of iodine in soil and water.

Cowan, Kassab, Silahian, and Shadarevian (1966) determined the daily iodine intake by composite food analysis in 10 families in each of the geographical regions of Lebanon—coastal, mountain, and valley. Their estimates of average daily iodine intake as given in Table 7 are much lower than the average values ranging from 150 to 230 μg per day found by ICNND by composite meal analysis in the Lebanese nonrefugee civilian families. The average values reported by Cowan et al. were about 50% or less than the generally accepted desirable intakes.

In another study covering the same regions but a larger number of villages, Cowan and coworkers (1967) reported the following distribution of iodine intake: less than 50 μg in 57.4%, 50 to 100 μg per day in 27.5%, and over 100 μg per day in 15.1% (Table 7).

The therapeutic observations of Najjar and Woodruff and the supplementation trial of Cowan et al. (1965) clearly indicate the beneficial effect of iodate (or iodide) administration in reducing the prevalence of goiter. Iodization of salt with iodide or iodate for the prevention of goiter is a comparatively simple procedure of proved efficacy in several countries. We understand that the WHO consultant had made a recommendation earlier to this effect. It has apparently not been implemented for reasons best known to the government of Lebanon.

TABLE 8
GOITER IN JORDAN[1]

	Nonrefugee Civilians				Refugee Civilians			
		Thyroid Enlarged				Thyroid Enlarged		
	Number	Grade I %	Grade II %	Total %	Number	Grade I %	Grade II %	Total %
Military	1528	4.3	0.2	4.5				
Males:								
0–4 years					246	0.4		0.4
5–9 years					467	3.4		3.4
10–14 years	290	15.5	0.7	16.2	295	9.8		9.8
15–44 years	271	5.2	0.7	5.9	199	5.0		5.0
> 45 years	225	2.2	—	2.2	128	1.6	0.8	2.4
Females:								
0–4 years					189	1.6		1.6
5–9 years					431	4.2	0.5	4.7
10–14 years	416	14.4	1.0	15.4	299	12.0	0.7	12.7
15–44 years	340	19.4	7.4	26.8	235	31.9	1.7	33.6
> 45 years	247	6.9	2.4	9.3	74	9.6	2.1	11.7
Pregnant	131	21.4	5.3	26.7	65	43.1	6.2	49.3
Lactating	273	20.1	7.3	27.4	136	32.4	4.4	36.8
Children (M & F)								
0–4 years					674	0.2		0.2
5–9 years					796	4.4	0.1	4.5

1. Source: ICNND Survey, 1962.

TABLE 9
GOITER IN JORDANIAN CHILDREN IN DIFFERENT AREAS[1]

Jordan	< 15 years	No.	Grade I	Grade II
Amman	Boys	114		
	Girls	106	0.9	
Ajloun	Boys	77	2.6	
	Girls			
Hebron	Boys	152	3.3	
	Girls	145	1.4	1.4
Jerusalem	Boys	361	6.1	
	Girls	360	10.0	0.3
Nablus	Boys	185	6.5	
	Girls	159	6.3	
Shore area	Boys	97	5.2	
	Girls	67	11.9	1.5

1. Source: ICNND Survey, 1962.

Jordan. In Jordan the prevalence of simple goiter is much less than in Lebanon. Tables 8 and 9 summarize the findings of the ICNND survey done in 1962. A prevalence of about 15% was reached in 10–14-year-old boys and girls. Thereafter goiter occurred more frequently in women of child-bearing age, primarily in pregnant and lactating women. As in Lebanon, the prevalence among refugee women was higher than in nonrefugee women. A survey among the boys and girls below 15 years in age showed that goiter was more common in the hilly area on the west bank of Jordan than on the east bank, although in the south (Ma'an district) of Jordan, goiter prevalence was comparable to that on the west bank.

The estimated iodine intake for the military varied between 142 to 312 μg/capita/day with an average of 206 μg. The intake of iodine among the civilians, based on a few food-composite analyses, was estimated to be 435 μg/capita/day. In the Jerusalem area iodine intake was 434 μg/day, in Amman 408 μg, and among refugees 474 μg/capita/day. In view of this, it is difficult to understand the reason for the prevalence rates of up to 10% reported in the ICNND survey.

REFERENCES

Abdou, I. A. 1965. *Nutritional Status in the New Valley* (in Arabic). Cairo, Egypt: National Documentation Center.

Cowan, J. W., S. S. Najjar, Z. I. Sabry, R. I. Tannous, and F. S. Simaan. 1965. Some Further Observations on Goiter in Lebanon. *Amer. J. Clin. Nutr.* 17: 164.

Cowan, J. W., G. Kassab, A. Silahian, and S. Shadarevian. 1966. Iodine Intake and Excretion in Three Different Areas of Lebanon. *Lebanese Med. J.* 20: 213.

Cowan, J. W., G. Kassab, J. P. Salji, and V. Djibelian. 1967. *A Study of Iodine Intake in Lebanon Villages: Third Symposium on Human Nutrition and Health in the Near East.* Beirut, Lebanon.

Cowan, J. W., A. Silahian, and V. Djibelian, 1968. Iodine Content of Selected Lebanese Foods. *Lebanese Med. J.* 21: 3–8.

Dolby, R. V. and M. Omar. 1924. A Note Concerning the Incidence of Goiter in Egypt: An Analysis of 216 Cases. *Lancet* ii: 549.

Follis, R. H., K. Vanaprapa, and D. Damrong-Sakdi. 1962. Studies on Iodine Nutrition in Thailand. *J. Nutr.* 76: 159.

Ghalioungui, P. 1955. A Short Medical Survey of the Kharga and Dakhla Oases. *Bull. Clin. Sci. Soc. Abbassiah Faculty of Medicine, Cairo* 6: 1.

———. 1965. Thyroid Enlargement in Africa with Reference to the Nile Basin. Cairo, Egypt: The National Information and Documentation Center.

Ibrahim, A. 1932. Endemic Goiter in the Dakhla Oasis of Egypt. *J. Egypt. Med. Assoc.* 15: 401.

Najjar, S. S., and C. W. Woodruff. 1963. Some Observations on Goiter in Lebanon. *Amer. J. Clin. Nutr.* 13: 46.

Perez, G., N. S. Scrimshaw, and J. A. Munoz. 1960. Technique of Endemic Goiter Surveys. *Endemic Goiter,* Monograph Series No. 44. Geneva, Switzerland: World Health Organization.

Sallam, F., M. Gabr, and M. Saadani. 1961. The Role of Defective Organification of Iodine in the Etiology of Nontoxic Goiter in Egypt. *Gaz. Egypt. Pediat. Assoc.* 9: 141.

Stanbury, J. B. 1960. Physiology of Endemic Goiter. *Endemic Goiter,* Monograph Series No. 44, Geneva, Switzerland: World Health Organization.

6 | Xerophthalmia, Rickets, and Scurvy

Vitamin A Deficiency and Xerophthalmia

Vitamin A is a fat-soluble vitamin. It is found in some, not all, fats of animal origin. Milk fat, fat in the yolk of egg, and fat contained in liver are good sources of vitamin A. Body fats such as mutton fat, beef suet, and lard do not contain vitamin A. Fish liver oils, commonly not used as food, are rich in vitamin A and until the advent of synthetic vitamin A were used as medicinal sources of the vitamin.

Although vitamin A does not occur as such in vegetable foodstuffs, its precursors, carotenoids, are found in green leafy vegetables, carrots, sweet potatoes, certain fruits such as mango, papaya, tomato, and apricot, and the cereal, yellow maize. Some of these carotenoids are converted in the body into vitamin A, β-carotene being the most potent in this respect. There are several other carotenoids which have biological activity varying from 10 to 60% of that of β-carotene in terms of their capacity for conversion into vitamin A. Red palm oil derived from the fruit of a palm tree (*Elaeis guineensis*) is very rich in β-carotene. In certain countries of West Africa and in Brazil, where the oil is used for cooking purposes, red palm oil forms a convenient rich source of vitamin A activity in food.

Intake of Vitamin A

The intake of vitamin A in human dietaries occurs through the ingestion of both the animal and vegetable foods. In poor communities which cannot afford such animal foods as milk, butter, cheese, and eggs in sufficient quantities in their daily diets, man depends to a large extent on the supply of vitamin A in the form of its precursors through such articles of food as green and yellow leafy vegetables and some fruits rich in vitamin A. One can estimate the total vitamin A activity of the diet if one knows the foodstuffs of which it is composed and the average amounts consumed. Such information is obtained through diet surveys.

Abdou and Mahfouz (1965) found in two villages in Kaliubieh Province in Egypt that the average per capita daily intake of eggs was 3 g per day and of milk 29 g per day, thus providing extremely small amounts of preformed vitamin A. They estimated the average daily intake of vitamin A activity as 4,466 International Units (I.U.), which showed that in these villages the bulk of vitamin A was derived from the precursors contained in foodstuffs of vegetable origin. In another survey of the dietaries of pregnant and nursing women in Cairo, Abdou and Amer (1965) estimated the average daily intakes as 3,028 and 3,436 I.U. respectively, which in their opinion was 50% of the estimated requirements according to the recommendations of the National Research Council, U.S.A. Unfortunately, sufficiently extensive information on dietaries in other parts of Egypt is not available to evaluate the adequacy of vitamin A intake in Egyptian diets. Abdou found in his food and nutrition studies in Kharga and Dakhla oases that the average daily intake per head was less than 1,500 I.U., most of it being from vegetable sources.

In Lebanon the ICNND reported the intake of vitamin A as varying between 2,116 and 6,556 I.U. per capita per day among the refugee and nonrefugee civilians. In Jordan the variation in intake was even greater, the range being from 1,102 to 6,184 I.U. per capita per day. There was not much difference between the refugee and nonrefugee families as regards vitamin A intake in both these countries. In Lebanon and Jordan about 75% of the ingested vitamin A activity was derived from vegetable foodstuffs. Information from the ICNND survey in Libya, limited in scope as it is, indicated the average intake between 1,200 and 2,500 I.U. per day for personnel of the armed forces and constabulary. Yang (1963) later reported an almost similar range of intake (1,012 to 2,639 I.U. per capita per day) in a few families of low and medium economic status.

It seems therefore that in the countries under consideration vitamin A intake may vary from deficient to marginal or adequate levels. The economic condition of the family and the ready availability or otherwise of protective foods rich in vitamin A and/or its precursor would determine the level of habitual intake, which in turn would influence the vitamin A nutrition of the population.

Effects of Vitamin A Deficiency

The deficiency of vitamin A causes keratinization of the epithelia at various sites in the body, such as trachea, salivary gland, pelvis of the kidney, ureter, and bladder. The vaginal epithelium undergoes keratinization so early in the state of deficiency that a rat test was devised for it for a bio-assay of the vitamin. Certain changes in the skin resulting from the keratinization of the hair follicle and its plugging are also ascribed to the deficiency of vitamin A, and this condition, known as hyperkeratosis follicularis, is usually recorded during nutrition surveys. However, its etiology is uncertain.

The ocular manifestations of vitamin A deficiency are the most serious and hence the most important. These have been well described by McLaren, Oomen, and Escapini (1966). They consist of night blindness; xerosis of the bulbar conjunctiva, generalized and local; xerosis of the cornea; keratomalacia and its sequelae. Night blindness is the inability to see clearly in the dark. This is usually the earliest symptom of hypovitaminosis A. In this condition the regeneration of visual purple bleached by exposure to bright light is defective, causing impairment in the function of dark adaptation. Xerosis of the bulbar conjunctiva may be generalized; it is seen as dryness and unwettability, thickening, wrinkling, and patchy pigmentation. Bitot's spot is localized conjunctival xerosis. The shape of the spot varies, but generally it is oval with the horizontal long axis situated on the temporal side of the cornea in the interpalpebral fissure. The surface of the spot is foamy and is raised above the conjunctiva. The foaminess can be removed by wiping but forms again within a short time.

Xerosis of the cornea results in the loss of transparency. Later, cellular infiltration may increase the opacity of the cornea. Ulceration of the cornea may follow. Softening of the cornea, called keratomalacia, is a rapid process. The cornea perforates, and lens is extruded. These changes lead to the permanent loss of vision in the affected eye. One or both eyes may be involved.

If intensive therapy brings about the healing of keratomalacia, scars are left in the eye as leucoma, staphyloma, and phthisis bulbi. Such scars seen in children below 10 years of age are most probably the results of keratomalacia. The various conditions described above are illustrated in Figure 1.

There is reason to believe that vitamin A deficiency occurred in Pharaonic times. References in night blindness and its treatment with roasted ox liver or the liver of a black cock are to be found in ancient Egyptian medical literature such as Eber's Papyrus

(Aykroyd, 1959; Moore, 1957). In more recent times one finds that night blindness is well known as a disease among Arabs in the Near East. Several vernacular names are used to describe the condition: (a) *el hidbal* (stumbling), the most popular name, (b) *el asha* (blindness after dusk), one may recall the title of the famous old Arabic book by Qualqueshandi, *SUBH EL A'SHA FI SINA'ET EL INSHA*, denoting that the Arabs have known the disease for several centuries, (c) *ama eljaj* (chicken blindness), used less frequently in Egypt than in the neighboring Arab countries, (d) *el wutwat* (the bat). The bat hits objects during flight, and the people have used its name to describe the condition in which stumbling against objects in the dark is a feature.

The vernacular names for Bitot's spot are: (a) *kushour beid* (eggshell); (b) *kushour beida* (white scales); (c) *kushour samak* (fish scales).

The terms used to indicate corneal xerosis are: (a) *ghabash* or *ajaj* (fog); (b) *dukhan* (smoke); (c) *gizaz* (glass or white china). The term *rashga* describes the softening and ulceration of the cornea, whether due to vitamin A deficiency or to any other cause.

The recognition of the dietary origin of night blindness is reflected in certain traditional methods of treatment known to the people in Arab countries. They know that eating fatty foods protects sight—*"Akl el zafar yekawi el basar"*—and that lack of fatty foods (*zafar*) leads to night blindness. Cakes (*fatyr*) soaked in clarified butter (*samneh*) are fed to the nyctalopic child. They prescribe fatty foods, fatty meat, and the offals (*mi'laak*) of the sheep, cow, or goat. The liver, *el sawda* or *el zaida*, especially, has a very wide use for treatment of night blindness. They eat it almost raw, or boil it and get the vapor to the child's eyes and feed the child with boiled liver. For topic application they press the liver to get its juice or add oil to the liver, grind it well, and drop the oily juice into the eyes of the nyctalopic child. We are not certain whether the other manifestations of xerophthalmia for which vernacular names are given above were associated in the minds of the people also with the lack of fatty foods.

Occurrence in Egypt

The limited number of nutrition surveys reported from Egypt make no mention of the occurrence of the ocular signs of vitamin A deficiency. However, moderate to severe vitamin A deficiency must occur, for there are accounts reporting keratomalacia among the infants and children admitted to hospitals. Nor-el-Din (1944) mentions night blindness resulting from the low dietary intake of vitamin

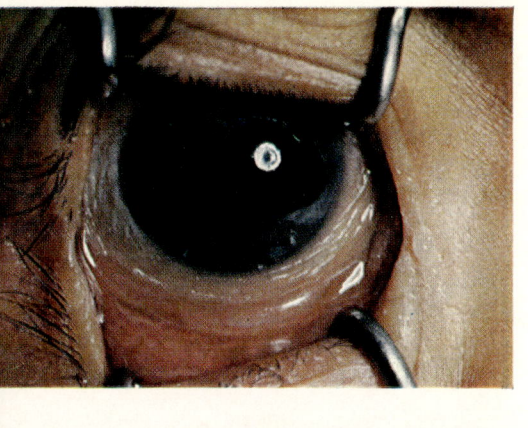
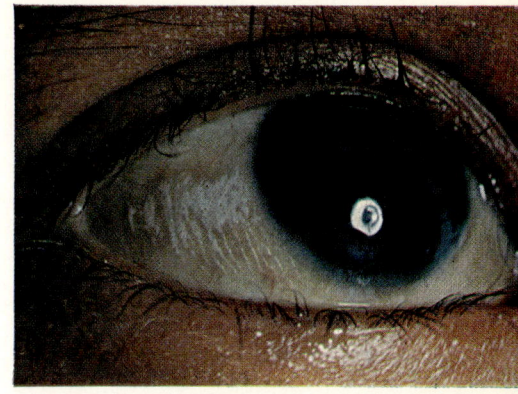
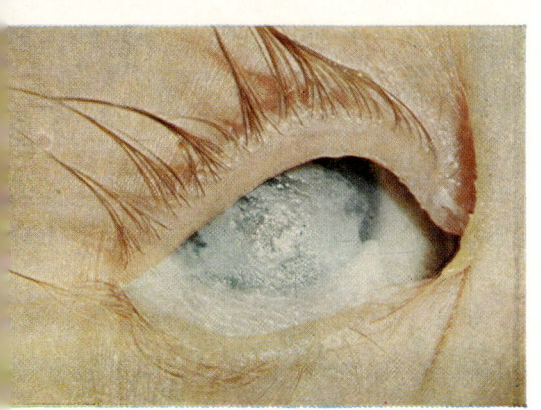
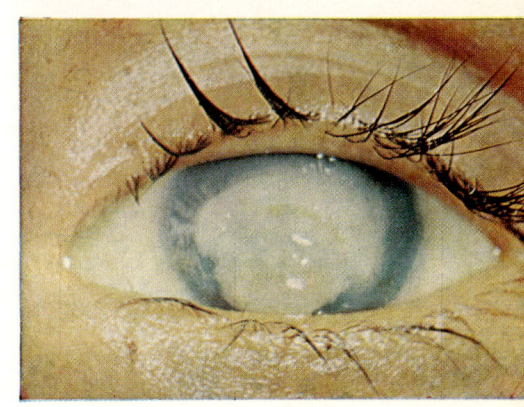

OCULAR MANIFESTATIONS OF VITAMIN A DEFICIENCY IN CHILDREN

A. Extensive xerosis of the conjunctiva with oedematous folds in the lower conjunctival sac. Distorted Bitot's spot visible. Male Indonesian child aged four years, right eye. Tests revealed blood-plasma vitamin-A level of 3 µg/100 ml, and a trace of carotene.

B. Biot's spot, striated, with hyperpigmentation and dryness surrounding conjunctive. Male Indonesian child aged three years, right eye.

C. Accumulation of debris in nine-month-old Jordanian male infant. The material has extended from the lower fornix on to the greater part of the cornia. Tests revealed blood-plasma vitamin-A level of 2 µg/100 ml and liver Vitamin-A level of 0 g/g liver.

D. Perforation of the cornea and extrusion of the lens in an eighteen-month-old Jordanian male child. Tests revealed blood-plasma vitamin-A level of 2 µg/100 ml.

Comparative values for healthy children: plasma vitamin-A 20-50 µg/100 ml; liver vitamin-A 50 µg/g.

A seen by him in only four cases, of which three were poor children in Cairo and one "a lady on a slimming diet." He, however, mentions the association of night blindness with liver disease. According to the information given by Oomen, McLaren, and Escapini (1964) there were 122 cases diagnosed and xerophthalmia or keratomalacia in a total of 430,000 children treated at the opthalmic hospitals in 1961. These authors also quote a pediatrician's opinion that 20 cases of xerophthalmia were seen annually in a children's hospital in Cairo. Hanafy (1947), in giving the first description of protein-calorie malnutrition in Egyptian infants and children, stated that vitamin A deficiency was associated in a high proportion of cases seen by him in Alexandria. He, however, gave no further details.

Other investigators refer to the cases of xerophthalmia only as subjects for serum vitamin A estimations. The questions of etiology and prevalence do not seem to have been touched upon. Taha and Emara (1959) determined serum vitamin A in 7 cases of night blindness and 6 of xerosis in Alexandria. Sandstead *et al.* (1965) found 3 cases of keratomalacia in 39 cases of kwashiorkor studied by them. Similarly Hammad (1966) refers to 6 cases of keratomalacia among 34 children with prekwashiorkor and kwashiorkor in whom he determined serum vitamin A. Quite recently El Tohamy (1968) collected 21 cases of xerophthalmia, 12 of which were, with keratomalacia, among 80 cases of protein-calorie malnutrition at Shebin-el-Kom in Menoufia Province. This is an unusually high proportion and can be explained on the assumption that the authors were looking for cases of xerophthalmia for special study on vitamin A deficiency associated with protein-calorie malnutrition.

The above account indicates that xerophthalmia is not rare in Egypt and is an indicator of the underlying vitamin A deficiency among the young child population. This is confirmed by the findings on serum vitamin A determinations in infants and children. Hammad (1966) reported an average serum retinol value of 24.2 μg/100 ml in 20 healthy children of 1 to 24 months in age; and in 16 healthy children 2 to 12 years the average serum retinol was found to be 25.5 μg/100 ml. Hammad did not determine the carotenoids. In 34 children with protein-calorie malnutrition, of age 2 to 40 months, the average serum retinol was 13.2 μg/100 ml. These latter values were almost identical with those found later by Tohamy in 81 cases of marasmus and kwashiorkor (12.8 and 12.7 μg/100 ml respectively) in Menoufia Province. He found in normal infants of 3 to 36 months the average values of 30.2 μg/100 ml for serum retinol and 99 μg/100 ml for carotenoids. The serum carotenoids were considerably reduced in marasmus and kwashiorkor, the average for the two groups being 38.3 µg/100 ml. The 12 cases with keratomalacia had even lower serum retinol, the average being 8.6 µg/100 ml. Tohamy further found that in 20 malnourished infants having chronic diarrhea, the average serum retinol was 8.6 µg/100 ml, comparable with that in children with keratomalacia. Tohamy concluded that diarrhea per se because of gastrointestinal hurry and impaired absorption may exacerbate the state of vitamin A deficiency.

Nor-el-Din (1944) determined the vitamin A content in the livers of premature and newborn infants. He does not mention the number of specimens examined but states that 15% of the livers had traces of retinol and the remaining 85% had an average of 48 µg/g. This latter value is much higher than the values ranging from 8 to 16 µg/g reported for livers of the newborn from Europe before 1940 (Kirk, 1962). Subsequent to 1940, however, the limited observations from Finland and U.S.A. indicate a higher range—from 40 to 91 µg vitamin A per g liver. Obviously this is an area in which more information is needed from the Near East countries, for it is important to know if liver reserves are low in populations in which xerophthalmia occurs.

Taha and Emara (1959) determined in Alexandria serum levels of vitamin A in healthy Egyptian subjects. Abboud, Osman, and Massoud (1968a) found fairly high levels of retinol in the serum in normal subjects from Cairo studied by them. The subjects were children and adolescents below 20 years of age from government schools, as well as adults, who were laboratory workers, policemen, and junior administrative, professional, and research staff. The average values reported from Alexandria were lower than those in the subjects from Cairo. The reasons are not clear. The results of the determination of vitamin A in serum among Egyptians reviewed thus far are given in Table 1.

According to Abboud *et al.*, there was a significant difference in serum retinol levels between the normal young and adult males and between adult males and adult females. They did not find this sex difference in the group below 20 years of age. Serum retinol in xerosis in the male and female subjects was significantly reduced. This interpretation of the findings would have been more convincing if the authors had demonstrated that the xerosis cases had responded to treatment with vitamin A. This group consisted of children, adolescents, and adults, the youngest subject being 6 years of age. In only 4 out of 54 cases of xerosis, reference is made to a complete cure on treatment with vitamin A.

TABLE 1
SERUM RETINOL AND CAROTENOIDS IN HEALTHY AND MALNOURISHED EGYPTIANS

Subjects	Sex	Age	No.	Retinol (μg per 100 ml Serum)		Carotenoids		Ref.
				Mean	S.D.	Mean	S.D.	
Healthy								
Infants and young children		1 to 24 m.	20	24.2				(1)
		2 to 12 yr.	16	25.5				(2)
		3 to 36 m.	25	30.2		99		(3)
Children and adolescents	M	6 to 19 yr.	45	45.0	18.6	72	27.4	
	F	6 to 19 yr.	32	41.3	12.8	79	25.5	
Adults	M	> 20 yr.	42	59.2	24.9	121	48.6	
	F	> 20 yr.	38	44.2	14.7	124	46.2	
	M	19 to 46 yr.	103	42		78		(4)
	F	16 to 40 yr.	20	37		78		
Malnourished								
Kwashiorkor (K)		2 to 40 m.	34	13.2				(1)
Kwashiorkor		12 to 36 m.	41	12.7		38.2		(2)
Marsmus (M)		12 to 36 m.	40	12.8		38.3		
K & M with keratomalacia		12 to 36 m.	12	8.6				(2)
Conjunctival xerosis	M	< 20 yr.	19	19.9	17.6	65	35.0	(3)
		> 20 yr.	25	29.1	18.6	73	31.4	
	F		10	25.6		101		

(1) Hammad, 1966.
(2) Tohamy, 1968.
(3) Abboud et al., 1968.
(4) Taha and Emara, 1959.

Occurrence in Libya and Lebanon

Some evidence regarding the occurrence of biochemical and mild clinical deficiency of vitamin A in the population in these two countries has been presented in the chapter on nutritional status. Not much information is available about the occurrence of the more severe forms of vitamin A deficiency in Libya and only a little more from Lebanon. Oomen, McLaren, and Escapini (1964) stated that xerophthalmia has not been previously reported from Lebanon. They found however that of the 300 malnourished children examined in Beirut and Saida, 40% had serum retinol levels of 10 µg/100 ml or less and another 42% had levels between 11 and 20 µg/100 ml; yet careful examination of the eye, including funduscopy, showed that the eyes of all these children were normal. Woodruff (1965) reported a mean serum retinol level of 8.9 µg/100 ml in 38 infants seen at the Government Hospital in Sindion in 1962 for acute gastroenteritis or pneumonia. In the following summer three cases of xerophthalmia were discovered in this group.

It appears therefore that although protein-calorie malnutrition is fairly common in Lebanon, the associated xerophthalmia seems to be rare. The rarity of xerophthalmia, in spite of the extremely low serum retinol levels, merits further careful investigation, particularly as xerophthalmia is not uncommon in the neighboring Arab countries such as Syria, Jordan, and Egypt.

Occurrence in Jordan

The results of serum retinol determinations in nearly 600 infants and children done in the Jordan Pediatric Survey (1964) and the WHO Xerophthalmia Study (1967) are given in Table 2.

The average values for serum retinol for the entire groups in the two studies were 21.9 and 20.3 µg/100 ml respectively. These were not very different, and there were minor differences in the average values for each age group. In the ICNND-ICNJ Pediatric Survey, 38 to 56% of children had serum retinol in the deficient and low ranges, whereas in the WHO study 51 to 76% were within this range. There is thus clear evidence of biochemical deficiency of vitamin A in Jordanian infants and young children.

In another series of 155 infants of 35 to 180 days of age observed in the WHO study, the average values for serum retinol considered at age intervals of one month were found even lower than the averages for all infants below one year grouped together. The reason for this difference probably was that the sample of infants below 6 months of age was from the poorer sections of the population in the rural areas.

TABLE 2
RETINOL AND CAROTENOIDS IN SERUM OF JORDANIAN INFANTS AND YOUNG CHILDREN

			μg/100 ml Serum				% Children With Serum Retinol < 20 μg/100 ml
			Retinol		Carotenoids		
Age		No.	Mean	S.D.	Mean	S.D.	
ICNND-ICNJ Pediatric Survey							
	< 1 yr.	21	24.9		33.6		38
	1 yr.	53	21.9		32.0		43
	2 yr.	61	21.2		43.1		47
	3 yr.	63	22.5		63.1		38
	4 yr.	52	19.7		56.7		56
	5 yr.	53	23.1		80.9		38
		303	21.9		53.6		
WHO Xerophthalmia Study							
	< 1 yr.	38	22.1	17.6	80	53.4	58
	1 yr.	54	20.4	20.0	103	47.3	76
	2 yr.	49	21.0	12.9	98	52.8	53
	3 yr.	49	23.5	17.0	127	55.4	51
	4 yr.	41	14.4	8.4	131	62.4	76
	5 yr.	55	19.8	12.1	128	56.0	54
		286	20.3	15.4	112	57.0	
	Days						
	35–60	22	19.1	10.26	107		
	61–90	43	15.1	10.54	103		
	91–120	39	15.3	11.60	97		
	121–150	23	16.7	11.54	111		
	151–180	28	14.8	10.35	78		

This does not appear to be the whole answer, however, for repeat observations on 42 of these children a year later gave an average value of 26.2 µg/100 ml for serum retinol. One could conclude from this that serum retinol levels in infants below 6 months of age are lower than those at one year and later, even though no vitamin A supplements are given during this period. Additional longitudinal observations on infants during the first year of life are necessary.

The very large difference in the serum carotenoid values found in the two studies deserves some comment. The average value in the Jordan Pediatric Survey Group was 53.6 µg/100 ml, whereas that in the WHO Xerophthalmia Study was 112 µg/100 ml, the latter being more than double the value found in the pediatric study. The two studies were done rather close together—only one year apart—and in both the children were examined in different seasons. We cannot offer any satisfactory explanation except to suggest that possibly in the year October 1963–September 1964 the consumption of carotenoid-rich foodstuffs could have been much higher. This explanation will not hold, however, for infants below 2 years of age. The matter must be left there until some further work throws more light on the situation.

One interesting point emerges from the pediatric study, in which it was observed that serum carotenoid values in children varied according to the season of the year. Peak values in each age group were found in the months of June–August. There were parallel changes in serum retinol, but these were less marked.

The prevalence of the ocular manifestations of vitamin A deficiency recorded in the report of the ICNND-ICNJ Jordan Pediatric Study was less than 1%. Xerosis of the conjunctiva and Bitot's spot were almost equal in distribution among the refugee and nonrefugee children. There is an additional entry, xerophthalmia, which, according to the ICNND *Nutrition Survey Manual* (1963) occurs "when the bulbar conjunctiva and cornea are dry and lustreless with a decrease in lacrimation." This is a much narrower definition than that suggested by McLaren, Oomen, and Escapini (1966) and that followed by Oomen throughout his investigations over a period of thirty years or more.

During the WHO Study on the Epidemiology of Xerophthalmia, Patwardhan and Kamel (1967) reported a prevalence of 8% in 1,180 children up to 6 years of age in a randomly selected population in Jordan. They found 95 cases of xerophthalmia (defined according to McLaren, Oomen, and Escapini) in 73 out of the 532 households surveyed. The distribution of ocular signs is given in Table 3. At the

TABLE 3
INCIDENCE OF SIGNS OF XEROPHTHALMIA IN JORDANIAN CHILDREN[1]

	Random Survey (95)	Notified (112)
Xerosis conjunctivae	77	72
Bitot's spot	7	20
Conjunctival pigmentation	15	10
Xerosis cornea	1	1
Corneal ulcer	1	0
Keratomalacia	0	10
Nebula	0	4
Leucoma	2	23
Staphyloma	0	10
Phthisis bulbi	0	2
History of night blindness	15	19

1. Source: Patwardhan and Kamel, 1967.

commencement of this study the government of Jordan had declared xerophthalmia a notifiable disease. This was preceded by discussions and seminars arranged at various centers to acquaint the physicians with the condition. As a result, 472 notifications were received in one year, of which 276 were in children of 6 years in age and below. Of these it was possible to follow up an appreciable proportion with visits to families and examination of siblings. The incidence of ocular signs of hypovitaminosis in these 112 children (which includes notified cases and their siblings) is also given in Table 3 for comparison with that found in the surveys in the randomly selected households.

There is a large difference between the prevalence rates found in the reports of the ICNND-ICNJ and WHO studies. The former was a general nutrition survey in which the eye may not have received special attention. On the other hand, in the WHO study careful examination of the eye was done with slit-lamp microscopy and funduscopy, according to a procedure agreed to by WHO experts. This was in addition to the clinical examination for other signs of malnutrition. This may be the reason for finding a higher prevalence of xerophthalmia.

The signs of xerophthalmia detected in the field survey were comparatively mild, only 4 cases with the involvement of the cornea being found. On the other hand, among the 112 cases from the notified group and siblings, 11 cases of active involvement of the cornea were found in addition to 35 others in which the sequelae of keratomalacia were revealed. In both groups the incidence was equal in boys and girls, and the peak incidence was between 3 and 4 years of age.

The WHO study brought out the following facts of interest:

1. Most xerophthalmia cases occurred in families economically classified as very poor.

2. The diets of the families were in general inadequate in vitamin A activity.

3. The weaning and supplementary feeding practices in Jordan were such that deficiencies of calories and protein and vitamin A were likely to occur among the infants. In families with xerophthalmia cases, a larger proportion—72 to 88%—of children received diets which were deficient in vitamin A as compared with 37 to 55% of children in families without xerophthalmia who received less than their estimated share of vitamin A through diet.

4. More children with xerophthalmia harbored intestinal parasites than those without.

5. The incidence of recurrent diarrheas and respiratory infections was greater in children with xerophthalmia than in those without.

It appears from the results of this study that the epidemiology of xerophthalmia in infants and young children is not dissimilar to that of the protein-calorie-deficiency disease. The conclusion is inescapable that both these conditions have a common origin and they thrive in the same socioeconomic, cultural, and unhygienic and unsanitary environment.

McLaren, Shirajian, Tchalian, and Khoury (1965) have reported on a clinical study of 31 cases of xerophthalmia in Jordan. Of these, 23 cases were infants and young children with associated kwashiorkor or marasmus. Eight older children with an average age of 7.55 years had only conjunctival lesions, and they did not suffer from protein-calorie-deficiency disease. In the younger age group there were 14 children with keratomalacia, and the remainder had only conjunctival lesions. The treatment for hypovitaminosis A consisted of: (a) a single intramuscular injection of an oily solution of retinyl palmitate, 50,000 I.U./kg body weight; or (b) 10,000 I.U./kg/day of a water-dispersible preparation given by nasogastric tube for five days. The ocular lesions responded well to either treatment, but mortality in children with xerophthalmia and protein-calorie-deficiency disease was 70% as compared with 15% in infants and children with kwashiorkor or marasmus but no xerophthalmia. The authors believe that when both conditions are present the prognosis is very poor, in spite of appropriate treatment. This level of mortality appears to be alarmingly high. There are practically no other published observations on mortality in xerophthalmia with or without associated protein-calorie-deficiency disease with the exception of that by De Haas

(1940) quoted by Oomen (1961). De Haas reported a mortality of 35% in his cases. This is an aspect on which more information is needed.

A review of the available information thus indicates that vitamin A deficiency occurs in the Arab countries in the Near East, although it is not so severe and so frequent as in Southeast Asia (Oomen, McLaren, and Escapini, 1964). The average serum retinol levels among Arab adults are not low, yet an appreciable proportion of the values lies within the low or deficient range. In infants and young children the ocular manifestations of moderate to severe degrees are not uncommonly seen. However, the situation may vary from country to country within the region. It is probable that infants are born with low vitamin A reserves; and since mother's milk in these countries is probably poor in retinol content and supplementary feeding is inadequate, there is not much chance of the vitamin A reserves of the infant being augmented. It is obvious that this situation ought to be remedied. The general remedial measures are discussed in Chapter Fifteen.

DEFICIENCY OF VITAMIN D—RICKETS

Vitamin D is fat soluble, and like vitamin A it occurs in eggs and in milk and milk products, such as cream, butter, and cheese. These are the only common foods in which vitamin D is found to occur naturally. Thus it will appear that only the rich can afford to eat foods which supply vitamin D in the diet. Obviously then man must obtain from extra-dietary sources vitamin D needed for the growth of bone and for the maintenance of its integrity. Fish liver oils which also contain vitamin D are not used as human food.

In 1919 Huldschinsky found that rickets could be cured by exposure to ultraviolet light. Hess and Unger (1921) showed that a similar effect could be obtained on exposure to sunlight. A convincing demonstration of the curative and protective action of sunlight against rickets was provided by Chick and collaborators (1922) in their investigations on rickets in postwar Vienna. These different classical studies explained in a satisfactory manner the wide occurrence of rickets in Europe and North America, which are the regions with long winters with comparatively little sunshine.

The antirachitic action of sunlight was later proved to be due to the fact that ultraviolet rays converted some naturally occurring sterols into compounds with vitamin D activity. The discovery provided a tool for the manufacture of vitamin D from ergosterol, a compound found in yeast and fungi. The skin of man, along with that of other animals, contains a related compound, 7-dehydrocholesterol, which under the influence of ultraviolet light is converted to vitamin D, thus satisfying the needs of the body for this vitamin.

Vitamin D promotes the absorption of dietary calcium from the intestine and thus makes it available for bone formation. Vitamin D also plays a direct role in bone formation in an as yet imperfectly understood manner. The ultimate effect of a deficiency of vitamin D is seen in defective mineralization of bone. During infancy and early childhood when bone is growing rapidly, the deficiency of Vitamin D leads to the formation of soft bones because of inadequate deposition of the mineral component, which is principally made up of calcium phosphates. When an infant crawls, sits, or walks, the weight of the body on long bones causes them to bend. Deformities of the skull, spine, and thoracic cage also occur.

It would appear that rickets should be rare in the tropics and subtropics, where there is plenty of sunlight. In fact, however, it is not so. Rickets has existed in Egypt from the Pharaonic times. Malformed persons depicted on Egyptian tombs at Beni Hassan dating from XI and XII dynasties of about 2000 B.C. show greatly deformed and bowed legs, which are typical of rickets. They also show flat feet, whereas the arches of other people depicted from the same area are high. There is little doubt therefore that, as Ruffer (1921) says, "We are in the presence of rickets."

Coming to more recent times, one finds a mention of rickets in Pruner's *Topography Medical du Caire* (1847) and in his *Die Krankheiten des Orients* (1847). Pruner reports seeing rickets in children of the higher classes of the society and in infants of mixed extraction (mulattoes). In rural areas he found it among the Copts but not the fellaheens. Rickets manifested itself a few months after birth by the swelling of the epiphyses and flaccidity of muscles and completed its entire development between 7 and 13 months of age. In some infants it was confined to the bones of the legs; in others it became more general and affected the thorax, giving the appearance of what is known as pigeon breast. Pruner did not believe that rickets was due to prolongation of breast-feeding, for it appeared early. He expressed the opinion, however, that the quality of breast milk might have something to do with its development.

In view of this early description of rickets in Egypt, it seems odd that Dick (1922) should write, "In Egypt, India and China where infants are brought up in the open air, and where they are bathed in daily sunshine from their birth onwards no errors of food will produce the disease." This is followed by the assertion, "Thus it can be taken as a general statement that in Egypt, Algeria, Morocco, West and East Africa, India, China and Japan, rickets is almost nonexistent at the present." One wonders what knowledge and experience and hence authority Dick had to make such a sweeping generalization.

As far as Egypt was concerned, Dick was very soon proved wrong. Shawky (1929) reported that rickets was common in Cairo and in other towns in Egypt. He made his diagnosis on clinical grounds when at least two signs of rickets were present. In an examination of 500 patients appearing at the children's out-patients departments of Kasr-el-Aini Hospital he found 45% with signs of rickets. Similarly in 1,000 of his private patients who presumably came from a higher socioeconomic group, 47% had signs of rickets. Shawky concluded that rickets was "very prevalent" in Egypt and that among the factors responsible were (a) relatively inefficient exposure to sunlight, (b) poverty of breast milk in vitamin D, and (c) frequency of gastrointestinal disturbances.

A few years later Sabri (1935) estimated that in Cairo 30% of infants between 6 months and 2 years of age suffered from rickets. He also observed that rickets was as common in Upper Egypt as it was in Cairo (Sabri, 1943). In spite of the reported high prevalence of rickets, there has been comparatively little interest in the study of the disease and its etiology.

Aboul-Dahab (1963) expressed the opinion that in recent years the prevalence of rickets in Cairo had decreased. In an analysis of 300 children of 4 months to 4 years in age attending the out-patients department in a hospital, he found an incidence of 26.6%, whereas among a comparable group of 358 patients attending private clinics the incidence was 10.6%. These figures are very much lower than those reported by Shawaki in 1929.

The figures for the incidence of rickets in hospital or private clinic patients does not give an idea of its prevalence in the community, for it is only sick children needing medical attention who go to these centers. There is some reason to believe that the prevalence of rickets in Egypt may be high, for Abdou, Ali, and Lebshtein (1965), who examined 1143 infants up to 2 years of age in four maternity and child health centers in Cairo, found clinical rickets in 13%. Similar figures from other centers in Egypt are not available, but judging by the past experience of Shawki (1928) and Sabri (1943) the prevalence outside Cairo is not likely to be different.

Despite the reports on the high prevalence of vitamin D deficiency rickets in infants, there are practically no references, as far as we know, in published literature to osteomalacia in Egypt. The only exception is one report by Giffen and Naguib (1939) who described 5 cases from a hospital in Assiut. It is possible that the cases of osteomalacia have been few and sporadic in occurrence, and a study was not considered worthwhile.

The Egyptian observers have attempted to examine the causes for the high prevalence of rickets in Egypt. Most of them seem to agree with the suggestions made by Shawky. Among these a deficiency of vitamin D in breast milk was considered important. Breast milk, even in the well-nourished communities, is not a rich source of vitamin D. There have been comparatively few assays, but the available information would place the vitamin D content of mature human milk between 0.4 and 2.5 I.U./100 ml (Kon and Mawson, 1950; Macy et al., 1953). Nor is the cow milk much richer unless the cows are fed irradiated yeast or vitamin D itself, or the milk is irradiated to increase its vitamin D content. The Food and Nutrition Board of the National Academy of Sciences, U.S.A. (1968) recommends 400 I.U. of vitamin D per day as a level of intake which will protect all normal children from deficiency. It is known, however, that as little as 100 I.U. of vitamin D per day can prevent rickets in a full-term infant. One liter of breast milk will supply between 4 to 25 I.U. of vitamin D per day. Thus it should be quite clear that breast milk alone will not satisfy even the minimum vitamin D needs of the growing infant in any country, and Egypt is no exception. In fact it will be correct to say that an adequate supply of vitamin D cannot ordinarily be obtained through diet unless foods are fortified with vitamin D. The major proportion of the body's vitamin D need is met through voluntary or involuntary exposure to sunshine or skyshine.

Omar (1932) examined the incidence of sunshine and especially the intensity of the ultraviolet component in Cairo. Using the technique developed at the National Institute of Medical Research, London, he found that the "biological activity" of ultraviolet light in Cairo was minimum in December. Thereafter it increased till the peak was reached in August and then declined. According to Omar, the biological activity of the ultraviolet light in Cairo sunshine during the months of November to February was almost identical with that determined for St. Ives in England. In summer the activity was much higher in Cairo than in St. Ives, in spite of the longer hours of sunshine at the higher latitudes. Omar made his measurements at rooftop level; at street level in Cairo the ultraviolet activity must be still lower. Furthermore, the frequent dust storms in the spring and early summer (April–May) and recently the smoke from incomplete combustion of the fuel in automobiles, buses, and trucks would cause a further diminution in activity in Cairo and other large cities. The question, however, has yet to be decided whether exposure to sunshine or skyshine at the time of the lowest ultraviolet activity in the year in an atmosphere laden with moisture, dust, and smoke would prevent rickets from developing. It is felt that infants in Egypt are protected from almost any exposure to sunlight by swaddling and confinement indoors. Although the Egyptian pediatricians have denied the significance of this practice as a contributory factor for the prevalence of rickets in Egypt, the problem does not seem to have been systematically investigated.

Information on the occurrence of rickets in Libya, Lebanon, and Jordan is extremely scanty. Ferro-Luzzi (1958) mentioned that rickets was frequent among Libyan infants. The other recent reference to Libya occurs in the *Seventh Report* of the Joint FAO/WHO Expert Committee on Nutrition (1967). A WHO consultant who made an extremely rapid and hence superficial survey in Algeria, Libya, Morocco, and Tunisia in 1965 found rickets to occur in all these countries. On the basis of the examination of infants and children in hospitals and dispensaries in towns and villages, the consultant found that 45 to 60% of children examined presented at least two of the following four signs of rickets—craniotabes, rachitic rosary, epiphyseal enlargement, and characteristic thoracic deformity. Severe rickets was found in only 3 to 18% of the children examined. Puyet and Budeir (1961), in their survey of infant nutrition in Palestine refugees living in Lebanon, found 9 infants out of 507 (1.8%) presenting beaded ribs. They mentioned in their report that many other infants showed isolated signs such as craniotabes, frontal bossing, large fontanelles, and delayed dentition. However, they did not consider these isolated signs specific enough to be classed as rickets. Harfouche, in a longitudinal study on 300 Lebanese infants starting from birth, stated that rickets constituted 2.3% of all illnesses seen during the 18 months for which the infants were under observation. Woodruff (1965), in his review of nutrition in Lebanese children, does not even mention rickets.

In the Jordan Pediatric Study rickets was found in about 1% of infants below 2 years of age and in nonrefugee male children up to 4-1/2 years of age (1.2% at 36–41 months and 2% at 48–53 months). Patwardhan and Kamel (1967) found 21 out of 1,050 children aged six years and below showing signs of rickets, which gives a prevalence rate of 2%. Obviously more information is necessary before a considered opinion can be given on the prevalence of rickets in these countries. However the available limited evidence indicates that this deficiency disease is less common in Lebanon and Jordan than in Egypt and possibly Libya.

DEFICIENCY OF ASCORBIC ACID—SCURVY

Scurvy is a nutritional disease resulting from the deficiency of vitamin C, also known as ascorbic acid. A prolonged absence of fresh foods, especially vegetables and fruits, from the diet leads to a deficiency of this vitamin. Ascorbic acid is relatively unstable, and much of it is destroyed in cooking, particularly prolonged cooking which is usually practiced to keep the food hot till the meal is taken.

The early signs of scurvy are seen in the gums, which are swollen, purplish in color, and bleed on slight pressure. Infections of the gum are often superimposed, causing the development of offensive odor in the breath. Other signs of advanced scurvy are bleeding in the skin, mainly around the orifice of the hair follicle and under the periosteum of long bones. In severe deficiency, bleeding may occur in any part of the body and in soft tissues. The alveolar bone atrophies; the teeth may become loose and drop out.

Swelling of gums, purple or red color, spongy appearance, and tendency to bleed are the signs which have often been used to indicate ascorbic acid deficiency in nutrition surveys. All gingivitis is not due to scurvy. In regions of the world where the dental hygiene is poor, gingivitis of infective origin often makes the diagnosis of early scurvy difficult and uncertain. The levels of ascorbic acid in plasma may help. They indicate the level of intake of this vitamin through food. With an adequate intake of ascorbic acid, the plasma levels are usually 0.4 mg/100 ml and above. It has been well established however that even with the plasma levels of ascorbic acid as low as 0.1 mg/100 ml, scurvy may not appear. The white blood corpuscles also contain ascorbic acid; when its level in the white corpuscles falls below 2 mg/100 ml, a presumptive diagnosis of scurvy may be made.

Scurvy seems to be a rare occurrence in Egypt. Pruner (1847a; 1847b) stated that scurvy occurred only in times of famine. Curiously enough his reference is to the flooding by the sea of the lowland lying near the coast, which affected the production of fresh food in those areas. Pruner mentions that the French army in Alexandria suffered from scurvy under the most unfavorable and artificial circumstances. He does not, however, amplify his statement regarding the situation which caused the outbreak of scurvy among the French troops. He was of the opinion, however, that scurvy did not ordinarily occur among the Egyptian population.

We have been unable to find any reference to scurvy in the modern Egyptian medical literature, which strengthens our view that scurvy must occur only rarely and under exceptional circumstances. This is probably due to the fact that the Egyptians, like other Arabs, are fond of eating a variety of fresh vegetables and hence their intake of ascorbic acid must be liberal, thus protecting them from scurvy.

Khalil and Waly (1949) determined plasma ascorbic acid in normal men, nonpregnant women, and pregnant and nursing women and their infants. The average values found for men and nonpregnant women (numbers not given) were 0.9 and 0.95 mg/100 ml plasma respectively. In 45 pregnant women followed through the course of pregnancy till term, the authors found a continuous fall in the average plasma ascorbic acid levels; the value at term was 0.56 mg/100 ml plasma. The average level in the newborn was 0.76 mg/100 ml plasma. It showed a fall up to the fifth day after birth, which was followed by a rise, reaching the maximum average value of 0.8 mg/100 ml at 18 days. The curve for plasma ascorbic acid in infants was generally at a higher level than that for plasma of the mothers of these infants, although the two ran parallel over this period.

Khalil and Waly also studied the plasma ascorbic acid levels in 57 other infants of one month to two years and their mothers. In infants plasma ascorbic acid levels fell between two and six months and then rose again. From four months on, the plasma ascorbic acid in mothers was slightly higher than that in infants. At 24 months, the plasma ascorbic acid in mothers had reached the prepregnancy levels and that of the infants was in the neighborhood of 0.9 mg/100 ml. At no stage during this study did the average levels fall below 0.5 mg/100 ml. This means that few infants and mothers had plasma ascorbic acid levels which could be interpreted as low or deficient according to the ICNND criteria.

The finding by Khalil and Waly of a large decrease (40%) of plasma ascorbic acid during pregnancy is difficult to explain, since there are no supporting dietary data to indicate whether there had been a decrease in the intake of vitamin C as pregnancy advanced. In the Vanderbilt Co-operative Study on Pregnancy, Darby et al. (1953) had also observed a fall of about 30% between 8 and 36 weeks of pregnancy. Their observations on dietary intake of ascorbic acid indicate only a small difference in the median values. It is possible that a diminished intake and increasing demand of pregnancy together brought about the lowering of plasma ascorbic acid levels observed in Egyptian pregnant women.

In Lebanon and Jordan scurvy seems to be rare. The mean

TABLE 4
PLASMA ASCORBIC ACID AND GUM LESIONS

Particulars	No.	Bleeding Gums %	Atrophic Papillae %	No.	Plasma Ascorbic Acid mg/100 ml Median	Sex and Age
Libya						
Police and Defense Forces	198	9.1	14.6	77	0.07	
Army	244	7.4	15.6	67	0.10	
Civilian Men	164	2.4	5.5	97	0.26	
Women						
nonpregnant	228	16.7	54.8	37	0.16	
pregnant	61	26.2	9.8	35	0.33	
			Swollen Red Papillae		Mean	
Lebanon						
Military	394		7.9			
Civilians						
nonrefugees	206		2.4	79	0.98	M & F below 15 yr.
	305		1.0	69	0.57	M & F > 15 yr.
refugees	1031		1.1	63	0.76	M & F < 15 yr.
	147		3.4			M & F > 15 yr.
Jordan						
Military	396		6.8	112	0.39	
Civilians						
nonrefugees	720		11.9			M & F all ages
refugees	575		11.6			M & F all ages
Refugees				54	0.98	< 1 to 5 yr.
				82	0.62	M & F < 15 yr.
				67	0.46	M & F > 15 yr.
Nonrefugees				156	0.89	M & F < 1 to 5 yr.
				96	0.81	M & F < 15 yr.
				117	0.49	M & F > 15 yr.

plasma ascorbic acid levels at all ages are in the elevated range (Table 4). According to Woodruff (1965), infantile scurvy is essentially unknown in Lebanon. In both these countries the frequent consumption of uncooked fresh green vegetables and citrus fruit by almost all segments of the population must protect the majority against scurvy. It is true that in the ICNND Survey swollen red papillae of the gums have been recorded in from nil to 12% of the population groups examined. Since the specificity of the sign is in doubt and no therapeutic trial was made, it is difficult to establish its significance with certainty. However, a comparison with the situation in Libya is revealing. A much higher frequency of bleeding gums and atrophic dental papillae has been recorded among the Libyan military and civilian population (See Table 4) together with unusually low average values for plasma ascorbic acid. As the table shows, a large proportion of the surveyed population had ascorbic acid values in the deficient and low ranges. We feel that this would be an ideal country to undertake a special clinical, biochemical, and therapeutic study for vitamin C nutrition. As mentioned earlier, the low levels of plasma ascorbic acid are not necessarily indicative of ascorbic acid deficiency bordering on clinical survey. However they undoubtedly reflect a habitual low intake of ascorbic acid and marginal state of vitamin C nutrition among the Libyans.

REFERENCES

Abboud, I. A., H. G. Osman, and W. H. Massoud. 1968a. Blood Serum Vitamin A and β-Carotene Contents in Normal Egyptians. *Med. J. Cairo Univ.* 36: 1.

Abboud, I. A., H. G. Osman, and W. H. Massoud. 1968b. Vitamin A and Xerosis. *Exptl. Eye Res.* 7: 388.

Abdou, I. A., and A. K. Amer. 1965. A Study of the Nutritional Status of Mothers, Infants, and Young Children Attending Maternity and Child Health Centers in Cairo. Part I—The Nutritional Status of Infants and Young Children. Part II—Dietary Intake and Nutritional Status of Pregnant and Nursing Mothers. *Bull. Nutr. Inst. UAR* 1: 9, 21.

Abdou, I. A., and A. H. Mahfouz. 1965. A Survey of the Diet in the Egyptian Village, and its Seasonal Variation. *Bull. Nutr. Inst. UAR* 1: 51.

Aboul-Dahab, Y. W. 1963. Clinical Studies on Rickets in Cairo. *J. Egypt. Pub. Hlth. Assoc.* 38: 203.

Aykroyd, W. R. 1958. In Hypovitaminosis A. *Federation Proc.* 17: 102.

Chick, H., E. J. Dalyell, M. Hume, H. M. M. Mackay, and H. Henderson-Smith. 1922. The Aetiology of Rickets in Infants: Prophylactic and Curative Observations at the Vienna University Kinderklinik. *Lancet* ii: 7.

Darby, W. J., and 13 others. 1953. The Vanderbilt Cooperative Study of Maternal and Infant Nutrition. IV—Dietary, Laboratory, and Physical Findings in 2,129 Delivered Pregnancies. *J. Nutr.* 51: 565.

Diek, L. 1922. *Rickets.* London: Heinemann.

Ferro-Luzzi, G. 1958. Report to the Government of Libya on Nutrition. FAO Report No. 920. Rome, Italy: Food and Agriculture Organization of the United Nations.

Food and Nutrition Board, National Academy of Sciences. 1968. *Recommended Dietary Allowances.* Washington, D.C.: National Research Council.

Giffen, H. K., and A. Naguib. 1939. Osteomalacia. Report of Five Cases. *J. Egypt. Med. Assoc.* 22: 129.

Hammad, Salah el Dine. 1966. Studies on Vitamin A in Health and Disease in Infancy and Childhood. Thesis for Faculty of Medicine, Alexandria University (M.D. Pediatrics).

Hanafy, M. 1947. The Subacute Subnutritional Syndrome in Infants. *J. Egypt. Med. Assoc.* 30: 440.

Harfouche, J. K. 1966. *Growth and Illness Patterns of Lebanese Infants (Birth–18 months).* Beirut, Lebanon: Khayats.

Hess, A. F., and L. J. Unger. 1921. Cure of Infantile Rickets by Artificial Light and by Sunlight. *Proc. Soc. Exptl. Biol. Med.* 18: 298.

Huldschinsky, K. 1919. *Vitamins: A Survey of Present Knowledge.* Medical Research Council, U.K. Special Report Series No. 167, London, 1932. Quoted in *Deutsch. Med. Wschr.* 45: 712.

Interdepartmental Committee on Nutrition for National Defense. 1963. *Manual of Nutrition Surveys.* 2nd ed. Bethesda, Md.: National Institutes of Health.

Interdepartmental Committee on Nutrition for National Defense. *Reports of Nutrition Surveys in Libya 1957; Lebanon 1962; Jordan 1963.*

Joint FAO/WHO Expert Committee on Nutrition. 1967. Seventh Report. Published by FAO and WHO. World Health Organization Technical Report Series.

Khalil, A., and G. Waly. 1949. Vitamin C in the Nutrition of Infants, Pregnant and Lactating Women. *J. Egypt. Med. Assoc.* 32: 158.

Kirk, J. E. 1962. Variations with Age in the Tissue Content of Vitamins and Hormones. *Vitamins and Hormones* 20: 67.

Kon, S. K., and E. H. Mawson. 1950. *Human Milk: Wartime Studies on Certain Vitamins and Other Constituents.* Special Report Series No. 269. London: Medical Research Council, U.K.

McLaren, D. S., H. A. P. C. Oomen, and H. Escapini. 1966. Ocular Manifestations of Vitamin A Deficiency in Man. *Bull. Wld. Hlth. Org.* 34: 357.

McLaren, D. S., E. Shirajian, M. Tchalian, and G. Khoury. 1965. Xerophthalmia in Jordan. *Amer. J. Clin. Nutr.* 17: 117.

Macy, I. G., H. J. Kelly, and R. E. Sloan. 1953. The Composition of Milks. National Research Council Publ. 254. Washington, D.C.: National Academy of Sciences.

Moore, T. 1957. *Vitamin A.* Amsterdam, Holland: Elsevier Publ. Co.
Nor-el-Din, G. 1944. Studies on the Carotene and the Vitamin A. *J. Egypt. Med. Assoc.* 27: 251.
Omar, W. 1932. Measurements of the Biologically Active Ultraviolet Rays of Sunlight in Cairo. *J. Egypt. Med. Assoc.* 15: 828.
Oomen, H. A. P. C. 1961. An Outline of Xerophthalmia. *Internat. Rev. Trop. Med.* 1: 179.
Oomen, H. A. P. C., D. S. McLaren, and H. Escapini. 1964. A Global Survey of Xerophthalmia: Epidemiology and Public Health Aspects of Hypovitaminosis A. *Trop. Geogr. Med.* 16: 271.
Patwardhan, V. N., and W. W. Kamel. 1967. *Studies on Vitamin A Deficiency in Infants and Young Children in Jordan.* Geneva, Switzerland: World Health Organization.
Pruner, F. 1847a. *Topographie medicale du Caire avec le plan de la ville et des environs.* Munich: Aux frais de l'auteur.
Pruner, F. 1847b. *Die Krankheiten des Orients vom stanpunkte der vergleichenden nosologie.* Erlangen: Verlag won J. J. Palm und Ernst Enke.
Puyet, J., and R. Budeir. 1961. *Infant Nutrition Survey among Palestine Refugees Living in Lebanon.* Beirut, Lebanon: United Nations Relief and Works Agency for Palestine Refugees.
Sabri, I. 1935. The Consideration of the Possible Causes of the Prevalence of Rickets in Egypt. *J. Egypt. Med. Assoc.* 18: 138.
Sabri, I. A. 1943. Rickets in Egypt. *J. Egypt. Med. Assoc.* 26: 166.
Shawky, I. 1929. Rickets in Egypt. *Compt. rend. Congr. Internat. Med. Trop. Hyg.* Tome II. Cairo: Imprimerie Nationale.
Ruffer, M. A. 1921. *Studies in Paleopathology of Egypt.* Edited by R. L. Moodie. Chicago, Ill.: The University of Chicago Press.
Sandstead, H. H., S. Shukry, A. S. Prasad, M. K. Gabr, A. Hifney, N. Mokhtar, and W. J. Darby. 1965. Kwashiorkor in Egypt. I-Clinical and Biochemical Studies, with Special Reference to Plasma Zinc and Serum Lactic Dehydrogenase. *Amer. J. Clin. Nutr.* 17: 15.
Taha, M. M. and H. H. Emara. 1959. Studies on Vitamin A in Diseases. *Alexandria Med. J.* 5: 187.
Tohamy, M. F. 1968. Estimation of Vitamin A and β-Carotene in Blood Serum of Malnourished Egyptian Children. Thesis for Faculty of Medicine (M.D. Pediatrics), Cairo University.
Woodruff, C. A. 1965. Growth and Nutrition of Lebanese Children. *Nutr. Rev.* 23: 97.
Yang, Y. H. 1963. *Food and Nutrition Policy: Report to the Government of Libya.* Rome, Italy: Food and Agriculture Organization of the United Nations.

7 THE ZINC-DEFICIENCY SYNDROME

Growth retardation and delayed genital maturation in patients with hookworm was described in detail in 1910 (Lemann). Its occurrence in many parts of the world, including the Middle East, has since been recognized. It affects both sexes (Billings *et al.*, 1968; Sandstead, unpublished) but appears to have its most striking effects on young men. A similar clinical syndrome may occur in young patients who practice geophagia (Prasad *et al.*, 1961) or are infected with *S. Japonium* (Chao-Ling *et al.*, 1959) or malaria (Nocht and Mayer, 1937). The nutritional etiology of this type of "dwarfism" was clarified beginning in 1963, in studies which grew out of the suggestion by Prasad *et al.* (1961) that Egyptian patients with the syndrome were deficient in zinc (Prasad *et al.*, 1963c). Later their responsiveness to zinc therapy was demonstrated (Sandstead *et al.*, 1967). The recognition that zinc deficiency may occur in man was largely due to these studies in the Middle East (Egypt, Iran) and constitutes a milestone in the understanding of the role of trace elements in human nutrition.

HISTORY

Zinc is an essential nutrient for both plant and animal life. Since Raulin's report in 1869 of a zinc requirement of *Aspergillus niger*, knowledge of the role of zinc in biology has gradually broadened. Maze in 1914 and Somner and Lipman in 1926 established its importance in plant nutrition. Their contributions have had immeasurable influence on the productivity of modern agriculture.

Preparation of a zinc-deficient diet by Todd in 1934 made it possible to study zinc deficiency in small rodents. Knowledge of these early investigations led Tucker and Salmon (1955) to recognize porcine parakeratosis as a zinc-deficiency syndrome. Since their pioneering studies in swine, zinc deficiency has been observed to occur in cattle (Legg and Sears, 1960) and has been produced experimentally in several species, including fowl (O'Dell et al., 1958) and lower primates (Macapinlac et al., 1967).

Eggleton in 1939 first reported that patients with protein-calorie malnutrition, pellagra, or beriberi may have decreased concentration of zinc in the serum and skin. His observations were confirmed twenty-four years later in studies by the staff of Vanderbilt University, Division of Nutrition, working at NAMRU-3 in Cairo, UAR. The latter found that infants (Sandstead et al., 1965) and adolescents (Prasad et al., 1963a) with severe protein-calorie malnutrition and/or pellagra (see patients 2 and 4, Prasad et al., 1963a) may have reduced levels of plasma zinc and other findings consistent with decreased body stores of this element.

HUMAN ZINC DEFICIENCY

Although the work of Eggleton (1940) on patients with protein malnutrition and the observations of Vallee et al. (1959) on patients with cirrhosis of the liver indicated that zinc deficiency might occur in man, the pathological effects of the deficiency were largely speculative until Prasad et al. (1961) observed that patients with a syndrome of growth failure, hypogonadism, iron deficiency, and geophagia had clinical features reminiscent of porcine parakeratosis and experimental zinc deficiency in the rat.

Subsequently Prasad and his associates (1963, 1963c) established by biochemical and therapeutic studies (Sandstead et al., 1967) that similar Egyptian patients were indeed deficient in the element. These individuals came from the low socioeconomic level. Their diets consisted primarily of cereal products and vegetables and contained little animal protein. Patients from the Nile Delta were infected with *Ankylostoma duodenale* and either *Schistosoma hematobium* or *mansoni*, while patients from Kharga Oasis (Prasad et al., 1963a) in the western desert were nonparasitized.

The major clinical features of zinc deficiency in these patients are illustrated by the patient in Figure 1. Growth retardation is severe, and genital development is delayed. Bone development is also retarded, as shown in Figure 2. The maturation of the carpal bones is

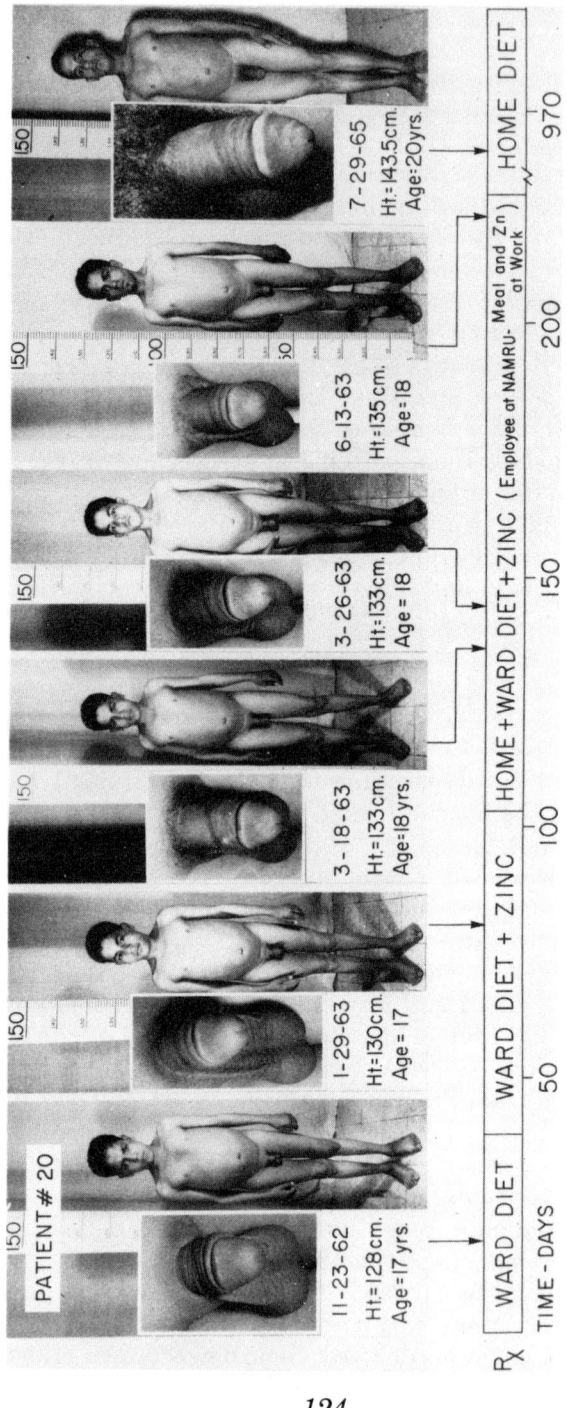

Figure 7.1. Zinc-deficient male age 17 years. Zinc therapy was promptly followed by an increase in size of the genitalia and appearance of pubic, facial, axillary and extremity hair. Two years after initial treatment sexual function was apparently normal.

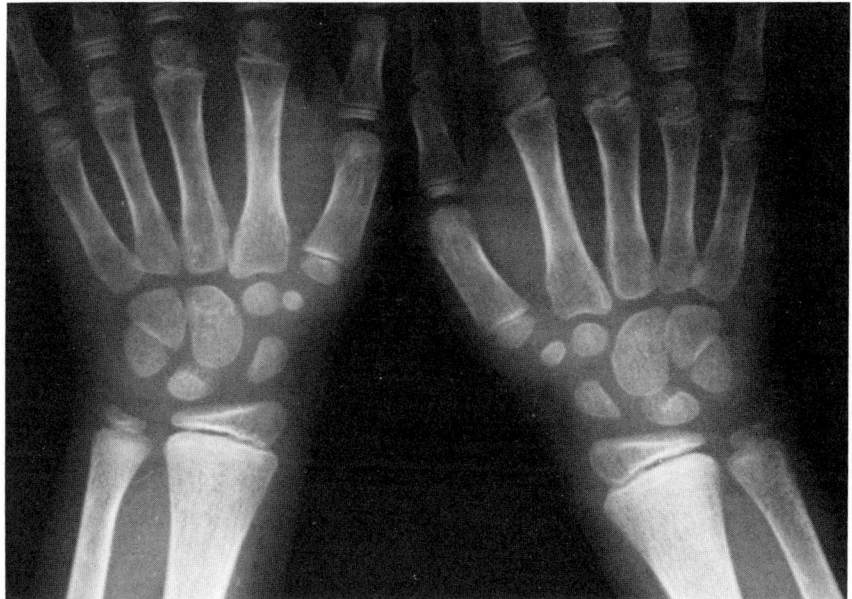

Figure 7.2. Wrist X-ray of a 16-year-old zinc-deficient male. The estimated bone age is 8 years. The epiphyses of the radius and metacarpal bones are open.

severely delayed, as is the closure of the radial and metacarpal epiphysis. Tooth growth and eruption may also be retarded. Figure 3 shows the presence of deciduous teeth in the mouth of the same sixteen-year-old whose wrists are illustrated in Figure 2.

Laboratory examination (Sandstead et al., 1965), as indicated in Table 1, has shown low plasma concentrations of zinc and iron deficiency to be extremely common in patients from the Nile Delta. Serum albumin also is decreased in patients who are deficient in protein. Deficiencies in other nutrients occur sporadically. Their occurrence is a reflection of the general poor quality of the village diet. Tests of liver function are usually normal to mildly deranged, even though schistosomal granulomata of the liver are common and severe fibrosis is sometimes present (Prasad et al., 1963).

Studies of zinc kinetics (Prasad et al., 1963c) have shown that the exchangeable pool of zinc is decreased while the rate of disappearance of injected ^{65}zinc from the blood is rapid, and the turnover rate is increased (Table 2). Urinary (Prasad et al., 1963) and sweat (Prasad et al., 1963b) losses of zinc are decreased (Tables 3 and 4). Of interest

TABLE 1
REPRESENTATIVE LABORATORY STUDIES ON 22 ZINC-DEFICIENT PATIENTS[1]

	Hgb g%	Plasma Zinc μg%	Serum Iron μg%	BUN mg%	BSP % Retained in 45 Min.	Alk P'tase B.U.	Serum Albumin g%	Serum Protein g%
Range	3.4–15.0	35–81	11–51	4.4–14.5	0.0–8.8	2.2–14.8	0.8–4.9	5.7–9.4
Median	9.4	65.0	25.0	10.5	1.6	8.1	3.9	7.7
Mean	9.1	64.7	26.8	10.0	2.3	8.4	3.8	7.6
S	2.9	12.4	12.5	2.8	2.2	3.6	0.88	0.81
"Normal"	11.2–16.5	102 ± 13	75–175	10–20	< 5	2–4.5	3.5–5.5	6–8

1. Source: Sandstead et al., 1967.

Zinc Deficiency

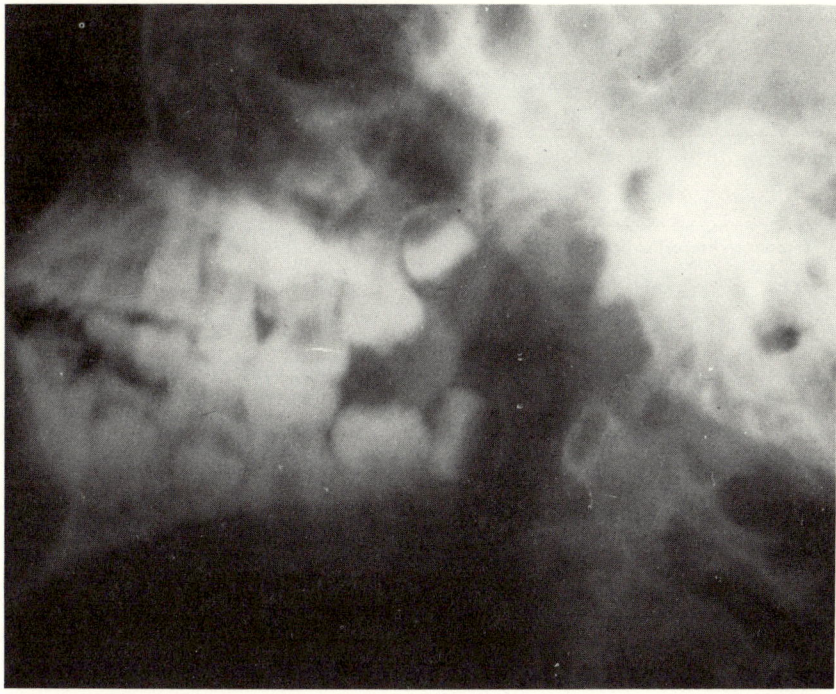

Figure 7.3. Teeth of a 16-year-old zinc-deficient male. Deciduous teeth are still present.

is the observation that while total urinary zinc excretion is low in these patients, their excretion in relation to body size is increased. Observations in a nonparasitized North American patient with zinc deficiency indicate that urinary zinc excretion can be markedly restricted by the normal kidney (Sandstead, unpublished) when gastrointestinal absorption of the cation is small. These findings raise the question as to whether the urinary losses of zinc which occurs in

TABLE 2
FRACTIONAL RATE OF DISAPPEARANCE OF ^{65}ZN FROM
THE PLASMA OF ZINC-DEFICIENT AND CONTROL SUBJECTS[1]

Phase	Controls	Patients	P
30–60 minutes	.0165	.0239	< .01
2–10 hours	.0592	.0912	< .01
1–7 days	.1412	.1174	< .01

1. Source: Prasad et al., 1963c.

TABLE 3
ZINC IN URINE OF ZINC-DEFICIENT AND CONTROL SUBJECTS[1]

	µg/Day	µg/gm Creatinine	µg/kilo Body Weight
Controls	613 ± 93	447 ± 108	9.8 ± 2.4
Patients	395 ± 46	679 ± 203	14.3 ± 2.9
P	< .01	< .01	< .01

1. Source: Prasad et al., 1963.

TABLE 4
ZINC IN SWEAT OF ZINC-DEFICIENT AND CONTROL SUBJECTS[1]

	Whole Sweat	Cell Free Sweat
Control	115 ± 30 µg%	93 ± 26 µg%
Patients	48 ± 12 µg%	29 ± 13 µg%
P	< .01	< .01

1. Source: Prasad et al., 1963b.

TABLE 5
ENDOCRINOLOGIC FINDINGS IN ZINC-DEFICIENT ADOLESCENT BOYS[1]

Measurement	Finding
Height	Retarded
Bone Age	Retarded
Genital Development	Retarded
Secondary Sexual Development	Retarded
Body Proportions	Normal
Growth Hormone Following Insulin Hypoglycemia	Low
Gonadotropin Excretion	Low
17 Ketosteroid Excretion	Low
17 Hydroxysteroid Excretion	Low to Normal
Response to Intravenous ACTH	Decreased
ACTH Reserve (Intravenous Metyrapone Test)	Decreased
Plasma Immunoreactive ACTH Following Oral Metyrapone	Normal
Thyroid Uptake of Iodine	Normal
Serum Protein-Bound Iodine	Normal
Testosterone Response Following Exogenous Gonadotropin	Low
Oral Glucose Tolerance Test	Impaired Absorption
Intravenous Glucose Tolerance Test	Normal

1. Sources: Sandstead et al., 1967; Coble, unpublished.

Zinc Deficiency

Egyptian patients may be in part related to *S. hematobium* infection of the urogenital tract. Is the zinc lost into the urine in exudative fluid produced by the ureteral and bladder mucosa in response to injury by *S. hematobium*?

The laboratory assessment of the endocrine status of these individuals is consistent with "hypopituitarism" (Sandstead *et al.*, 1967). These are summarized in Table 5. Initial and follow-up observations on the patient shown in Figure 1 are charted in Figure 4.

The adrenal cortical response to ACTH (AC) and metyrapone (SU) (Figure 4) is not well understood (Sandstead *et al.*, 1967). Responses are quite variable among patients. The finding of a normal rise in plasma immunoreactive ACTH (Table 5) in some of them (Coble, unpublished) in response to oral metyrapone suggests that low excretions of urinary 17 hydroxysteroids (17 OHCS) which follow ACTH or metyrapone administration may be in part attributable to impaired adrenal cortical function. Urinary excretion of 17 OHCSs reflects the over-all responsiveness of the adrenal gland and pituitary, and in view of the subsequent failure of the metyrapone test to improve (Figure 4) following treatment with zinc (in contrast to the improved responsiveness to ACTH) it appears that the pituitary ACTH reserve may have been severely depressed in certain of these patients and slow to recover.

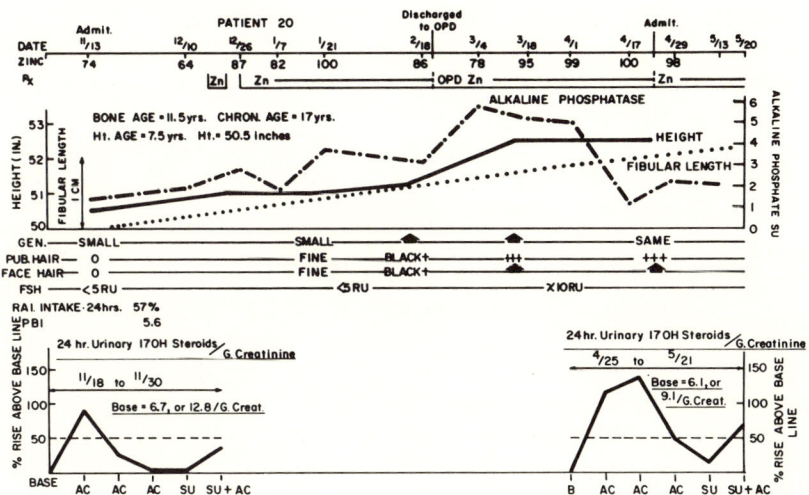

Figure 7.4. Clinical course of the 17-year-old patient illustrated in Figure 1. Treatment with zinc was followed by improvement in all parameters except the metyrapone test (SU).

TABLE 6
GROWTH OF ZINC-DEFICIENT ADOLESCENT MALES FOLLOWING THERAPY[1]

Therapy	Number of Patients	Duration of Therapy (Days)	Average Growth Increment for One Year
Village Diet	2	300 and 400	0
Hospital Diet	10	40 to 110	1.8
Hospital Diet Plus Iron	4	125 to 210	2.9
Hospital Diet Plus Zinc	9	80 to 210	5.0

1. Source: Sandstead et al., 1967.

Therapeutic trials (Sandstead et al., 1967; Ronaghy et al., in press) with diet alone, diet plus iron, or diet plus zinc have shown that growth (Table 6) and genital development subsequent to zinc administration is far out of proportion of changes which occur following treatment with either diet alone or diet plus iron. Figures 1, 4, and 6 illustrate the changes in growth and genital development which occurred in an Egyptian patient following zinc supplementation. Similar dramatic effects have been found in zinc-deficient adolescent girls (Ronaghy et al., in press) and in a recently studied 20-year-old North American male with regional enteritis of long standing (Sandstead, unpublished). Of interest was the rise in serum alkaline phosphatase activity which followed zinc administration (Figure 4) to the patient shown in Figure 1. Similar increases in serum activity of this zinc metalloenzyme have been observed when parakeratotic swine are treated with zinc.

The prognosis of zinc-deficient patients without treatment is unknown. Many probably eventually mature sexually but never achieve their genetic potential for growth. This supposition is based on the outcome of follow-up observations on the untreated patients from Kharga Oasis (Coble et al., 1966). They exhibited sexual maturation two years after the initial study. Ronaghy has found that after 300 days some of his patients matured sufficiently to have nocturnal emissions (Ronaghy et al., in press), although those getting zinc experienced emissions some 40 days after supplementation was initiated. It seems likely in the case of the Egyptian patients that growth and sexual development occurred following an improvement in their dietary intake due to achieving some seniority in the family. Thus they probably were given the more desirable animal proteins and coincidentally a greater intake of available zinc and other essential nutrients.

Zinc Deficiency

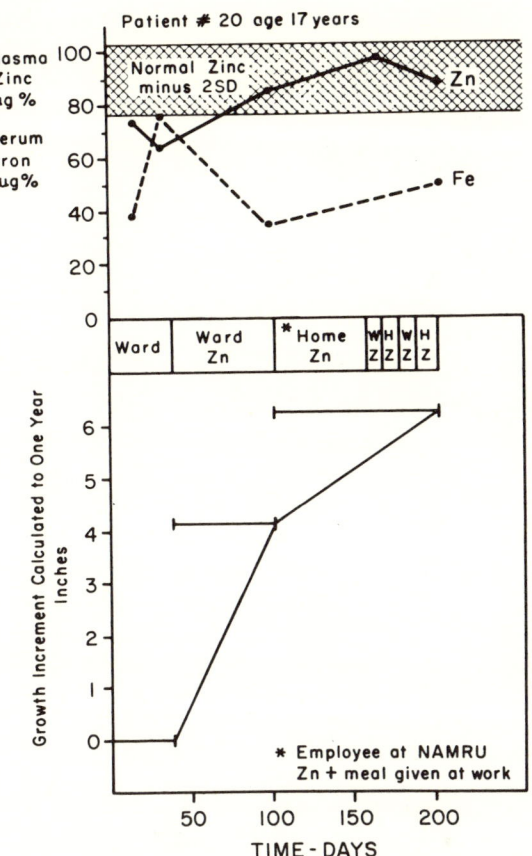

Figure 7.5. Growth response of patient in Figure 1 to zinc. Striking growth acceleration occurred.

Treatment with zinc alone is not sufficient to produce acceleration of growth of puberty in growth-retarded village school boys (Carter *et al.*, 1969). When a dietary supplement containing all essential micronutrients and essential amino acids is given along with zinc, iron, or a placebo (Ronaghy *et al.*, 1969), genital development is significantly increased in the boys given zinc in comparison to changes which occur subsequent to administration of iron or a placebo.

Protein-calorie malnutrition (PCM) is common among infants in the Middle East. Studies of infants with PCM from Cairo, UAR, have shown that these patients have extremely low concentrations of plasma zinc (42 ± 14.5 μg%; normal = 100 ± 13 μg%) (Figure 7)

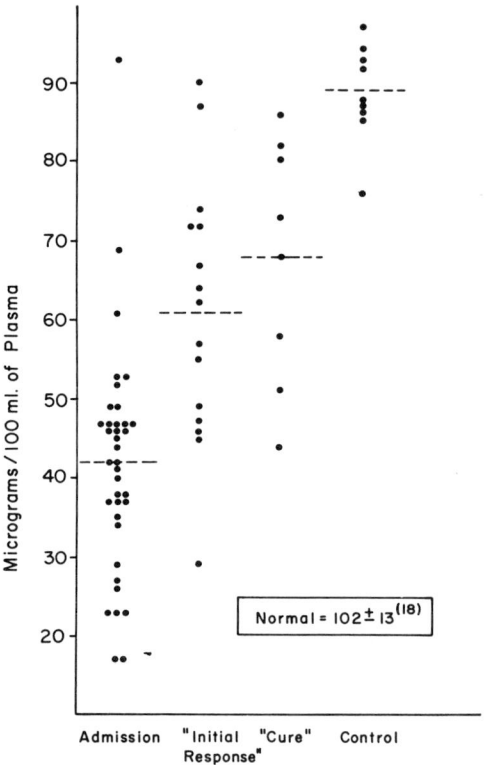

Figure 7.6. Plasma zinc concentrations in patients with protein-calorie malnutrition. Note the failure of the plasma zinc to return to normal subsequent to conventional therapy (17).

(Sandstead et al., 1965). Following conventional therapy, plasma zinc did not return to normal levels in these infants by the time of "clinical recovery." This finding suggests that their body stores of zinc were insufficient to permit recovery of their plasma zinc levels to normal without added dietary zinc and that the therapeutic regimen did not provide sufficient zinc to fulfill these needs. It is likely that the diets of these infants are low in zinc prior to the onset of acute PCM; their usual home diets are low in animal protein (milk) and high in cereals (phytate). Growth failure is relatively common in infants and young

Zinc Deficiency

children in areas of the world where PCM occurs. It seems possible that zinc lack may contribute to this retardation.

Low plasma concentrations of zinc have been found in neopartum Iranian women (Sarram et al., 1969). The significance of this observation has not as yet been established. In view of the teratogenic, aborting, and growth-retarding effects *in utero* (Dreosti et al., 1968; Hurley, 1969; Sandstead and Glasser, 1969) of zinc deficiency and the neonatal growth retardation (Lema and Sandstead, 1970) which results from zinc deficiency of the lactating mother rat, it is reasonable to speculate whether these low plasma concentrations of the cation may indicate actual or potential injury due to maternal zinc deficiency in man. This clearly is an important area for investigation.

PHYSIOLOGY OF ZINC

That dietary factors affect the availability of zinc from food was documented during the early 1960s (O'Dell, 1969). Phytic acid was shown to decrease the availability of dietary zinc for experimental animals, while added calcium aggravated the deficiency which occurred when diets were high in phytate. Apparently calcium and phytate form an insoluble complex with zinc, thus decreasing its absorption. Calcium and zinc are apparently not antagonistic, as this effect does not occur in the absence of phytate. Recent studies have shown that phytate in unleavened bread decreased the availability of zinc for rats (Reinhold, unpublished).

Other chelating substances which presumably bind dietary zinc include alkaline clays and phaeophytin (a degradation product of chlorophyll). Clay-eating (geophagia) is believed to be a major pathogenic factor in the development of iron and zinc deficiency described from Iran (Prasad et al., 1961; Minnich et al., 1968). Demonstration of the binding of zinc by phaeophytin (Mills, 1964), a potent chelator of copper, has not as yet been reported.

Of the animal protein foods ingested by infants and children, colostrum (roughly 20 mg/l) and milk (3-4 mg/l) are among the most important sources of dietary zinc (Berfenstam, 1952). For older individuals, meat and other animal proteins provide much of the available metal.

While the quantitative zinc requirements of man are not established, studies by Engel et al. (1966) suggest that growing children probably need to absorb 2 mg or more of zinc per day if they are to retain the 0.25 mg per day estimated essential for growth. Engel found that a mixed diet containing 6 mg of zinc was sufficient to meet this requirement in young school girls. Studies in college women consuming 13 mg to 15 mg zinc daily have shown that they may retain as much as 6 mg of the element (Tribble and Scoular, 1954). In contrast to the studies in normal individuals, balance studies in a patient with long-standing regional enteritis and malabsorption syndrome have shown that he absorbed only 10% (1.2 mg) of his dietary zinc and had developed zinc deficiency (Sandstead, unpublished). These data suggest that dietary requirements are related to growth rate, body size, and losses. Normal losses occur in sweat, urine, stool, menstrual blood, milk, desquamated epithelial cells, and hair. Abnormal loss occurs with gastrointestinal bleeding, proteinurea, failure to reabsorb zinc in intestinal secretions, severe catabolic states, and cirrhosis of the liver (urinary).

Zinc in bone and soft tissue of experimental animals does not appear readily available for mobilization or transport when increased needs arise (Dreosti et al., 1968; Mills et al., 1969). These findings suggest that rats and presumably man are relatively dependent on their daily intake of zinc to meet physiological needs. Observations on human wound-healing support this concept (Pories et al., 1967; Husain, 1969). The implications of this concept for human pregnancy have been referred to previously.

BIOCHEMISTRY

Zinc is essential for function of approximately twenty metalloenzymes including carbonic anhydrase, carboxypeptidase, several phosphatases, dehydrogenases, and transaminases (Parisi and Vallee, 1969). In experimental animals it has been shown that the activities of pancreatic carboxypeptidase (Mills et al., 1969) and intestinal alkaline phosphatase (Prasad et al., 1967) are decreased in zinc deficiency. These effects may in part be due to decreased synthesis of apoenzyme, as well as formation of an abnormal tertiary structure of the enzyme (Reinhold and Kfoury, 1969). The physiologic significance of these enzyme abnormalities is unknown. The apparent decrease in synthesis of apoenzymes which occurs in zinc deficiency may be a manifestation of impaired amino acid utilization (Hsu et al., 1969).

In addition to its role as an activator of metalloenzymes, zinc is involved in those processes which regulate protein and nucleic acid synthesis and turnover. Knowledge of this function is incomplete. Studies using *E. gracillus* (Schneider and Price, 1962; Wacker, 1962) or *Mycobacterium smegmatus* (Winder and Dinneny, 1959) have shown that DNA replication is inhibited and concentrations of RNA and protein are decreased when these organisms are zinc deficient. In physiologic concentrations (10^{-4} M) zinc inhibits yeast ribonuclease (Ohtaka et al., 1963). In support of these findings zinc-deficient plants have been shown to have increased ribonuclease activity in their leaves (Kessler and Monselise, 1959), and the activity of this enzyme is increased in testes of zinc-deficient rats (Somers and Underwood, 1969). The concentrations of nucleic acids and protein also are decreased in testes of zinc-deficient animals (Somers and Underwood, 1969), while the incorporation of amino acids into protein or orotic acid into nucleic acids of this tissue is not decreased (Macapinlac et al., 1968), implying an increased rate of degradation. In contrast, other tissue from zinc-deficient rats has been found to have a decreased incorporation of amino acids into protein (Lema and Sandstead, 1970; Hsu et al., 1969), suggesting that protein synthesis is decreased.

Studies with ribosomes from *E. coli* (Tal, 1969) show that zinc is present on the ribosome and may have a role in maintenance of the tertiary structure of this intracellular organelle. If this finding is confirmed in mammalian tissue, the hypothesis of Schneider and Price (1962) that an abnormality in "RNA metabolism" is the primary lesion in zinc deficiency may indeed be true.

A nonenzyme, rapidly effected function for zinc, such as confirmation of ribosomal tertiary structure, would account for the rapidity of onset of such effects as decreased food utilization (Todd et al., 1934) and anorexia in experimental zinc deficiency. It would also explain the effects of the deficiency on DNA metabolism discussed below.

The importance of zinc for mammalian cell replication has been best shown by studies with tissue culture (Lieberman et al., 1963). Zinc-deficient rabbit kidney cells have decreased activities of thymidine kinase and DNA-polymerase and demonstrate decreased DNA synthesis. Partially hepatectomized rats (Fujioka and Lieberman, 1964) demonstrate a similar impairment of DNA replication when they are perfused with EDTA soon after hepatectomy. Zinc is the only metal found to reverse the effect of EDTA, while magnesium or iron will augment the effect of zinc. Dietary deficiency of zinc will also impair DNA synthesis in the liver (Sandstead and Rinaldi, 1969), epiphysis (Lema and Sandstead, 1970), neural tissue of twelve-day rat fetuses (Swenerton et al., 1969), and in the brain of eleven-day old nursing rat pups (Sandstead, unpublished).

These observations have suggested the following hypothesis (Lema and Sandstead, 1970): Zinc is essential for preservation of ribosomal tertiary structure. When zinc concentrations are decreased, ribosomes tend to "unfold." Associated with "unfolding" of ribosomes, the activity of ribonuclease is increased and the "unfolded" ribosomes are degraded. When zinc is adequate, synthesis of ribonuclease is suppressed at the level of DNA through feedback inhibition by a hypothetical "ribonuclease suppressor." Synthesis of "ribonuclease suppressor" is regulated by the conformation of ribosomes. When ribosomes "unfold," synthesis of "suppressor" is decreased and synthesis of ribonuclease is increased. "Unfolded" ribosomes do not function as templates for protein synthesis. Therefore, synthesis of proteins such as DNA polymerase, thymidine kinase, and proline hydroxylase, etc., is decreased. Nucleic-acid synthesis is impaired, cell replication inhibited, and growth fails.

PUBLIC HEALTH SIGNIFICANCE: AREAS FOR FUTURE INVESTIGATION

The significance of zinc deficiency in the Middle East at the present time is unknown. However, its importance in human nutrition and for basic processes such as the synthesis of protein and nucleic acid is clear. Speculation as to the significance of zinc in public health is therefore offered.

The widespread growth failure observed in children in many of the underdeveloped areas may in part be due to a dietary zinc lack. Because of the importance of zinc in protein synthesis, it seems conceivable that it may even play a role in the body defenses against infection. Certain experimental findings lead to asking whether it may be essential for the synthesis of immunoproteins and leucocyte function. In this connection it is of interest to note that in experimental animals zinc is essential for wound healing (Sandstead et al., 1970), which process is but a manifestation of the body's response to injury. Zinc deficiency results in atrophy of the thymus of rats (Sandstead, unpublished) and a decrease in certain plasma-globulin fractions of Japanese quail (Spivey Fox and Harrison, 1966). *In vitro* lymphocyte transformation requires the presence of zinc (Auford, 1970), and a patient with zinc deficiency has been reported who had impairment of this phenomenon (Caggiano et al., 1969). Thus zinc deficiency adversely affects certain biological functions which play a role in the body's defense mechanisms. Studies should be done in man to evaluate the possible role of zinc in infection.

The importance of zinc for fetal and neonatal growth (Dreosti et al., 1968; Hurley, 1969; Sandstead and Glasser, 1969; Lema and Sandstead, 1970) has been noted. There is reason to suspect that human populations subsisting on diets high in poorly refined cereal grains and small amounts of animal protein may be marginal in their zinc nutriture (Sarram *et al.*, 1969; O'Dell, 1969; Reinhold, unpublished). Attention should be given to the question as to whether low-birth-weight infants and abortions occurring in these populations may in part be due to maternal zinc deprivation.

REFERENCES

Auford, R. 1970. Metal Cation Requirements for Phytohemaglutinin Induced Transformation of Human Peripheral Blood Lymphocytes. *J. Immunol.* 104: 698.

Berfenstam, R. 1952. A Clinical and Experimental Investigation into the Zinc Content of Plasma and Blood Corpuscles with Special Reference to Infancy. *Acta Pediatr.* (Stockholm), Suppl. 87, 41:3.

Billings, F. T., H. H. Sandstead, L. K. Wallwork, and G. H. Booth. 1968. Appalachia: A Ghetto. *Trans. Am. Clin. Cli. Assoc.* 80: 82.

Caggiano, V., R. Schnitzler, W. Strauss, R. K. Baker, A. C. Carter, A. S. Josephson, and S. Wallach. 1969. Zinc Deficiency in a Patient with Retarded Growth, Hypogonadism, Hypogammaglobulinemia and Chronic Infection. *Am. J. Med. Sci.* 257: 305.

Carter, J. P., L. E. Grivetti, J. T. Davis, S. Nasiff, A. Mansour, W. A. Mousa, A. Atta, V. N. Patwardhan, M. A. Moneim, I. A. Abdou and W. J. Darby. 1969. Growth and Sexual Development of Adolescent Egyptian Village Boys. Effects of Zinc, Iron, and Placebo Supplement. *Am. J. Clin. Nutr.* 22: 59.

Chao-Ling, C., C. Shih-T'ao, C. Kuoch'en, Y. Lan-sheng, L. Sheng-Ch'ing, L. Chin-sen, K. Ching-yun, L. Yi-Fen, and H. Ching-Ya. 1959. Schistosomal Hypophyseal Dwarfism: Study of 72 Cases. *Chinese Med. J.* 79: 26.

Coble, Y. D. Unpublished observation.

Coble, Y. D., A. R. Schulert, Z. Farid, and W. J. Darby. 1966. Growth and Sexual Development of Male Subjects in an Egyptian Oasis. *Am. J. Clin. Nutr.* 18: 421-425.

Dreosti, I. E., S. H. Tao, and L. S. Hurley. 1968. Plasma Zinc and Leukocyte Changes in Weanling and Pregnant Rats During Zinc Deficiency. *Proc. Soc. Exptl. Biol. Med.* 128: 169.

Eggleton, W. G. E. 1940. The Zinc and Copper Content of Blood in Beriberi, in Conditions Associated with Protein Deficiency and in Diabetes Mellitus. *Chinese J. Physiol.* 15: 33.

Engel, R. W., R. F. Miller, and N. O. Price. 1966. Metabolic Patterns in Preadolescent Children: XIII. Zinc Balance. In *Zinc Metabolism,* compiled and edited by A. S. Prasad, Springfield, Ill.: Charles C. Thomas, p. 326.

Fujioka, M., and I. Lieberman. 1964. A Zn^{++} Requirement for Synthesis of Deoxyribonucleic Acid by Rat Liver. *J. Biol. Chem.* 239: 1164.

Hsu, J. M., W. L. Anthony, and P. J. Buchanan. 1969. Zinc Deficiency and Incorporation of ^{14}C-Labeled Methionine into Tissue Proteins in Rats. *J. Nutr.* 99: 425.

Hurley, L. S. Zinc Deficiency in the Developing Rat. *Am. J. Clin. Nutr.* 22: 1332.

Husain, S. L. 1969. Oral Zinc Sulfate in Leg Ulcers. *Lancet* 1: 1069.

Kessler, B., and S. P. Monselise. 1959. Studies on Ribonuclease, Ribonucleic Acid and Protein Synthesis in Healthy and Zinc-Deficient Citrus Leaves. *Physiologia* Pl. 12: 1.

Legg, S. P., and L. Sears. 1960. Zinc Sulfate Treatment of Parakeratosis in Cattle. *Nature* 186: 1061.

Lema, O., and H. H. Sandstead. 1970. Zinc Deficiency: Effect on Epiphyseal Growth. *Clin. Res.* 18: 458.

Lemann, I. I. 1910. A Study of the Type of Infantilism in Hookworm Disease. *Arch. Internal Med.* 6: 139.

Lieberman, I., R. Abrams, N. Hunt, and P. Ove. 1963. Levels of Enzyme Activity and Deoxyribonucleic Acid Synthesis in Mammalian Cells Cultured from the Animal. *J. Biol. Chem.* 238: 3955.

Macapinlac, M. P., G. H. Barney, W. N. Pearson, and W. J. Darby. 1967. Production of Zinc Deficiency in the Squirrel Monkey (Saimiri sciureus). *J. Nutr.* 93: 499.

Macapinlac, M. P., W. N. Pearson, G. H. Barney, and W. J. Darby. 1968. Protein and Nucleic Acid Metabolism in the Testis of Zinc-Deficient Rats. *J. Nutr.* 95: 569.

Maze, P. 1914. Influences Respective Des Eliments De La Solution Minerale sur Le Developpement Du Mais. *Ann. Inst. Pasteur* 28: 21.

Mills, C. F. 1964. Metabolic Interrelationships in the Utilization of Trace Elements. *Proc. Nutr. Soc. Engl. Scot.* 23: 38.

Mills, C. F., J. Quarterman, J. C. Chesters, W. B. Williams, and A. C. Dalgarno. 1969. Metabolic Role of Zinc. *Am. J. Clin. Nutr.* 22: 1240.

Minnich, V. A., A. Okçuoğlu, Y. Tarcon, A. Arcasoy, S. Cin, O. Yörükoğlo, F. Renda, and B. Demirağ. 1968. Pica in Turkey. II. Effect of Clay upon Iron Absorption. *Am. J. Clin. Nutr.* 21: 78.

Nocht, B. and M. Mayer. 1937. *Malaria.* London: *John Bale Medical Publ.* p. 21.

O'Dell, B. L. 1969. Effect of Dietary Components upon Zinc Availability: A Review with Original Data. *Am. J. Clin. Nutr.* 22: 1315.

O'Dell, B. L., P. M. Newberne, and J. E. Savage. 1958. Significance of Dietary Zinc for the Growing Chick. *J. Nutr.* 65: 503.

Ohtaka, Y., K. Uchida, and T. Sakai. 1963. Purification and Properties of Ribonuclease from Yeast. *J. Biochem.* (Tokyo) 54: 322.

Parisi, A. F., and B. L. Vallee. Zinc Metaloenzymes: Characteristics and Significance in Biology and Medicine. *Am. J. Clin. Nutr.* 22: 1222.

Pories, W. H., J. H. Henzel, C. G. Rob, and W. H. Strain. 1967. Acceleration of Healing with Zinc Sulfate. *Ann. Surg.* 165: 432.

Prasad, A. S., J. A. Halsted, and M. Nadimi. 1961. The Syndrome of Iron Deficiency Anemia, Hepatosplenomegaly, Hypogonadism, Dwarfism and Geophagia. *Am. J. Med.* 31: 532.

Prasad, A. S., A. R. Schulert, A. Miale Jr., Z. Farid, and H. H. Sandstead. 1963a. Zinc and Iron Deficiency in Male Subjects with Dwarfism and Hypogonadism but without Ancylostomiasis, Schistosomiasis or Severe Anemia. *Am. J. Clin. Nutr.* 12: 437.

———. 1963b. Zinc, Iron and Nitrogen Content of Sweat in Normal and Deficient Subjects. *J. Lab. Clin. Med.* 62: 84.

———. 1963c. Zinc Metabolism in Patients with the Syndrome of Iron Deficiency Anemia, Hepatosplenomegaly, Dwarfism, and Hypogonadism. *J. Lab. Clin. Med.* 61: 537.

Prasad, A. S., H. H. Sandstead, A. R. Schulert, and A. S. El Rooby. Technical Assistance of Richard P. Koshakji. 1963d. Urinary Excretion of Zinc in Patients with the Syndrome of Anemia, Hepatosplenomegaly, Dwarfism, and Hypogonadism. *J. Lab. Clin. Med.* 62: 591.

Prasad, A. S., A. Miale, Jr., Z. Farid, H. H. Sandstead, A. R. Schulert, and W. J. Darby. 1963e. Biochemical Studies on Dwarfism, Hypogonadism and Anemia. *Arch. Int. Med.,* 111: 407.

Prasad, A. S., D. Oberleas, P. Wolf, and J. P. Horwitz. 1967. Studies on Zinc Deficiency: Changes in Trace Elements and Enzyme Activities in Tissue of Zinc-Deficient Rats. *J. Clin. Invest.* 46: 549.

Raulin, J. 1869. Etudes cliniques sur la vegetation. *Ana Sci. Nat'l. Botan. Biol.* Ser. 5, 11:93.

Reinhold, J. G. Unpublished Observations.

Reinhold, J. G. and G. A. Kfoury. 1969. Zinc-Dependent Enzymes in Zinc-Depleted Rats; Intestinal Alkaline Phosphatase. *Am. J. Clin. Nutr.* 22: 1250.

Ronaghy, H. A., R. Barakat, A. S. Prasad, J. G. Reinhold, M. Haghshenas, P. Abadee, and J. A. Halsted. 1970. A Preliminary Report on Zinc Supplementation. *Pahlavi University Med. J.,* in press.

Ronaghy, H., M. R. Spivey Fox, S. N. Garn, H. Israel, A. Harp, P. G. Moe, and J. A. Halsted. 1969. Controlled Zinc Supplementation for Malnourished School Boys. *Am. J. Clin. Nutr.* 22: 1279.

Sandstead, H. H. Unpublished Observations.

Sandstead, H. H., and S. R. Glasser. 1969. Fetal Growth and ^{65}Zinc Uptake in Zinc Deficient Rats. *Clin. Res.* 17: 549.

Sandstead, H. H., V. C. Lanier, G. H. Shepard, and D. D. Gillespie. 1970. Zinc and Wound Healing: Effects of Zinc Deficiency and Zinc Supplementation. *Am. J. Clin. Nutr.* 23: 514.

Sandstead, H. H., A. S. Prasad, A. R. Schulert, Z. Farid, A. Miale, Jr., S. Bassilly, and W. J. Darby. 1967. Human Zinc Deficiency, Endocrine Manifestations and Response to Treatment. *Am. J. Clin. Nutr.* 20: 422.

Sandstead, H. H., and R. A. Rinaldi. 1969. Impairment of Deoxyribonucleic Acid Synthesis by Dietary Zinc Deficiency in the Rat. *J. Cell Physiol.* 73: 81.

Sandstead, H. H., S. Shukry, A. S. Prasad, M. K. Gabr, A. El Hifney, N. Mokhtar, and W. J. Darby. 1965. Kwashiorkor in Egypt. I. Clinical and Biochemical Studies with Special Reference to Plasma Zinc and Serum Lactic Dehydrogenase. *Am. J. Clin. Nutr.* 17: 15.

Sarram, M., M. Younessi, P. Khorvash, G. A. Kfoury, and J. G. Reinhold. 1969. Zinc Nutrition in Human Pregnancy in Fars Province, Iran. Significance of Geographic and Socioeconomic Factors. *Am. J. Clin. Nutr.* 22: 726.

Schneider, E., and C. A. Price. 1962. Decreased Ribonucleic Acid Levels: A Possible Cause of Growth Inhibition in Zinc Deficiency. *Biochem. Biophys. Acta* 55: 406.

Somers, M., and E. J. Underwood. 1969. Ribonuclease Activity and Nucleic Acid and Protein Metabolism in the Testis of Zinc-Deficient Rats. *Aust. J. Biol. Sci.* 22: 1277.

Somner, A. L., and C. B. Lipman. 1926. Evidence on the Indispensable Nature of Zinc and Boron for Higher Green Plants. *Plant Physiol.* 1: 231.

Spivey Fox, M. R., and B. N. Harrison. 1966. Zinc Deficiency and Plasma Proteins. In *Zinc Metabolism,* compiled and edited by A. S. Prasad. Springfield, Illinois: Charles C. Thomas, p. 187.

Swenerton, H., R. Schrader, and L. S. Hurley. 1969. Zinc-Deficiency Embryos: Reduced Thymidine Incorporation. *Science* 166: 1014.

Tal, M. 1969. Metal Ions and Ribosomal Conformation. *Biochem. Biophys. Acta* 195: 76.

Todd, W. R., C. A. Elvehjem, and E. B. Hart. 1934. Zinc in the Nutrition of the Rat. *Am. J. Physiol.* 107: 146.

Tribble, H. M., and F. I. Scoular. 1954. Zinc Metabolism of Young College Women on Self-Selected Diets. *J. Nutr.* 52: 209.

Tucker, H. F., and W. D. Salmon. 1955. Parakeratosis or Zinc Deficiency Disease in the Pig. *Proc. Soc. Exptl. Biol. Med.* 88: 613.

Vallee, B. L., W. E. C. Wacker, A. F. Bartholomay, and F. L. Hoch. 1959. Zinc Metabolism in Hepatic Dysfunction. *Ann. Int. Med.* 50: 1077.

Wacker, W. E. C. 1962. Nucleic Acids and Metals. III. Changes in Nucleic Acids, Proteins, and Metal Content as a Consequence of Zinc Deficiency in *Euglen gracilis*. *Biochemistry* 1: 859.

Winder, F. and J. M. Denneny. 1959. Effect of Iron and Zinc on Nucleic Acid and Protein Synthesis in *Mycobacterium smegmatis*. *Nature* 184: 742.

8 PROTEIN-CALORIE DEFICIENCY DISEASE

The syndrome which is commonly known as kwashiorkor was described by Cicely Williams from the Gold Coast (now Ghana) in 1933. The clinical features were: "oedema chiefly of hands and feet, wasting, diarrhea, irritability, sores chiefly of the mucous membranes and desquamation of areas of skin in a constant and unique manner." Williams noted that infants and young children between 1 and 4 years of age suffered from the disease, the onset of which was preceded by a history of abnormal dietary. Breast-feeding was inadequate, and supplementary food consisted of preparations made from fermented maize dough. Williams found that dietetic treatment effected a cure. In view of the poor dietary history and response to dietetic treatment, she considered the syndrome to result from dietary deficiency. The term kwashiorkor first used for the syndrome by Williams (1935) was the local name in Ghana "for the disease that the deposed baby gets when the next one is born." In this latter publication reporting on 60 cases of kwashiorkor, Williams found the age range of patients wider than in her original report. Her youngest patient was 9 weeks and the oldest 5 years of age; the majority were between 6 months and 4 years.

The syndrome described by Williams came gradually to be recognized as the commonest form of severe infant and child malnutrition seen in a large number of developing countries. Knowledge about its distribution, clinical features, pathology, biochemistry, and treatment, which accumulated in the next twenty years after the original report of Williams, contributed to an improved understanding of its etiology and pathogenesis. It is recognized that the syndrome had earlier been recorded from many areas and under a variety of terms. This has been ably summarized by Trowell, Davis, and Dean in their book entitled *Kwashiorkor* (1954).

The global importance of the disease came to be recognized largely as a result of the interest of the World Health Organization and the Food and Agriculture Organization of the United Nations from the year 1950 and the number of studies promoted and supported by them. The predominant role of protein deficiency in the development and occurrence of the syndrome was recognized as a result of enquiries into the dietary history, biochemical studies, and therapeutic effects of diets containing insufficient protein of high biological value. It soon became clear that unsatisfactory feeding of infants involved inadequacy of calories as well as of protein in quality and quantity. Whereas sometimes calorie intake was disproportionally large in relation to the insufficient intake of protein, in other situations protein and calories were both inadequate and there were stages in between. Depending upon these differences in diets, how early in life defective diets were started, and the occurrence and the nature of infectious diseases, especially diarrheal disease, a final clinical picture emerged. It ranged from kwashiorkor at one end to nutritional marasmus characterized by emaciation on the other, with intermediate stages in between. Professor J. F. Brock of Cape Town was the first to suggest that this was a spectrum of the same syndrome. Jelliffe (1959) later gave it the name "protein-calorie-malnutrition." Accepting the concept and realizing that the deficiency of calories in varying degrees accompanying the deficiency of protein resulted in the range of clinical pictures constituting the spectrum, the 6th Joint FAO/WHO Expert Committee on Nutrition (1962) gave the generic classification as protein-calorie-deficiencies under which were included: (a) kwashiorkor (including marasmic kwashiorkor); and (b) marasmus (e.g., athrepsia, cachexia, extreme wasting). The two together became the protein-calorie-deficiency disease. This term with its subclasses is used in the following discussion.

The clinical features of kwashiorkor are as follows:

The child is small for his age. The weight is usually about 60% or even less than that expected for his age. The height too is less—but not to the same extent. Edema is always present; it may be restricted to lower extremities, or it may be generalized. Hair is usually discolored, brittle, easily pluckable, and sparse. Hyperpigmented desquamating lesions may be present, usually on the legs, thighs, perineum, and over other parts of the body. Liver is often enlarged.

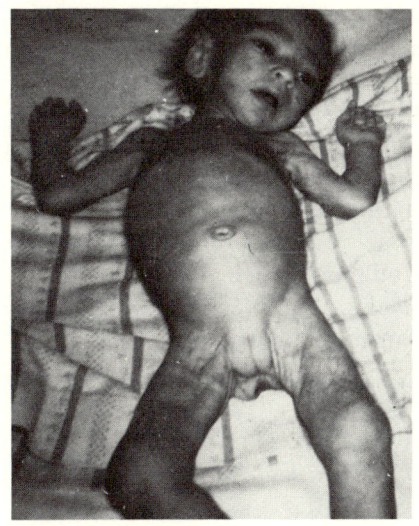 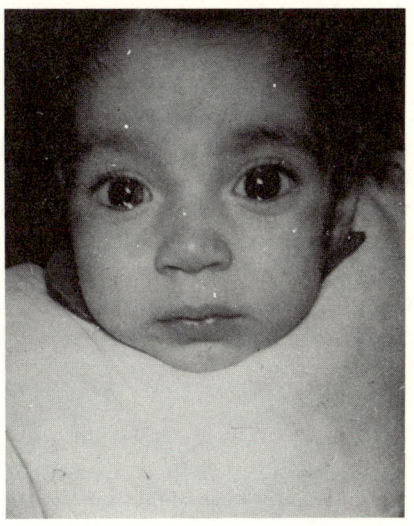

Plate 8.1. A case of marasmic kwashior-kor on admission.

At discharge from the hospital.

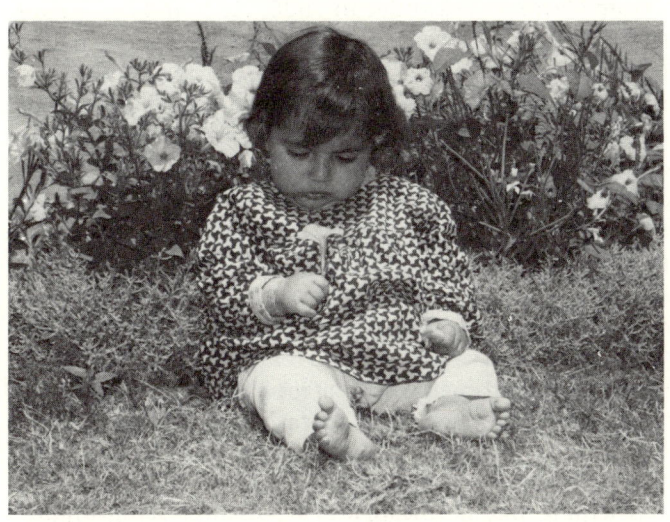

After sixteen months at home following discharge.

Mental apathy and peevishness are invariably seen. Signs of associated vitamin deficiencies are not uncommon.

In marasmus, growth failure is more evident than in kwashiorkor. Emaciation may be extreme. The skin loses its turgor and elasticity. Subcutaneous fat is practically absent, and the skin is thrown into folds. Diarrhea is often present. There is no edema; there are no changes in hair and no dermal lesions. Liver is not enlarged. The child is apathetic but irritable.

An intermediate stage in which edema, dyschromotrichia, and dermatosis are superimposed on a background of emaciation is also encountered not infrequently. It is usually described as marasmic kwashiorkor.

EGYPT

Recognition of Kwashiorkor as a Nutritional Disorder

The occurrence of protein-calorie-deficiency disease among Egyptian infants and children was but slowly recognized. At about the same time, however, it attracted the attention of physicians in other developing countries, mainly because of the efforts of the two specialized United Nations Agencies, WHO and FAO. A condition not unlike it was described from Cairo by Iskander in 1935. He found in 10 children between 20 to 36 months in age the condition which he called "post dysenteric oedema in children." In these cases the average total serum protein was 4.29 g per 100 ml. He excluded on clinical grounds other causes of edema, such as nephritis and pyelitis. His observation that edema disappeared and serum proteins increased on hospital diet is revealing. The author, however, missed the significance of this phenomenon and failed to recognize the primary role of malnutrition in the condition which he was studying. Abboud (1937), while discussing the cause of "dystrophies in infants," considered underfeeding as an important cause. He further referred to the prolonged periods of absolute or relative starvation in the treatment of gastrointestinal disturbances as contributing to the dystrophy. Abboud studied 8 cases, 4 of which were due to unspecified dietetic errors alone, 3 with chronic infections, and 1 of coeliac disease. Shukry, Mahdi, and Gholmy (1938) published also from Cairo an account of 18 cases of edema in children which, in the absence of cardiac or renal abnormalities, they attributed to malnutrition. Sixteen out of the eighteen cases were between 1-1/2 and 3 years in age. Like Abboud, Shukry *et al.* also found prolonged dietary restriction during the attacks of diarrhea and in convalescence preceding the appearance of edema. Total serum protein and serum albumin were reduced in almost all cases.

Hanafy (1947) was the first to describe the syndrome from Alexandria. Under the appropriate title "The Subacute Subnutritional Syndrome in Infants" he reported a series of 197 cases of malnutrition in children, 90% of whom were between 1 and 3 years of age. In addition to describing the various manifestations of protein-calorie deficiency as we know them today, he drew attention to a high incidence of signs attributable to the deficiencies of riboflavin and vitamin A. He also found rickets associated with a condition in which growth failure or arrest was a characteristic feature. Hanafy's description reminds one of the "syndrome pluricarencial" of Latin America, the basis of which is, of course, protein-calorie deficiency.

Hanafy found that a high protein diet with various vitamin supplements was effective in treatment. The information which he obtained on the past medical history of his cases and his observations on the associated infections led him to recognize a role of chronic diarrhea and of measles against a background of inadequate child-feeding practices as important factors contributing to the condition.

Badr el Din (1964) described cases of infantile wasting which comprised, according to him, 16.5% of total admissions to the University Hospital for Sick Children in Alexandria. Underfeeding and inappropriate feeding were the principal causes for the condition. Wishahy (1958) from Cairo analyzed 30 cases of "pellagra"[1] in infants and children. He devotes considerable attention to dermal lesions, lesions of the mouth and tongue, and nervous manifestations, but not to much else. The ages of the patients are not stated, nor is there mention of the treatment given and its results. Wishahy referred to the occurrence of parotid enlargement in his cases and rightly believes that he was dealing with a multiple-deficiency syndrome. It is probable that most, if not all, of these cases were suffering from protein-calorie deficiency.

Paucity of Information on Prevalence

In 1959, Nabawy reviewed the studies on kwashiorkor in Egypt. He stated that in 1957-58, marasmus and nutritional edema cases formed 15.4% of total pediatric admissions in the Mounira Children's Hospital. Awwaad, Eissa, and Attia (1961) reported that during the five years 1948-52 a yearly average of 9,081 "marasmic" infants

1. The term infantile pellagra was widely used in referring to protein-calorie malnutrition during the 1950s. This arose from the presence of skin lesions and of diarrhea, but the term should not be interpreted to indicate any necessary relationship to true pellagra that results from a deficiency of niacin.

attended the Outpatients Department of the Mounira Children's Hospital in Cairo. In the same period an average of 222 infants annually were in-patients at the hospital; of these 146 cases were of marasmus, and 37 were of nutritional edema. Sheikh (1962) reports on 62 cases of post-diarrheic edema; 44 children were underweight and showed signs of malnutrition such as rickets and "deficiency of vitamin B group" (signs and symptoms for this latter not mentioned). Sheikh believes that these were not cases of kwashiorkor.

Evidently interest in protein-calorie malnutrition must have been great among the pediatricians in recent years, for meetings of a special section on Nutritional and Gastrointestinal Disorders were held at the First Regional Middle East and Eastern Mediterranean Pediatric Conference convened in Cairo in March 1960. This interest has continued unabated to date, and much information is available on the protein-calorie-deficiency disease as it occurs in Egypt. This information is derived mainly from reports from the Pediatrics Departments of Cairo and Ein Shams Medical Faculties and of Alexandria University Medical Faculty. A search of the published and unpublished information reveals that more than 700 cases have been studied from different angles and reported upon by investigators mainly in Cairo and Alexandria teaching hospitals. NAMRU-3 in Cairo participated in some of these studies, and its staff is continuing an active interest and participation in further investigations organized in collaboration with Professor Gholmy and his colleagues in the Pediatrics Department of the Ein Shams University Medical Faculty in Cairo. On the other hand, information on protein-calorie-deficiency disease from Upper Egypt is practically nonexistent.

Recent Investigations

The etiology and course of the protein-calorie-deficiency disease in Egypt (as also in the neighboring Arab countries) is similar in general to that obtaining in most developing countries of the world. Growth retardation commencing at 5 or 6 months after birth; inadequate, unsatisfactory, and unhygienic infant feeding practices (Hanafy 1947; Badr el Din, 1954; Gholmy 1960; Abdou *et al.*, 1964; Carter *et al.*, 1968); gastrointestinal disturbances, measles, and respiratory infections as a precipitating cause (Iskandar, 1935; Sandstead *et al.*, 1965; Carter *et al.*, 1968), and prolonged food restriction during convalescence from the frequent illnesses are among the characteristic phenomena which have been observed in Egypt as well as in other countries in which protein-calorie-deficiency disease occurs.

It is the infants and preschool age children who suffer most, as

Protein-Calorie Malnutrition

usual. More than 90% of 197 cases reported by Hanafy were between 1 and 3 years of age; Gholmy et al. (1960) have reported cases of protein-calorie-deficiency disease, most of whom were between 4 months and 3-1/2 years of age. The cases studied by Sandstead et al. (1965) were between 1 and 3 years of age, and of 105 cases in the series of Carter et al. (1969) all but 2 ranged between 6 months and 3 years in age. There does not seem to be any appreciable difference in sex incidence, boys and girls being affected with almost equal frequency.

Clinical Features of Kwashiorkor in Egypt

Awwaad (1961) has given a good clinical description of kwashiorkor as seen in Cairo, based on his experience of 200 cases. Since this is in general the experience of other investigators in Egypt, it will be worth while to give a brief description of Awwaad's observations.

The cases were derived mostly from the poorer sections of the community, 96% being from families in which the income per head per month was two L.Eg. or less. The incidence of kwashiorkor was found to reach a peak in the summer months of the year; only a small number of cases occurred in winter. Children under three years formed 99% of Awwaad's cases. All 39 cases described by Sandstead et al. (1965) were between 1 and 3 years of age. Our own recent experience is similar, as Table 1 will show.

There was little difference in sex incidence, boys and girls within the susceptible ages being equally affected.

Retarded growth was found in all cases, the patients being underweight by 20 to 40% in spite of edema. Lengths were 1/2 to 1-1/2 inches below the expected length for age.

Since these were cases of kwashiorkor and included also marasmic kwashiorkor as defined in Egypt, edema was present in all. In moderate cases it was confined to dorsa of the feet, legs, hands, and arms. In

TABLE 1
AGE INCIDENCE OF KWASHIORKOR IN EGYPT

Age	Awwaad (1961) 200 Cases	Carter et al. (Unpublished) 105 Cases
	%	%
6 months	1	5
6–12 months	12	14
13–24 months	70	56
25–36 months	16	23
37–48 months	1	1
49–60 months		1

more severe cases genitalia, abdomen, and face were involved, together with both the extremities. Only one of Awwaad's cases showed ascites. Awwaad classified his cases as mild, moderate, and severe, mainly on the degree of edema. Skin lesions were found in 90% of the severe, 60% of the moderate, and 5% of the mild cases. The lesions started in the napkin area and spread to buttocks, thighs, and legs. Usually the lesion was of the variety described as crazy-pavement dermatosis. Hair changes consisted of sparseness, lack of luster, easy pluckability, and dyspigmentation and were seen in almost all cases.

In 18% of Awwaad's cases lesions of the mucous membrane occurred chiefly as redness of oral mucosa, atrophy of mucosa of the tongue, and fissuring at the angles of the mouth and the lower lips. The occurrence of norma has not been reported from Egypt.

Liver was enlarged one to two fingers below costal margin in 62% and more in 8% of cases. Absence of liver enlargement was found in severely wasted cases. Spleen was enlarged in only 5% of cases.

Anemia occurred in almost all cases. The hematological status of the patients did not return to normal on high protein diet and control of infections, suggesting the coexistence of associated deficiency of hemopoietic factors. Rickets was found in 3% of the cases. The lesions of the mucous membrane mentioned already were probably the sign of ariboflavinosis. No other nutritional deficiency as associated with kwashiorkor has been recorded by Awwaad.

The above description, which can be considered fairly typical, will show that if marasmus is excluded the clinical features of kwashiorkor seem to be similar to those described from other countries. There may be minor differences in some aspects, such as age incidence, and frequency of liver enlargement, of skin lesions, and of the associated deficiencies; but these do not indicate any definite trends.

It is difficult to form an opinion on the relative frequency of marasmus and kwashiorkor in Egypt. Hospital records are unreliable guides in this respect, and the reports of special investigations are more so because of a bias in the selection of cases depending upon the particular interest of the investigator and the need of the specific aspect under study. It would appear from the analysis of a 5-year record of admissions to the Mounira Children's Hospital that the proportion of marasmus to kwashiorkor would be 4 : 1. On the other hand, in the cases of Gholmy (1960), this ratio was a little less than 2 : 1. A survey on a randomly selected population group would be the only method of obtaining reasonably correct information on this aspect. Before making such a survey, however, it will be advisable to define the criteria for marasmus. An infant with wasting and no edema is usually classified as marasmic, even in the absence of other clinical features characteristic of this condition. It should be simpler, however, if one adopts the classification suggested by Gomez, Galvan, Cravioto, and Frenk (1955), which is based on the deviation of the actual from the expected body weight for a given age as a mean of classifying the protein-calorie-deficiency disease with the presence or absence of edema noted.[2] In this way much uncertainty about the meaning of the word marasmus, confusion about its interpretations, and controversy about frequency will be avoided.

The usually accepted signs and symptoms of protein-calorie-deficiency disease are found in Egyptian cases with varying frequency. Growth failure resulting in an underweight and undersized child is a feature of every case. Dyspigmented, sparse, and easily pluckable hair; dermatosis in the regions of perineum, groin, axialla, lower abdomen, and extremities; edema of varying severity and extent; enlarged liver, apathy, and irritability are found in the majority of cases. The occurrence and frequency of signs and symptoms of protein-calorie-deficiency disease in Egypt do not indicate that it differs there from that occurring in other parts of the world.

The nomenclature recently used by the investigators in Egypt is kwashiorkor for cases with edema, marasmus for cases of emaciation without edema, and marasmic kwashiorkor to include cases which are emaciated and also have edema. In this they accept the concept that marasmus and kwashiorkor are but two ends of a continuous spectrum of the syndrome of protein-calorie-deficiency disease.

Marasmus

Unlike kwashiorkor, there are comparatively few detailed studies on marasmus, although the number of marasmus cases in children's hospitals outnumber those with kwashiorkor by at least 2 : 1 if not more. Awwaad, Eissa, and Attia (1961) studied 20 cases of marasmus aged 4 months to 2 years mainly for serum proteins, so the authors

---

2. Gomez *et al.* classify malnutrition in three degrees as follows:

Degree of Malnutrition	Deviation of actual body weight from average theoretical body weight for age in per cent.
1st	10 to 25
2nd	25 to 40
3rd	over 40

give no clinical details except to say that they were cases of "third degree" marasmus, that they had no skin and ear infections, and that their chests and hearts were free of signs of disease. Liver was palpable one finger below the costal margin in 3; in the rest it was not palpable. Our own studies on marasmus are limited. It must be admitted, however, that owing to the greater frequency with which marasmus occurs in Egyptian infants as compared to kwashiorkor, the condition is of considerable importance and deserves more detailed attention than has been bestowed on it so far.

Before the Egyptian physicians classified their cases into kwashiorkor, marasmic kwashiorkor and marasmus, the description of nutritional dystrophies or infantile malnutrition included cases of all three types and the clinical and biochemical data given were usually lumped together. This makes the task of describing nutritional marasmus in Egypt extremely difficult.

Biochemical Investigations

Awwaad et al. (1961) found the following values for serum proteins in 22 cases of marasmus: total protein, 5.66 g per 100 ml with a range of 4.7 to 6.5 g, and serum albumin, mean 3.51 g per 100 ml with a range of 2.26 to 4.37 g. They also found blood amino acid N elevated with a mean of 11.9 mg per 100 ml (range 10.0–13.7 mg) as compared with 6 to 8 mg per 100 ml, which Awwaad and Eissa (1959) had found in normal children of comparable age. Our own values for serum proteins in 13 marasmus cases ranged between 4.0 and 8.6 g for total protein and between 1.3 and 5.4 g for serum albumin, with the averages of 6.6 and 3.7 respectively. Similarly, Gholmy et al. (1962) found in 12 cases of marasmus the average total serum protein 5.47 g per 100 ml and serum albumin 2.18 g per 100 ml, whereas in the same series the corresponding values for kwashiorkor were 3.61 and 1.06 g per 100 ml respectively.

The values for total serum proteins and their fractions in protein-calorie-deficiency disease (including kwashiorkor and marasmus) reported by several workers have been summarized in Table 2. Similar determinations made on apparently healthy children of comparable age reported by several of these workers are given in Table 3 for comparison. The serum albumin values were considerably lower in kwashiorkor, as is to be expected. In the two sets of comparable observations which record values after "clinical recovery" or "clinical cure," serum albumin had risen markedly but was still below the reported normal for Egyptian children. In this connection it may be noted that the value of 3.32 g per 100 ml reported by Gholmy et al. in

TABLE 2
SERUM PROTEINS AND FRACTIONS IN EGYPTIAN CHILDREN WITH KWASHIORKOR

Reference	No. of Cases	Total Protein g/100 ml	Serum Protein Fractions g/100 ml							
			Albumin	Globulins						
				α_1	α_2	β	γ	Total		
Nabawy (1959)	24	4.0	1.6							
Awwaad & Abdel-Wahab (1960)	47	4.99	1.86	0.25	0.56	0.41	1.34	2.56		
Gholmy et al. (1960)	19	3.92	1.42	0.40	0.50	0.60	1.10	2.60	On admission	
		6.80	3.08	0.60	0.78	0.91	1.56	3.85	After treatment	
Ismail et al. (1960)	55	5.35	2.12	0.45	0.67	0.67	1.26	3.05		
Shehata et al. (1966)	12	4.22	1.46	0.47	0.57	0.71	1.02	2.77		
Sandstead et al. (1965)	39	4.12	1.17	0.35	0.58	0.53	1.49	2.95	On admission	
	10	7.20	3.92	0.28	0.72	0.76	1.51	3.27	After treatment	

TABLE 3
SERUM PROTEINS AND FRACTIONS IN HEALTHY EGYPTIAN CHILDREN OF 1 TO 4 YEARS

Reference	No. of Cases	Total Protein g/100 ml	Serum Protein Fractions g/100 ml						
			Albumin	Globulins					
				α_1	α_2	β	γ	Total	
Awwaad & Abdel-Wahab (1960)	13	7.37	4.37	0.25	0.88	0.70	1.17	3.00	1–3 years
Gholmy et al. (1960)	10	7.17	3.32	0.51	0.67	0.83	1.84	3.85	
Ismail et al. (1960)	31	7.38	4.66	0.42	0.62	0.62	0.91	2.57	
Shehata et al. (1966)	10	7.29	4.84	0.33	0.63	0.61	0.86	2.43	1–4 years
Sandstead et al. (1965)	19	7.50	4.77	0.24	0.62	0.67	1.13	2.66	1–3 years

10 healthy children is markedly lower than those reported by all other observers. Furthermore, the average value for γ-globulin reported by Gholmy et al. is much higher than the other reported values.

There are a few other observations on other blood or serum constituents in kwashiorkor and marasmus, the most comprehensive being those published by Sandstead et al. Gholmy and his group have been active in this field as well. It was considered desirable for the sake of completeness to summarize most of the reported values in a single table (Table 4). Those dealing with serum iron, TIBC, and serum copper will be described when discussing the anemias associated with kwashiorkor.

It will be clear from the table that most of the observed blood and serum constituents show a slight to a marked fall in the stage of active disease and that they tend to return to the normal levels on "clinical cure." Zinc in serum stands out in this respect. According to Sandstead et al., it was still much lower at "clinical cure" than the normal observed values. It is interesting to note that the serum albumin levels of their patients at the "clinical cure" stage had also not reached the normal value. It is obvious that at this stage the cure was not complete in the sense that the composition of tissues had not fully returned to normal during the comparatively brief period over which the observations were made.

With regard to the serum enzymes such as LDH, SGOT, and SGPT the values were higher in the active stage of the disease, indicating some derangement in liver function. The values tended to return to normal when liver responded to treatment. The lower values of serum alkaline phosphatase could be ascribed to the arrest of bone growth contributing to growth failure, which is characteristic of protein-calorie-deficiency disease.

The findings of Sandstead et al. (1965) on the reduction of activity of the above-mentioned enzymes in serum is in keeping with several observations on other serum enzymes in kwashiorkor in different parts of the world. These have been summarized by Waterlow (1960). Choline esterase, esterase, lipase, amylase, alkaline phosphatase in serum were all reduced in activity in malnourished infants. A 200- to 300-percent increase in activity resulted on treatment. According to Waterlow, the lowering of enzyme activity in protein-calorie deficiency is a reflection of the depression of protein synthesis in the body, which is a common factor in this condition.

Eissa et al. (1967a) have confirmed the oft-repeated observation that in protein-calorie-malnutrition fasting, blood glucose level is

TABLE 4
SOME BLOOD CONSTITUENTS AND SERUM ENZYMES IN PROTEIN-CALORIE-DEFICIENCY DISEASE AS OBSERVED IN EGYPT

Particulars	On Admission	"Clinical Cure"	Control Normal	Reference
Plasma zinc µg/100 ml	37 42 ± 14.5	8 68 ± 15.5	9 89 ± 6.0	Sandstead et al. (1965)
Plasma magnesium mEq/L	10 1.63 ± 0.35	5 1.92 ± 0.245	10 1.77 ± 0.34	Sandstead et al. (1965)
Serum calcium mg/100 ml	33 7.4 ± 1.35	9 9.8 ± 0.85	13 10.8 ± 0.80	Sandstead et al. (1965)
Blood Glutathione mg/100 ml	16 9.8	8 22.5	21 24.4	Gholmy et al. (1960)
Blood sugar mg/100 ml	34 51	11[1] 68		Carter et al. (1969)
Serum Inorg P mg/100 ml	39 2.8 ± 1.10	10 4.7 ± 1.10	—	Sandstead et al. (1965)
SGOT (Sigma Units)	37 36 ± 11.0	9 41 ± 16	12 23 ± 10	Sandstead et al. (1965)
SGOT Units/100 ml	15 12.6	10 9.6	17 10.0	Gholmy et al. (1960)
SGPT (Sigma Units)	38 22 ± 12.5	9 15 ± 6.5	12 9 ± 6	Sandstead et al. (1965)
Serum LDH (Sigma Units)	37 642 ± 197	10 510 ± 176	13 388 ± 90	Sandstead et al. (1965)
Alk. P-ase (Bodansky Units)	39 6.0 ± 1.95	10 9.9 ± 4.0	6 9.7 ± 2.4	Sandstead et al. (1965)

NOTE: The first row of figures represents the number of patients examined, the second row the mean ±1 standard deviation.
1. On disappearance of edema.

lower than normal. They also found that the levels of α-ketoacids in blood (both pyruvic and α-ketoglutaric acid) were increased. All these values returned to normal on recovery. Eissa *et al.* (1967b) further reported that the intravenous glucose tolerance in kwashiorkor was impaired, as compared to that in healthy children of comparable age. Carter *et al.* (1968) reported a more severe impairment in intravenous glucose tolerance in kwashiorkor. Glucose utilization returned to normal on treatment with protein-rich diets.

Shehata *et al.* (1964) determined by single-dimensional paper chromatography 6 nonessential and 4 essential amino acids in serum of 12 kwashiorkor cases and of 10 normal children. They observed a marked reduction in leucine and valine, less so in lysine; on the other hand threonine showed a 50% increase over the normal. This last finding is not in line with those reported in a careful study by Holt, Snyderman, Norton, Roitman, and Finch (1968) on plasma specimens from 64 kwashiorkor cases obtained from 9 different countries. These authors found a decrease in all the essential acids in plasma; the degree of reduction depended upon the degree of severity of kwashiorkor. Furthermore they observed a more or less uniform alteration in the serum amino acid patterns, using their precise methods; their observations had included cases from Egypt as well.

Whitehead and Dean (1964) had observed that in protein-calorie-deficiency disease the serum concentration of essential amino acids was reduced much more than those of nonessential amino acids. Using simple single-dimensional paper chromatography, they found that the ratio of nonessential amino acids (glycine, serine, glutamine, and taurine) to essential amino acids (leucine, isoleucine, valine, and methionine) increased in protein-calorie-deficiency disease. According to them such ratios were between 3.5 and 8 in kwashiorkor; the ratios decreased with treatment and clinical improvement, approaching the values of 2 and below as observed by them for the serum of healthy children, African and European. In a study currently in progress at NAMRU-3, serum amino acid ratios were determined on admission in 19 cases of kwashiorkor and 9 cases of marasmus. Although the numbers are relatively small, the highest ratio that we observed was 8.0 for kwashiorkor and 2.4 for marasmus, the average values for the two groups being 3.65 and 1.3, respectively. It is puzzling why such high ratios as those recorded by Whitehead and Dean are comparatively rare in the Egyptian children with kwashiorkor. McLaren, Kamel, and Ayyoub (1965) have reported from Beirut, Lebanon, low serum amino ratios in kwashiorkor and marasmus. Furthermore, in a field study in which they determined the serum amino acid ratios in 260 infants and children mainly from Jordan, they concluded that ratios between 2.1 and 4.0 did not correlate with the weight deficit and would not be helpful in identifying potential cases of malnutrition, as Whitehead and Dean had suggested in their report.

It would be interesting to speculate on the reasons for this difference between the findings in Uganda on the one hand and Egypt and Lebanon on the other. Since the ratios will be influenced by the relative alterations in the concentrations of either the essential or the nonessential amino acids or both, a closer study of the actual amino acid concentrations under question will be worth-while. Relative differences in amino acid concentration could possibly be ascribed to the previous dietary history of the cases in the two situations. A satisfactory explanation must, however, await further study. On the other hand, the urinary hydroxyproline-creatinine index later developed by Whitehead (1965) seems to be reliably predictive of the degree of malnutrition in infants and young children. In our studies on kwashiorkor and marasmus patients, the hydroxyproline-creatinine index was correlated with the deficit in weight of the patient as compared with the expected weight for age with a correlation coefficient of 0.61 ± 0.14 (n = 49). This index has, in our hands, proved more reliable than the serum amino acid ratio as an indicator of malnutrition.

Liver

Observations on the enlarged liver in kwashiorkor have been reported upon by a few Egyptian workers. Alfi (1956) and Gholmy et al. (1960) obtained biopsy specimens from 50 and 58 cases respectively. On histological examination they found fatty change more marked in the periportal region than in the central zone. Alfi mentions that on clinical improvement fat receded from central and midzonal areas before it did so from the periportal area. Nabawy et al. (1964) have published a detailed histological and histochemical study of serial liver biopsies in 80 cases of kwashiorkor. Three biopsies were done on each case, the first on admission, the second after the edema had disappeared, and the third after a further period of three weeks. On first biopsy they found varying degrees of fatty infiltration, more in the periportal than in the central zone, with frequent pseudocyst formation owing to rupture and coalescence of fat-laden cells. Round cell infiltration in the portal tract was found in half the cases and in some a fibroblastic reaction in the same location. At the second biopsy fatty infiltration was less marked; in some cases fat had disappeared although the cells were still vacuolated. At the third biopsy, i.e., at the time of the estimated clinical cure, the liver looked normal in 90% of the cases. Thickening of the portal tract and residual inflammatory cells were found in some. The results of histochemical studies on biopsy material indicated marked reduction in RNA and DNA. Phospholipid and lipoprotein were also reduced. The cells contained a fair amount of glycogen. No stainable iron was found in parenchymal cells. On recovery these changes were reversed. The observations of Nabawy et al. (1964) that in three clinically cured cases fat in liver reappeared after an attack of colitis, although the nutritional state was not much disturbed, are worth noting.

In 18 post-mortem specimens of liver in kwashiorkor, Nabawy et al. (1964) found fatty infiltration of varying severity, mild fibrosis in three cases outlining the lobular pattern with no evidence of cellular regeneration. They also found no association between the atrophic changes in the exocrine portions of pancreas and fatty infiltration of the liver. It will be clear from the above description that the histopathology of liver in Egyptian kwashiorkor resembles that described from most other parts of the world with comparable response to treatment.

Other Tissues

Histopathological changes in other tissues in Egyptian cases of protein-calorie-deficiency disease include observations on skin and adrenals. Shukry, Safouh, Fayed, and Elwi (1963) examined seventeen surgically removed skin biopsies from kwashiorkor patients and ten scalp specimens obtained at post mortem. They found that hyperkeratosis and parakeratosis constituted the most important lesions of the corneal layer. In stratum granulosum abnormalities in the amount of pigment and its distribution were noted. There were no marked changes in the dermis apart from keratosis and cystic changes in hair follicles. The scalp showed loss of hair pigment, degeneration and fusion of hair sheaths, and cystic changes.

Shukry, Safouh, and Fayed (1964) examined the adrenal glands removed at autopsy from 14 cases of kwashiorkor. The glands were atrophic and showed histopathological changes. Diffuse or focal lipoid depletion was a constant feature. Mild hemorrhages in the cortical and medullary areas were occasionally seen. Cortical atrophy and necrosis, particularly in the zone fasciculata, were found in five cases. How far these changes were characteristic of protein-calorie-deficiency disease and to what extent they were modified by the associated infections was not certain.

Abbassy, Mikhail, Zeitoun, and Ragab (1967) studied the adrenocortical function in kwashiorkor. They found 17-hydroxycorticosteroids (17-OHCS) in plasma elevated; the mean value in 30 cases was 24.1 ± 7.15 µg/100 ml on admission. It decreased during treatment, and after 2 months a mean value of 11.64 ± 3.01 µg/100 ml was found in 14 cases. During the active stage of the disease the administration of ACTH had no effect on the plasma level of 17-OHCS, whereas after recovery it caused an increase of over 100%. Eosinophil count was low in kwashiorkor and was not responsive to ACTH; on recovery eosinophil count was high, and it was lowered on ACTH administration. The authors conclude from these observations that the adrenal gland, in response to the skin of malnutrition, increases its glucocorticoid secretion and functions at maximum capacity, returning to its normal state after recovery.

Associated Conditions

Awwaad (1961), unfortunately, does not describe in detail the associated conditions other than vitamin deficiencies. He, however, mentions that "in the majority of the cases enterocolitis either persists or becomes intermittent during the course of the disease." Sandstead *et al.* found diarrhea in 56%, broncho-pneumonia in 41%, and infections of the eye such as conjunctivitis, blepharitis, and trachoma in 5 to 10% of their cases. In our own experience (Carter *et al.*, 1968) a variety of associated infections, including those of gastrointestinal, respiratory and urinary tracts, and skin, have occurred in a majority of cases. Five of 62 cases had pulmonary tuberculosis, and one had *cancrum oris*. Such findings are indicative of the very low resistance to infection in kwashiorkor. Among the cases which had diarrhea, 12 were found to exhibit lactose intolerance which was transitory in that it responded to treatment. Bade el Din and Aboul Wafa (1960) had earlier demonstrated the presence of galactose intolerance in 10 kwashiorkor cases. They considered it responsible for intractable diarrhea in kwashiorkor. However they also recognized its transient nature.

Gabr, Abdel Salam, and Malek (1968) have studied lactose intolerance in marasmic infants. They compared the effect on blood sugar levels of lactose, glucose, and an equimolecular mixture of glucose and galactose given orally at the level of 2 g/kg. The tolerance curves were indicative of delayed absorption and impairment in utilization. In cases with diarrhea they found a greater delay in reaching the peak and return to fasting level after lactose than after glucose and galactose. On the other hand, in marasmic infants with no diarrhea, all three sugars behaved identically. Gabr *et al.* conclude that it is probably diarrhea per se rather than lactose deficiency that causes an impairment in the absorption of lactose. These observations do not explain the intolerance for galactose observed by Badr el Din and Aboul Wafa, as mentioned above. Furthermore, direct evidence on lactose deficiency would have been more appropriate. It may be stated here that Bowie, Barbezat, and Hansen (1967) have found such evidence in malnourished children in South Africa through disaccharidase assays in mucosal biopsies. Lactase, maltase, and sucrase all were found deficient.

The incidence of parasitic infestation in our series of 100 cases was found to be surprisingly small; *Giardia lamblia* occurred in 17 cases and Ascaris in one. *Entamoeba nana* occurred in 3, *Entamoeba coli* in 3, and *Trichomonas hominis* and *Chilomastix mesnili* in one case each. Sandstead *et al.* also found only 2 out of 39 cases harboring Ascaris or *Giardia lamblia*. This picture of comparative freedom from intestinal parasites, if confirmed by further observations, appears to be different from the experience reported in kwashiorkor from many other areas of the tropics and subtropics. This may partly be due to the fact that in Egypt most cases of protein-calorie-deficiency disease (PCDD) are below three years in age and the chances of intestinal parasitism in this age group are smaller as compared to the older age groups of PCDD cases in many other countries. For example, Gopalan (1956) had earlier observed that the incidence of Ascaris infection in cases of PCDD in Uganda was much less than in India. He also mentioned that in India a significantly high proportion of cases occurs in children above 3 years of age in contrast to the situation in Uganda, which is not unlike that in Egypt. Few other Egyptian investigators on PCDD provide information regarding this particular aspect, which is much to be regretted.

Treatment

The importance of high protein diet in the treatment of protein-calorie-deficiency disease has been recognized since Hanafy's (1947) observations on the "subacute subnutritional syndrome in infants." Fresh whole milk and reconstituted whole or skimmed milk have formed the sheet anchor of the dietary management in the early stages of hospitalization as advocated by various workers in Egypt. Hanafy (1951) found that fermented whole milk gave better results than reconstituted skim milk, half-cream cow milk, or buttermilk. Diluted buffalo milk, according to him, gave poor results. Nabawy

(1959) found that acidified half-cream milk fortified with casein to provide 3–5 g protein per kg body weight proved very successful. He also found that an unspecified vegetable oil homogenized with milk was well tolerated and mentions that from the second week onwards adequate calorie intake ought to be ensured so as to be between 100–150 Cal/kg/day. When the patient's appetite is restored under this initial treatment, other foods, about which the Egyptian investigators are usually vague when describing treatment, are added to the diet. Awwaad (1961) treated mild cases with high protein and low salt diets. For infants up to 8 months the diet was made up from a "dried protein milk," whereas for older patients mashed beans, sweet cheese, egg yolk, minced chicken and rice, and vegetables (both without added salt) were also given. This regimen is somewhat similar to that followed by Sandstead et al. (1965) in their study. Carter et al. (1968) have based the initiation of dietary treatment on reconstituted whole milk with added sucrose to provide between 3.5 to 5 g protein and 100–150 calories per kg body weight per day. As the appetite improves with the clinical improvement, and after edema disappears, they gradually introduce biscuits, bread, and local soft white cheese.

Although high protein diet has usually been stated to have been supplemented with multi-vitamin preparations, the quantities of these supplements and the duration for which they are given have not been specified. Blood transfusion (Badr el Din, 1954) and plasma transfusions (Awwaad, 1961) have also been given in severe cases. Awwaad found that with plasma transfusions in moderate and severe cases, the time of disappearance of edema was reduced by 3 to 5 days. Badr el Din, however, finds that weight gain in "infantile wasting" was no different in cases given dietary treatment alone or the same treatment with blood transfusions.

It is difficult to evaluate the efficacy of different treatments given or advocated in the absence of any set of objective criteria applied for their evaluation. We feel that it should not be difficult to define such criteria for this purpose. Investigators do not seem to have devoted sufficient attention to this aspect; perhaps they did not think it of sufficient importance.

Since a variety of infections is associated with protein-calorie-deficiency-disease cases admitted to hospitals, specific drug therapy of infections often accompanies dietary treatment. Apart from this, Badr el Din (1954) reports that in his cases of infantile wasting a daily oral supplement of 60 to 100 mg aureomycin in 4 divided doses caused an increase of body weight by 500 g per week. This was in comparison with a weekly gain of 150 g per week in cases treated with diet alone, which consisted of humanized buffalo milk and "protein milk."

Milk substitutes in treatment

The comparatively high cost of cow and/or buffalo milk and their relative unavailability, as well as the lack of milk preparations for artificial feeding of infants, led to a search for suitable substitutes based on vegetable products.

Wishahy (1958) describes a preparation called *el labat* made as follows: Sesame (50 g), roasted chick-pea (50 g), rice (20 g), all in powder form, and cane sugar (40 g) are added to 1 liter of water, boiled for 15 minutes, and flavored with rose water. The opalescent fluid which results has protein, 2.1%; fat, 3.2%; and carbohydrate, 7.8% and provides 71 calories per 100 ml. Wishahy found that babies tolerated it quite well. Ragab and Wishahy (1960) tested its digestibility in infants and children from 9 months to 14 years in age and found it to be better than buffalo milk. They recommend the use of *el labat* in infant feeding. Wishahy (1963) treated 7 cases of marasmus and 5 cases of kwashiorkor with *el labat* and found it acceptable. He reports that gains in body weight in marasmus were 10 to 50 g a day and in kwashiorkor (apparently after the loss of edema) 15 to 87 g a day. More extensive trials of this mixture are obviously needed.

Hanafy and Seddik (1960) first used a peanut preparation for the feeding of infants allergic to animal milk. They prepared it by roasting and decorticating peanuts, and homogenizing with water, with the addition of cane sugar. The preparation had 3% protein, 5.1% fat, 5.8% carbohydrates and provided 78 calories per 100 ml. Hanafy and Seddik treated 4 cases of milk allergy with the peanut preparation and also found it to be well tolerated in 15 other infants from a few days of age to twelve months old. The authors recommended its use in infant feeding as an animal milk substitute when the latter was not available. However further work by Hanafy, Ibrahim, Khateeb, and Seddik (1964) indicated that the peanut formula was not suitable for infants below four months in age, for it did not promote growth. A little later Hanafy, Ibrahim, and Khateeb (1965) reported that a preparation made from roasted peanut and roasted chick-pea after soaking in lime water in the proportion of 2 : 1 gave better nitrogen retention and growth than the peanut formula alone in infants older than 4 months.

Hassan, Morcos, and Zamzami (1960) tried out in young rats a mixture of peanut flour, sesame flour, and roasted chick-pea flour in the proportion of 2: 2: 1, incorporated in rat diets at approximately

15% protein level, and found it satisfactory. We are not aware of any attempts to test this mixture in infant feeding. We feel that the efforts in this direction initiated by such pediatricians as Wishahy and Hanafy should be further encouraged and properly organized for a complete biochemical, animal, and human testing program. Cheap and nutritious milk substitutes should be developed so as to provide suitable articles not only for the treatment of protein-calorie-deficiency disease but also for the feeding of infants and children. This subject is of importance not only to Egypt but also to the neighboring Arab countries and is therefore of general interest. It will be discussed in detail at the end of the chapter as one of the suggested measures for control and prevention of protein-calorie-deficiency disease.

Fatality

The reported fatality has varied from 5 to 28%, including the deaths which occurred in the first 24 to 48 hours after admission. Considering the fact that usually children are brought into the hospital not only with advanced symptoms of protein-calorie-deficiency disease but also with often severe manifestations of acute respiratory and gastrointestinal infections, the average fatality rate cannot be considered excessive. Table 5 summarizes the available information on the fatality experience in the hospitalized cases of protein-calorie-deficiency disease in Egypt.

The deaths often result from the associated or intercurrent infections such as bronchopneumonia or enterocolitis. In our series one patient died of tuberculous meningitis. Sudden deaths due to unaccountable causes occurring in later stages of treatment such as have been commented upon by Trowell, Davies, and Dean (1954) either did not occur in Egyptian cases or were not specifically mentioned by the investigators in this country. It is more likely to be the former, for Awwaad, Sandstead, *et al.* and Carter *et al.* in an over-all experience

TABLE 5
FATALITY RATE IN PROTEIN-CALORIE-DEFICIENCY DISEASE IN EGYPT

Authors	No. of Cases	Deaths	Fatality %
Alfi (1956)	24	4	16.7
Nabawy (1959)	—	—	5 to 20
Awwaad (1961)	200	16	8
Sandstead et al. (1965)	39	11	28.2
Carter et al. (1968)	110	18	16.3

of more than 300 cases of protein-calorie-deficiency disease treated by them have been able to account for the immediate causes of death in the cases which died in hospitals.

PROTEIN-CALORIE-DEFICIENCY DISEASE IN THE NEIGHBORING ARAB COUNTRIES

Libya, Sudan, Jordan, and Lebanon will be considered as neighboring Arab countries. A good deal of information is available from Jordan, somewhat less from Lebanon and Sudan, and unfortunately the least from Libya. Nutrition surveys in Libya (1957), Lebanon (1962), and Jordan (1963), sponsored by the U.S. Interdepartmental Committee on Nutrition for National Defense (ICNND) can be considered as starting points for later nutritional studies undertaken in Lebanon and Jordan.

Libya

The ICNND Team weighed, measured, and examined 102 infants and children up to the age of three years at a MCH Center in Tripoli. They found that heights and weights of these children approximated the lower percentiles in U.S. children. Kwashiorkor was suspected in four children, and marasmus was found in three. It is a pity that the recommendations of ICNND for investigations into infant and child malnutrition have not been followed up. A World Health Organization Nutrition Adviser has been working in Libya for about two years, but no reports are available.

Sudan

According to Hassan (1960), kwashiorkor in Sudanese children is not common. He, however, reported on 48 cases admitted to Khartoum Civil Hospital between June 1958 and December 1959 with a fatality of 15%. These were children between 10 months and three years; sex ratio was 4 : 3. All exhibited growth failure, edema, dermatosis, and dyschromotrichia. Serum proteins determined in 30 cases gave the average values for total protein, 4.01 g/100 ml and for albumin, 1.77 g/100 ml. Reconstituted skim milk with or without Casilan was used for treatment. Fatality was 15%, mainly due to bronchophenumonia or intractable gastroenteritis.

It is difficult to judge the validity of Hassan's statement about the frequency of the occurrence of protein-calorie-deficiency disease in Sudan without further investigation.

Smith (1954) had earlier deplored the lack of information on this subject. He however mentioned that several typical cases had been treated in the hospitals of Khartoum, Khartoum North, and Omdurman. Smith also refers to the observations of Hewer (1932) on a group of cases with retarded growth and hepatosplenomegaly which, according to Smith, may have been the late results of malnutrition in infancy.

Jordan

The ICNND Nutrition Survey carried out in Jordan in April–June 1962 covered only a small number of infants and children up to three years. Retardation of growth commencing at about six months was noticed; the lengths and weights after this period corresponded to the 16th percentile of the values found in U.S. children. Clinical evidence of protein-calorie-deficiency disease in an appreciable number of children was also seen. Suspecting the presence of protein-calorie-deficiency disease as a health problem in Jordan, ICNND recommended further investigation. This was undertaken in the following year jointly by ICNND and the Interdepartmental Committee for Nutrition in Jordan established by the government of Jordan. The results of this study reported by Pharaon, Darby, Shammout, Bridgforth, and Wilson (1965) are revealing, and some of these findings are summarized below.

The survey extended over the whole of Jordan, covering all its eight provinces. The sample consisted of 1563 boys and 1280 girls of 0 to 5 years of age from the rural and urban areas; the sample included 665 refugee children. Signs and symptoms of marasmus and kwashiorkor were found in 2.14 and 1.23% of the children, respectively. There were seasonal variations: the highest incidence was in September–November following the summer and lowest in March–May. In addition, a milder variety of protein-calorie-deficiency disease which the authors call pre-kwashiorkor was considered to exist to the extent of 4.8%. The authors emphasize the fact that marasmus and pre-kwashiorkor taken together occur far more frequently than kwashiorkor and hence deserve greater attention than they have so far received. Patwardhan and Kamel (1967) in a survey for vitamin A deficiency carried out in 1963–64, covering 1,257 infants and children of 0 to 6 years in age mainly from the rural and urban regions of the provinces of Amman and Jerusalem found signs of protein-calorie-deficiency disease in 5.8% of the children examined.

Thus there is little doubt that protein-calorie-deficiency disease is one of the major public health problems of malnutrition in Jordan.

Clinical studies on hospital patients have been reported by Majaj (1960) and Pharaon (1960) from Jerusalem and Amman, respectively. Majaj describes 183 cases of which 141 had edema among the Arab refugee children in Jordan. The age range was 2 months to 3 years; 82% of the cases were between 6 and 24 months of age. Forty-two cases had no edema and were presumably cases of wasting which could be called marasmus. Treatment was based on reconstituted skim milk fortified with Casilan and cane sugar. Fatality was 15%, including deaths which occurred on the first day of admission. Pharaon (1960) describes 216 cases from Amman. Most of these patients had been referred to the hospital for diarrhea with dehydration mainly in summer or for acute respiratory infection usually in winter. Only a few cases were sent to the hospital for under- and malnutrition. Ninety-five percent were between 4 months and 2 years in age; 45% came from towns, 34% from villages, and 21% were Bedouin children. Seventy-six cases had edema, and 90 were marasmic. The remainder had various grades of wasting not sufficient to be classified as marasmic. Treatment was initiated with half-strength fresh cow milk acidified with lemon juice. Later on, fermented milk with banana, sugar, olive oil, minced meat, fresh fruit juice, and a boiled egg daily were given. The fatality was comparatively high at 25%, deaths within 24 hours of admission accounting for 22% of the total fatality. Of the surviving patients, 66% had improved moderately or considerably before discharge, the remainder having left the hospital against medical advice.

The researches of Mertz and his colleagues in USA (reviewed by Mertz, 1967) had shown that the trace element chromium was essential in animal nutrition and that it was one of the factors involved in the efficient utilization of glucose in the body. Tests with chromium administration in adults with defective glucose utilization had brought about an improvement in glucose tolerance in a certain proportion of cases. Majaj and Hopkins (1966) in Jordan attempted to determine whether the impaired glucose utilization commonly found associated with protein-calorie malnutrition was due to chromium deficiency. They found that a single oral dose of 250 μg Cr (as $CrCl_3$) restored to normal the diabetic type of glucose tolerance curves in four infants from Jerusalem suffering from kwashiorkor. On the other hand five infants from Jericho also suffering from kwashiorkor had higher fasting blood glucose levels than the infants from Jerusalem and a normal intravenous glucose tolerance. They attributed this difference between kwashiorkor cases from Jerusalem and Jericho to a possible chromium deficiency in the former. The only evidence they have is the chromium content of drinking water; Jerusalem water had 0.4 to 0.5 µg/liter of chromium, whereas the Jericho water had 1.2 to 1.8 µg/liter. Carter et al. (1968) studied 34 cases of kwashiorkor in Cairo. Fasting blood glucose was low, and the intravenous glucose tolerance curve was of the diabetic type. The oral administration of 250 µg chromium (as $CrCl_3$) was without any effect. The glucose tolerance curves returned to normal on high protein high calorie diet without additional chromium. Carter et al. analyzed foods that they believed were consumed by the children before their hospitalization as well as foods and medicaments used in their study and found appreciable amounts of chromium in both. The plasma chromium in eight infants in whom it was determined was within the normal range. The authors concluded therefore that chromium deficiency did not appear to be responsible for the impairment in glucose utilization seen in kwashiorkor cases in Cairo, Egypt.

Hopkins, Ransome-Kuti, and Majaj (1968) have further reported a positive chromium response in 6 malnourished Nigerian infants from Lagos. Tap water in Lagos had less than 1 µg/liter of chromium, and the milk reconstituted from powdered milk gave chromium values comparable to those found in Jerusalem (18 µg/liter). There is not information on plasma chromium in Nigerian infants or Nigerian foods. It appears, therefore, that if the hypothesis of chromium deficiency as being responsible for impaired glucose utilization in kwashiorkor is to be substantiated, much more information on chromium intake and its effect on plasma chromium in healthy and malnourished infants will be needed.

Lebanon

The ICNND Survey Team measured and examined 193 children of 0 to 6 years of age from the refugee and nonrefugee population. In infants and preschool age children from the nonrefugee population, growth retardation became evident after the first year of life. Among the children from the refugee population, it probably started earlier. The report mentioned the possibility of mild protein-calorie deficiency among the nonrefugee infants, but it is more specific in describing the refugee children among whom they recorded finding dyspigmentation of hair, muscular wasting, and hepatomegaly in meaningful numbers as indicative of protein-calorie-deficiency. ICNND did not, however, record having found frank cases of kwashiorkor or marasmus in their Lebanon survey.

McLaren, Ammoun, and Houri (1964) have reported on 190 children with protein-calorie malnutrition of the marasmic type and their socioeconomic background in two locations in Lebanon—Beirut and Saida. In age, more than 90% were between 1 and 24 months. In the Beirut sample the male children exceeded female children by a ratio of over 2 : 1; however, in Saida the ratio was 3 : 4. Most of these cases came from the families belonging to the low socioeconomic group. In Beirut the average income of 86% of the families was $84 per year. All these children exhibited growth retardation to varying degrees; the majority were below the 3rd percentile compared with the growth chart of the Children's Medical Center, Boston. The majority of the cases came in an acute condition with diarrhea and dehydration. Others suffered from respiratory infections. The fatality in Beirut was 14.7% and much higher in Saida, 30%. These authors consider marasmus as the outstanding nutritional disorder of early childhood in all countries of the Near East and North Africa. They may be right, for the figures, inadequate though they are, quoted for Egypt indicate that so far as hospital admissions are concerned, marasmus cases outnumber those of kwashiorkor 2–4 to 1. Probably a similar situation exists in the community at large, as the survey of Pharaon et al. (1965) in Jordan indicates. Unfortunately similar information is not available for Egypt. McLaren (1966) is of the opinion that marasmus is on the increase in the developing countries of the world owing to earlier weaning and repeated gastrointestinal and respiratory infections, coupled with near starvation during illness and in convalescence imposed by traditional habits.

In view of the wide prevalence of protein-calorie-deficiency disease and the need for suitable infant-feeding preparations, workers at the American University of Beirut, Lebanon, have devoted attention to one of the important aspects of the situation, namely the development and testing of cheap and nutritious vegetable-protein-rich food mixtures suitable for infant feeding. The mixtures were made from locally available foodstuffs with a small supplement of dried skim milk, bone ash, and vitamins. Tannous et al. (1965) tested five such mixtures in rats for growth and Asfour et al. (1965) tested four of these in 24 apparently healthy infants between 5 and 12 months old. The tests in infants included acceptability, tolerance, nitrogen balance, and growth. The mixtures were fed at 100 g level as the only supplement to breast milk. The acceptability of the mixture was high, and all three gave position N balance. As a result of these tests the authors recommend the formula Laubina 103 as the most suitable. Its composition is as follows: Parboiled wheat (*burghul*), 60 parts; chick-pea flour, 20 parts; dried skim milk, 10 parts; vegetable oil, 5 parts; sugar, 2 parts; bone ash, 1 part; citric acid, 1 part; sugar containing vitamins A and D, 1 part. The nutrient composition per 100 g of Laubina 103 is as follows: Protein, 16 g; fat, 6 g; Ca, 629 mg; P, 602 mg; Fe, 11.4 mg; vitamin A, 5000 I.U.; thiamine, 0.4 mg; riboflavin, 0.27 mg; niacin, 3.4 mg; and vitamin D, 500 I.U. The Protein Efficiency Ratio of this mixture was found to be 2.30 (casein 2.85) and net protein utilization (NPU) 49%. The results of both the rat test and infant trials appeared promising. We are not aware, however, of any further developments in the production and popularization of this mixture for infant feeding in Lebanon.

PROTEIN-RICH WEANING FOODS

The development of nutritious and relatively cheap foods to be used as weaning foods for infants and young children up to the age of two years or a little over is important in developing countries, principally because milk is in short supply, hence expensive and relatively unavailable, not only to the poorer sections of the population but to the lower-middle classes as well. It is therefore desirable that attempts to formulate and list suitable milk substitutes prepared principally from locally available foodstuffs should be encouraged. In this context a brief account of parallel international developments in this field should prove of interest.

The specialized agencies of the United Nations, namely, World Health Organization, Food and Agriculture Organization, and United Nations Children's Fund (UNICEF), have devoted considerable attention to this important problem over the last 15 years. The Protein Advisory Group, established first by World Health Organization in 1956, which since 1960 has functioned under the joint auspices of the above-mentioned three organizations, has initiated investigations on and promoted the development of protein-rich food mixtures in such countries as India, Uganda, and Guatemala. Investigations in this field were considerably expanded under a program sponsored by the Committee on Protein Malnutrition of the Food and Nutrition Board of the United States National Academy of Sciences. The search for suitable protein-rich material ranged over a variety of products such as meals left after the extraction of oil from oil seeds, soya beans and other grain legumes, torula yeast, fish protein concentrates, and leaf protein.

The materials were analyzed for their protein content, the amino acid composition was determined, nutritive value of protein estimated by animal experiments, and observations made on freedom from toxicity. Finally tests of acceptability followed by nitrogen retention and growth tests were done in sick and healthy infants and children. The search for protein-rich foods was catching, and such a large number of investigators came up with a variety of results and suggestions for making preparations for infant and child feeding that there was danger of chaos reigning in the field.

There was obviously need for some basic guidelines for the testing and development of protein-rich food mixtures intended for application in programs for combatting protein-calorie deficiency. Some thought had been given to this aspect as early as 1955 at a conference on Human Protein Requirements and Their Fulfillment in Practice convened in 1955 in Princeton, New Jersey, U.S.A., under the joint auspices of Food and Agriculture Organization, World Health Organization, and Josiah Macy Jr. Foundation, New York; and suggestions had been made at the conference about the procedures for testing a new processed food. A knowledge of the source and nature of the material and of the processing to which it was subjected was considered essential. Its full chemical composition, including the amino acid content, had to be determined. The product had to be bacteriologically safe and free from toxicity as tested in animals. This was to be followed by tolerance and acceptability trials in adults, healthy children, and malnourished children, in that order. The product which successfully emerged from all the above tests would then be subjected to field trials. Of course, it had to be understood that the proposed product should be considerably less expensive than milk if it were to find popular application.

The Protein Advisory Group of WHO/FAO/UNICEF accepted the validity of these procedures. However in order to simplify the requirements for human testing while at the same time making the tests more meaningful, the Protein Advisory Group prepared in 1966 a memorandum on Human Testing of Supplementary Food Mixtures. The full text of this memorandum will be found in the Protein Advisory Group Bulletin No. 7, distributed from New York in October 1967. The salient points are as follows:

The need for the identification of the source of edible protein, the quantity available, and the study of its economic development is stressed. The knowledge of chemical composition of the original material as well as that of the proposed mixture in which it is to be formulated is considered essential, as is the effect of processing on the nutritive value of protein contained in the mixture. Suitable animal experiments should ensure freedom from toxicity. Only after the above information is made available can the product be considered ready for testing in children of the age group for which it is intended.

This last procedure will consist of tests for (a) acceptability and tolerance, (b) growth, (c) nitrogen balance, and (d) other parameters for determining the suitability of protein, if necessary.

Where protein-rich mixtures are made from foodstuffs which are already commonly used as human food and where processing is minimal, much of the above-mentioned preliminary information may already be available, and the need for human testing may be limited to tests for acceptability and tolerance.

The real problem arises after all the testing has been done and the product is found suitable for infants and young children. The acceptable product has to be manufactured in sufficient quantities at relatively low cost in order that poor people for whose children it is intended should be in a position to buy it. Furthermore, since the product would be something new, its popularization among the people, education about its use, and the benefits to be derived from such use are aspects which require considerable promotional effort. Large-scale production and promotion are activities which only the food industry can undertake. Understandably, the food industry is usually conservative in its approach to such problems, and there is need to educate the industry itself in order to ensure its co-operation. Success on these fronts can only be achieved by close co-operation between the scientists involved in testing and development of protein-rich food mixtures, the government of the country which is interested in protecting the health of infants and children, and the food industry which will be concerned with production and promotion. There is increasing evidence that such co-operative effort can be successful. A good example is INCAPARINA which was developed after considerable experimentation and testing by the Institute of Nutrition for Central America and Panama (INCAP), Guatemala City, Guatemala. The government of Guatemala was interested, and so also was the food industry. As a result of this tripartite co-operation the sale and use of INCAPARINA has been increasing in Guatemala over the last five years. What is more important is that the good news about the product has spread beyond the borders of Guatemala, and similar preparations are being manufactured in other countries in Latin America.

Another good example of the development and use of a protein-rich weaning food is FAFA (which means "to grow big and strong"), developed in Addis Ababa, Ethiopia, by the Ethio-Swedish Nutrition Unit. It is based on a locally produced cereal, teff (*Eragrostis abyssinica*). Chick-pea (*Cicer arietinum*), dried skim milk (10%), sugar, iodized salt, and vitamins are other constituents. FAFA has 15% protein and provides 350 calories per 100 gm and is a complete food in itself. After preliminary chemical, animal, and clinical testing, the product was used as supplementary feeding of infants and found satisfactory. It is now produced on a fairly large scale; free distribution is discouraged if not completely stopped. The production is marketed at 8 U.S. cents per 300-gram bag through retail trade, and sales have been reported to be good.

Somewhat similar developments have occurred independently in India, but because of the reluctance of the food industry so far to get involved, the large-scale production of protein-rich foods has been delayed. There are signs, however, that this bottleneck will be overcome, and cheap nutritious protein-rich food will soon be made available for Indian infants and children.

The reason for going into so much detail in this question is that appropriate weaning foods are needed in this region where also protein-calorie deficiency is a public health problem. The isolated efforts of scientists and pediatricians described in this chapter need to be followed up on a properly organized scale, and the industry as well as the governments of the countries concerned need to interest themselves in ensuring that cheap, nutritious infant foods are produced and made available for use to the population. This is one important development which will effectively contribute to the control if not prevention of protein-calorie deficiency in infants and young children of the region.

REFERENCES

Abbassy, A. S., M. Mikhail, M. M. Zeitoun, and M. Ragab. 1967. The Suprarenal Cortical Function as Measured by the Plasma 17-Ketohydroxy Steroid Level in Malnourished Children. *J. Trop. Pediat.* 13: 154.

Abboud, M. A. 1937. Dystrophies in Infants. *J. Egypt. Med. Assoc.* 20: 17.

Abdou, I. A., A. K. Lebshtein, and T. A. Kassim. 1964. A Study of the Nutritional Status of Mothers, Infants, and Young Children Attending Maternity and Child Health Centers in Cairo. J. Egypt. Publ. Hlth. Assoc. 39: 241.

Alfi, O. 1956. Studies on Kwashiorkor Disease in Egyptian Infants. *Gaz. Egypt. Pediat. Assoc.* 4: 140.

Asfour, R. Y., R. I. Tannous, Z. I. Sabry, and J. W. Cowan. 1965. Protein-Rich Food Mixtures for Feeding Infants and Young Children in the Middle East. II—Preliminary Clinical Evaluation with Laubina Mixtures. *Amer. J. Clin. Nutr.* 17: 148.

Awwaad, S. 1961. Kwashiorkor in Egyptian Children: A Clinical Study of 200 Cases. *Bull. Clin. Sci. Soc. Abbassia Fac. Med.* 12: 10.

Awwaad, S., and E. M. Abdel-Wahab. 1960. Electrophoretic Studies of Serum Proteins in Nutritional Oedema in Egyptian Children. *Gaz. Egypt. Pediat. Assoc.* 8: 494.

Awwaad, S., and E. A. Eissa. 1959. Studies on Blood Amino Acid Nitrogen in Normal Egyptian Infants and Children and in Cases of Nutritional Oedema. *Arch. Pediat.* 76: 395.

Awwaad, S., E. A. Eissa, and O. Attia. 1961. Studies on Blood Proteins and Blood Amino Acid Nitrogen in Marasmic Infants. *J. Egypt. Med. Assoc.* 44: 437.

Badr el Din, M. K. 1954. Management of Food Intolerance in Infantile Wasting. J. Egypt. Med. Assoc. 37: 93.

Badr el Din, M. K., and M. H. Aboul Wafa. 1960. Galactose Intolerance in Kwashiorkor. *Gaz. Egypt. Pediat. Assoc.* 8: 458.

Bowie, M. D., G. O. Barbezat, and J. D. L. Hansen. 1967. Carbohydrate Absorption in Malnourished Children. *Amer. J. Clin. Nutr.* 20: 89.

Carter, J. P., and others. 1969. Kwashiorkor in Egypt. Unpublished.

Carter, J. P., A. Ghattab, M. Abdel-El-Hadi, J. T. Davis, A. Gholmy, and V. N. Patwardhan. 1968. Chromium (III) in Hypoglycemia and in Impaired Glucose Utilization in Kwashiorkor. *Amer. J. Clin. Nutr.* 21: 195.

Eissa, E. A., A. S. Shukry, I. M. Fayed, D. M. Metwally, and S. M. Ismail. 1967a. Some Aspects of Carbohydrate Metabolism in Protein Malnutrition in Children (I) *Gaz. Egypt. Pediat. Assoc.* 15: 9.

———. 1967b. Some Dynamic Aspects of Carbohydrate Metabolism in Protein Malnutrition (II). *Gaz. Egypt. Pediat. Assoc.* 15: 132.

Gabr, M., E. Abdel Salam, and A. Malek. 1968. Lactose Tolerance in Marasmic Infants. *Med. J. Cairo Univ.* 36: 23.

Gholmy, A. 1960. In Round Table Conference on Kwashiorkor. *Gaz. Egypt. Pediat. Assoc.* 8: 397.

Gholmy, A., Y. M. Aboul Dahab, M. Essawi, Y. A. Abdel-Rahman, and A. Malek. 1962. Biochemical Studies on Anemia in Malnourished Infants: A Comparison of Marasmus and Kwashiorkor Cases. *J. Trop. Med. Hyg.* 65: 64–67.

Gholmy, A., M. Nabawy, M. Khattab, A. S. Shukry, M. K. Gabr, B. Sabaie, S. Aidoros, and L. Soliman. 1960. Fatty Liver in Childhood (An Analysis of 93 Cases). *Gaz. Egypt. Pediat. Assoc.* 8: 383.

Gholmy, A., M. Nabawy, A. S. Shukry, S. Ismail, and M. F. Hawary. 1960. Biochemical Studies on the Serum Proteins in the Kwashiorkor Syndrome in Egyptian Infants. *Gaz. Egypt. Pediat. Assoc.* 8: 399.

Gholmy, A., M. Nabawy, A. S. Shukry, S. Ismail, and M. F. Hawary. 1960. Studies on the Blood Glutathione in Kwashiorkor of Egyptia Infants. *Gaz. Egypt. Pediat. Assoc.* 8: 443.

Gholmy, A., M. Nabawy, A. S. Shukry, S. Ismail, F. Hawary, and M. Khattab. 1960. Serum Transaminase Study in Kwashiorkor. *Gaz. Egypt. Pediat. Assoc.* 8: 450.

Gomez, F., R. R. Galvan, J. Cravioto, and S. Frenk. 1955. Malnutrition in Infancy and Childhood with Special Reference to Kwashiorkor. *Advances in Pediat.* 7: 131.

Gopalan, C. 1956. Kwashiorkor in Uganda and Coonoor (A Comparison of Some Salient Aspects). *J. Trop. Pediat.* 1: 206.

Hanafy, M. 1947. The Subacute Subnutritional Syndrome in Infants. *J. Egypt. Med. Assoc.* 30: 440.

Hanafy, M. 1951. Malnutrition in Egyptian Infants. *J. Egypt. Med. Assoc.* 34: 470.

Hanafy, M., and Y. Seddik. 1960. A Peanut Milk Substitute for the Feeding of Infants Allergic to Milk. *Gaz. Egypt. Pediat. Assoc.* 8: 524.

Hanafy, M., A. H. Ibrahim, and S. Khateeb. 1965. Trials on Vegetable Milk-Substitutes. II-Growth of Infants Feed on a Modified Peanut Milk Substitute. *Alexandria Med. J.* 11: 241.

Hanafy, M., A. H. Ibrahim, S. Khateeb, and Y. Seddik. 1963. Trials on Vegetable Milk Substitutes: Growth and Nitrogen Retention in Infants Fed on a Peanut Milk Substitute. *Alexandria Med. J.* 9: 477.

Hassan, A., S. R. Morcos, and S. Zamzami. 1960. A Protein-Rich Plant Food for the Young: Rat Feeding Experiments Demonstrating Its Nutritive Value. *Gaz. Egypt. Pediat. Assoc.* 8: 487.

Hewer, T. F. 1932. Splenomegaly and Infantilism. *Trans. Roy. Soc. Trop. Med. Hyg.* 26: 139.

Holt, L. E., S. E. Snyderman, P. M. Norton, E. Roitman, and J. Finch. 1963. The Plasma Aminogram in Kwashiorkor. *Lancet* ii: 1343.

Hopkins, L. L., O. Ransome-Kuti, and A. S. Majaj. 1968. Improvement of Impaired Carbohydrate Metabolism by Chromium (III) in Malnourished Infants. *Amer. J. Clin. Nutr.* 21: 203.

Human Protein Requirements and their Fulfillment in Practice: Proceedings of a Conference in Princeton, N.J. Edited by J. C. Waterlow and J. M. L. Stephen. Rome: F. A. O. 1957.

Interdepartmental Committee on Nutrition for National Defense. *Reports of Nutrition Surveys in Libya 1957; Lebanon 1962; Jordan 1963.*

Iskandar, F. 1935. Post-Dysenteric Oedema in Children. *J. Egypt. Med. Assoc.* 18: 134.

Ismail, A. A., A. Abdel Hay, G. Kamel, and F. Behery. 1960. Blood Proteins in Nutritional Oedema. *Gaz. Egypt. Pediat. Assoc.* 8: 475.

Jelliffe, D. B. 1959. Protein-Calorie Malnutrition in Tropical Preschool Children: A Review of Recent Knowledge. *J. Pediat.* 54: 227.

Joint FAO/WHO Expert Committee on Nutrition. 1962. Sixth Report. Geneva, Switzerland: Wld. Hlth. Org. Tech. Rep. Ser. 245.

Majaj, A. S. 1960. Protein Malnutrition and Macrocytic Anemia among Palestine Refugees in Jordan. *Gaz. Egypt. Pediat. Assoc.* 8: 610.

Majaj, A. S., and L. L. Hopkins. 1966. The Response of Hypoglycemia and Impaired Glucose Utilization to Chromium (III) Treatment in Protein-Calorie-Malnourished Infants. *Lebanese Med. J.* 19: 177.

McLaren, D. S. 1966. A Fresh Look at Protein-Calorie Malnutrition. *Lancet* ii: 485.

McLaren, D. S., C. Ammoun, and G. Houri. 1964. The Socioeconomic Background of Marasmus in Lebanon. *J. Med. Liban.* 17: 85–96.

McLaren, D. S., W. W. Kamel, and N. Ayyoub. 1965. Plasma Amino Acids and the Detection of Protein-Calorie Malnutrition. *Amer. J. Clin. Nutr.* 17: 152.

Mertz, W. 1967. Biological Role of Chromium. *Federation Proc.* 26: 186.

Nabawy, M. 1959. Study of Kwashiorkor in Egypt. *Gaz. Egypt. Pediat. Assoc.* 7: 79.

Nabawy, M., A. S. Shukry, M. Safouh, and I. Fayad. 1964. The Liver in Kwashiorkor. *Gaz. Egypt. Pediat. Assoc.* 12: 1.

Patwardhan, V. N., and W. W. Kamel. 1967. *Studies on Vitamin A Deficiency in Infants and Young Children in Jordan.* Geneva: World Health Organization.

Pharaon, H. M., W. J. Darby, H. A. Shammout, E. B. Bridgforth, and C. S. Wilson. 1965. A Year-Long Study of the Nutriture of Infants and Preschool Children in Jordan. *J. Trop. Pediat. Afr. Child Hlth.* 2: Monograph No. 3, 1–39.

Ragab, M. M., and A. G. Wishahy. 1960. Clinico-Radiological Study on the Digestibility of Vegetable and Animal Milks. *J. Egypt. Med. Assoc.* 43: 1934.

Sandstead, H. H., A. S. Shukry, A. S. Prasad, M. K. Gabr, A. Hifney, N. Mokhtar, and W. J. Darby. 1965. Kwashiorkor in Egypt. I—Clinical and Biochemical Studies, with Special Reference to Plasma Zinc and Serum Lactic Dehydrogenase. *Amer. J. Clin. Nutr.* 17: 15.

Sandstead, H. H., M. K. Gabr, S. Azzam, A. S. Shukry, R. J. Weiler, O. Mohy el Din, N. Mokhtar, A. S. Prasad, A. Hifney, and W. J. Darby. 1965. Kwashiorkor in Egypt. II—Hematologic Aspects (The Occurrence of Macrocytic Anemia Associated with Low Serum Vitamin E and a Wide Range of Serum Vitamin B_{12} Levels). *Amer. J. Clin. Nutr.* 17: 27–35.

Shehata, A. H., A. A. Hay, G. Kamel, B. Kammah, M. Safouh, and M. Talaat. 1965. Biochemical Studies in Kwashiorkor. II-Serum Proteins and Amino Acids. *J. Endocrinol. Metabolism* 11: 11.

Sheikh, A. 1962. Post-Diarrheic Oedema in Children and Its Treatment by the Newer Corticoids. *J. Egypt. Med. Assoc.* 45: 96.

Shukry, H., M. A. Mahdi, and A. A. El Gholmy. 1938. Nutritional Oedema in Children in Egypt. *Arch. Dis. Childhood* 13: 254.

Shukry, A. S., M. Safouh, and I. M. Fayad. 1964. Histopathological Study on the Adrenals in Kwashiorkor. *Gaz. Egypt. Pediat. Assoc.* 12: 21.

Shukry, A. S., M. Safouh, I. M. Fayad, and A. Elwi. 1963. Histopathological Study on the Skin and the Hair in Kwashiorkor. *Gaz. Egypt. Pediat. Assoc.* 11: 33.

Smith, D. A. 1954. *Food and Society in the Sudan.* Khartoum: McCorquodale and Co. (Sudan) Ltd.

Tannous, R. I., J. W. Cowan, F. Rinner, R. J. Asfour, and Z. I. Sabry. 1965. Protein-Rich Food Mixtures for Feeding Infants and Preschool Children in the Middle East. I-Development and Evaluation of Laubina Mixtures. *Amer. J. Clin. Nutr.* 17: 143.

Trowell, H. C., J. N. P. Davies, and R. F. A. Dean. 1954. *Kwashiorkor.* London: Edward Arnold.

Waterlow, J. C., J. Cravioto, and J. M. Stephen. 1960. Protein Malnutrition in Man. Advances in Protein Chemistry 15: 220.

Whitehead, R. G., and R. F. A. Dean. 1964. Serum Amino Acids in Kwashiorkor. I-Relationship to Clinical Condition. II-An Abbreviated Method of Estimation and Its Application. *Amer. J. Clin. Nutr.* 14: 313 and 320.

Williams, C. D. 1933. Nutritional Disease of Childhood Associated with Maize Diet. *Arch. Dis. Childhood* 8: 423.

———. 1935. Kwashiorkor: Nutritional Disease of Children Associated with Maize Diet. *Lancet* ii: 1151.

Wishahy, A. G. 1958a. El Labat, an Egyptian Vegetable Milk: Review of Literature on Vegetable Milk. *J. Egypt. Med. Assoc.* 41: 433.

———. 1958b. Clinical Studies on Pellagra in Infants and Children. *J. Egypt. Med. Assoc.* 41: 553.

———. 1963. The Use of Egyptian Vegetable Milk (El Labat) as Food in Diseases of Infants and Children. *J. Egypt. Med. Assoc.* 46: 415.

9 | Treatment of Kwashiorkor and Marasmus

The treatment of kwashiorkor and marasmus varies at present from one hospital to the next throughout the Middle East. Many physicians fail to recognize the syndromes, especially when edema is absent and symptoms of infection predominate. Infants who are hospitalized usually receive a better diet than they have at home, though not necessarily a therapeutically adequate one. It is the general practice to permit mothers to stay with the patients while they are in the hospital, and they frequently bring in food from the outside. The treatment given, therefore, depends on the physician's knowledge of the underlying role of malnutrition, of the synergism between nutrition and infection-producing illness in his patient, and on the available facilities.

Gastroenteritis is a frequently associated infection. The loss of electrolytes and water from recurrent diarrhea leads to hypotonicity and disorganized cell composition and function. Intracellular water and sodium concentration are increased, while the concentration of potassium in the cell is significantly decreased (Metcoff *et al.*, 1966).

Two excellent rehydration programs were instituted in this region by Drs. Majaj and Karakashian, both working in Jordan. Dr. Majaj gives intravenous fluids on admission to the hospital, using scalp-vein infusions that are started and maintained by trained nurses. The solutions are:

        1/6 M sodium lactate
        Normal saline

5% Dextrose in water
KCL (14.9%, injection, U.S.P.)

He routinely gives 200 ml/kg of fluid during the first 24 hours, providing 9.5 meq Na/kg, 9 meq Cl/kg, and 10 meq K/kg. The amount of sodium lactate given is usually of the order of 100 ml.

Nothing is given by mouth during the first 6 hours. Afterwards, water and tea are given, and reconstituted milk powder is started as soon as tolerated. The milk is started gradually, one ounce being offered every three hours.

Dr. A. Karakashian organized a large out-patient rehydration center at Akabat Jaber, the refugee camp in Jericho. The patients were treated by continuous nasogastric drip. They were given 200 ml/kg/24 hours, 50 ml/kg being administered during the first 6 hours. If vomiting and diarrhea were severe, the solutions used were 1/2 as 5% Dextrose in saline, and 1/2 as Najjar's solution.

Najjar's salt packet contains:

sodium citrate	50 g
sodium chloride	10 g
sodium biphosphate	25 g
KCL	25 g
glucose	890 g

15 g of the mixture are added to
250 ml of water to make the solution.

If there is diarrhea and no vomiting, only Najjar's solution is given in the first 6 hours.

Chlorpromazine, 0.5 mg/kg, is given 15 minutes before starting the drip, which is run slowly at 60–70 ml/hr. The patients go home after 6 hours of treatment. The mother is given 2 tablets of Luminal, 0.015 g each, and instructed to give the child one in the afternoon and one in the evening. The tablets are crushed and given by mouth. She also is instructed to give orally to the child Najjar's packets dissolved in water as above before she returns with the child to the rehydration center the following morning. Najjar's packets are given according to the following dosage schedule:

Age 3 months	1 Najjar's packet (15 g of mixture)
Age 3 mth.–1 year	2 packets
Age more than 1 year	3 packets

The 6-hour intragastric drips are continued until there is no more vomiting and diarrhea and the patient's hydration is considered satisfactory. If the patient is considered to be well nourished at this time, he is discharged in a few days.

If, on the other hand, after vomiting and diarrhea have ceased and the patient's hydration is satisfactory he is judged to be malnourished, he is referred to a post-diarrhea feeding center.

At the center nutritious meals are given once a day. Infants under 4 months of age are given milk feedings: 50% skim milk, 50% whole milk. Infants and children over 4 months of age are given cooked rice and carrots, sour milk with olive oil, and bananas. The average stay in the post-diarrheal feeding center is 2 weeks to 1 month.

Both Dr. Majaj's ward and Dr. Karakashian's center were closed in the wake of the June 1967 Arab-Israeli War. Rehydration and nutrition rehabilitation centers have been opened in Amman and elsewhere in East Jordan and are patterned along the same lines.

Infections, though incompletely diagnosed, are usually adequately treated in these children because antibiotics are given freely. Often a patient may be receiving several different antibiotics at once and his dietary management almost completely ignored. In our experience at NAMRU-3, the most effective therapeutic regimen is one which simultaneously treats both infectious disease and malnutrition.

Proper diagnosis of an infection is a prerequisite to proper treatment. Proper diagnosis depends on clinical assessment, routine blood, urine, and stool examinations, and the taking of cultures for bacteriologic diagnosis. Almost every child with kwashiorkor or marasmus has some associated infection, frequently gastrointestinal, respiratory, including tuberculosis, or genitourinary. Multiple infections are not uncommon; multiple diagnoses are the rule and not the exception.

The etiologic agents responsible for gastroenteritis are a case in point. Northway, Cahill, Davies, Kawaguchi, and Miller (1965), working at NAMRU-3 in Cairo, were able, by taking repeated rectal swabs over a two-week period of observation, to identify a specific bacterial pathogen in 72% of cases of infantile gastroenteritis. The pathogens identified were *Shigella,* enteropathogenic *E. coli,* and *Salmonella,* in that order of frequency.

The implications for treatment are obvious. These patients should be cultured once and treatment started soon afterwards. If a patient is seriously ill, we do not even wait 48 hours for the report of the culture. In Cairo, *Shigella* is usually sensitive to tetracycline, and pathogenic *E. coli* to neomycin. In the case of *Salmonella,* we rely more on antibiotic disc sensitivities, although chloromycetin or ampicillin are good drugs to start with empirically if needed. When a specific bacterial pathogen has been identified, there can be a choice of antibiotics based on the organism and its sensitivities.

The simultaneous treatment of infection and malnutrition is based on the understanding of the synergism between nutrition and infection. The nutritional status of the host often must be improved before recovery from infection can be hastened by appropriate treatment. Patients with diarrhea, for example, may have to be fed in spite of their diarrhea. The studies of Chung et al. (1948, 1950) have shown that feeding such patients increases the frequency and bulk of the stools but does not lengthen the time required for recovery, if intravenous fluids are given simultaneously when indicated to treat dehydration. Patients with vomiting and diarrhea often can be fed by continouus intragastric drip, which, if done slowly, is well tolerated.

Dietary management should begin by correcting the existing nutritional deficiencies. Protein and calories are the most common ones, but they are by no means the only ones. Deficiencies of vitamin A, iron, folic acid, riboflavin, vitamin D, iodine, vitamin E, zinc, and other trace elements are also common in that order of importance in the Middle East region.

Protein repletion can be successfully begun by starting with a protein of high biological value, usually cow's milk, at 3.5 g protein/kg of body weight. As the child's appetite improves, he will consume more than this amount, sometimes as much as 8–10 g protein/kg. Tube feeding has rarely been necessary, although anorexia is common initially in many patients.

Calorie intake varies initially from 90–100 Cal/kg and as appetite improves may go as high as 150–200 Cal/kg. Additional calories are usually supplied as "biscuits," but other local foods, some of them high in calories and low in protein, are given after the edema disappears and the child is recovering. Some of these foods, especially carotene-containing vegetables, help to correct some of the other associated nutritional deficiencies.

Dr. Raja Asfour, working with marasmic infants in a metabolic unit at the Department of Pediatrics of the American University of Beirut, has found it advantageous to initiate feedings at low caloric level, 60 Cal/kg, and gradually to increase over a one-week period to an *ad libitum* schedule. By this time the marasmic infant's tolerance and appetite have improved so much that he may take up to 200 Cal/kg/day. Dealing with marasmic infants below one year, Dr. Asfour provides all of the calories required for the repleted infant from cow's milk in the standard dilution. In the first few days of repletion, some infants show intolerance to the milk by having persistent severe diarrhea. He also limits the fluid intake of the marasmic infants during the initial hydration period. Based on his studies showing an increased total body water with an increased extra-cellular compartment in marasmics (who have no clinical signs of edema), he limits the total fluid intake to 120 ml/kg. To selected cases of marasmus with severe gastroenteritis and acute dehydration and on the verge of shock, he gives 20 ml/kg of blood or plasma slowly and at least 5 meq K/kg/24 hr. in the subsequent infusions.

Vitamin A is given routinely at NAMRU-3, usually orally in a water-miscible form, 10,000 I.U. daily. Oleum A liquid (5,000 I.U./drop) is used. Higher doses are given when signs of xerophthalmia are present (25,000–50,000 I.U. daily). Not many suitable parenteral preparations of vitamin A are readily available.

Vitamin B complex is given routinely to all of our patients. We use a local preparation called Varolex Syrup which contains in one teaspoon:

vitamin C	33 mg
vitamin B_1	1.7 mg
vitamin B_2	1 mg
vitamin B_6	0.7 mg
calcium pantothenate	1.7 mg
nicotinamide	7 mg

One teaspoon is given daily from the day of admission.

Intramuscular iron is given routinely on admission to all patients with hemoglobin less than 10 g per 100 ml. One ml of imferron (50 mg elemental iron) is given intramuscularly daily for 4 days. If the patient has not responded within 2 weeks after this initial therapy, he is subsequently treated with folic acid. Blood smears and reticulocyte counts are done routinely.

While vitamin D deficiency rickets is common in preschool children in the Middle East, it is not commonly associated with kwashiorkor and marasmus, perhaps because it takes a growing child to produce the deformities. When rickets is associated with marasmus, tuberculosis is a possibility. This is in spite of the fact that many protein-calorie-malnourished infants with tuberculosis have a negative tuberculin test. They may or may not show hilar node enlargement and/or tuberculosis pneumonia on the chest film because of bronchogenic spread. Frequently, the only symptom of tuberculosis in these children is a failure to gain weight and to do well in spite of appropriate therapy.

Other therapeutic problems, transient in nature, are those of lactose intolerance and the nutrition recovery syndrome. The former is especially common when skim milk is the source of protein. For a period of a few days after initiating therapy, reducing sugars are often present in the stools. These stools are pasty and yellowish in color and resemble those of a breast-fed infant. They react acid to litmus paper. The presence of reducing sugars can be demonstrated by doing a Clinitest on the stools (Kerry and Anderson, 1964). This "diarrhea" is transient in nature and does not result in significant calorie wastage or prevent positive nitrogen balance, as indicated by continued weight gain. Infective gastroenteritis can also be associated with the transient lactose intolerance.

The nutrition recovery syndrome is also an apparently harmless phenomenon consisting of abdominal distention with a venous pattern over the abdomen, progressive liver enlargement, and splenomegaly in the majority of cases.

The syndrome develops several weeks after admission, after the edema has disappeared and the child is gaining weight and shows an increase in serum albumin. The child continues to make an uneventful recovery in spite of what appears to be clinically portal hypertension. Liver function tests are normal except for SGOT and SGPT, the levels of which are higher than the upper limits of normal. Histological examination of tissue obtained by serial needle liver biopsies shows fat on admission with subsequent clearing on treatment.

All the above changes regress over a period of several months. The average duration of the syndrome is 10 weeks. Some livers regress and then become enlarged again and remain enlarged for as long as a year or more.

Hypoglycemia as a cause of death has been described from other parts of the world, for example, by Kahn and Wayburne (1961) in South Africa. In our experience in Cairo, we have not seen it, in spite of the fact that fasting blood sugars are low. We have not fasted our children for longer than 4 hours, however, for laboratory investigations.

We believe whole blood transfusions are seldom indicated because of the increase in plasma volume which occurs in kwashiorkor in the first few days of treatment. Blood transfusions and other plasma expanders are indicated and are better tolerated in patients with profuse diarrhea and peripheral circulatory collapse. The difficulty, however, is in diagnosing dehydration and shock in patients with kwashiorkor and marasmus. If these patients are not in shock or dehydrated, transfusions may further increase the blood volume and overhydration, and congestive heart failure may develop. The slow transfusion of packed red cells is indicated in cases of severe anemia. Blood transfusions are given by some physicians as a source of protein and as a tonic or general body-builder. This practice is to be deplored.

Lastly, these severely protein-calorie-malnourished infants need daily tender, loving care, which only a dedicated, competent nurse working with the mother can provide. No fancy therapeutic maneuver nor a mere understanding of the intricate errors of metabolism associated with this condition and attempts to correct them individually can substitute for that. These children will not survive if any of the members of the team concerned with their care have a carefree attitude, or do not consider them worth saving in the first place. Their parents, too, must also be willing to learn how to feed a growing child properly and to invest the time and whatever money they can afford to ensure the survival and normal growth and development of their children.

REFERENCES

Chung, A. W., and L. E. Holt, Jr. 1950. Place of Oral Feeding in Infantile Diarrhea. *Pediatrics* 5: 421.

Chung, A. W., and B. Viscorova. 1948. Effect of Early Oral Feeding Versus Early Oral Starvation on Course of Infantile Diarrhea. *J. Pediat.* 33: 14.

Kahn, E., and S. Wayburne. 1961. Hypoglycemia in Patients Suffering from Advanced Protein Malnutrition (Kwashiorkor). *Proc. Nutr. Soc. S. Afr.* 1: 21.

Kerry, K. R., and C. M. Anderson. 1964. A Ward Test for Sugar in Feces. *Lancet* i: 981.

Metcoff, J., S. Frenk, T. Yoshida, R. T. Pinedo, E. Kaiser, and J. D. L. Hansen. 1966. Cell Composition and Metabolism in Kwashiorkor (Severe Protein-Calorie Malnutrition in Children). *Medicine* 45: 365.

Northway, J. D., K. Cahill, J. Davies, P. T. Kawaguchi, and L. F. Miller. 1965. A Study of "Infantile Diarrhea" in Egypt. Unpublished.

10 | Infant Feeding Practices

Breast-feeding of infants in the Arab countries has probably followed the tenets of the sacred book *el Qura'an* with little apparent change since the spread of Islam. The following is an English version of the passage taken from Sûrah II, paragraph 233.

Mothers shall suckle their children for two whole years, (that is) for those who wish to complete the suckling. . . . If they desire to wean the child by mutual consent and (after) consultation, it is no sin for them; and if ye wish to give your children out to nurse, it is no sin for you, provided that ye pay what is due from you in kindness.[1]

The Arab physicians of the ninth and tenth centuries, who greatly influenced the teaching and practice of medicine during the Middle Ages through their medical writings, were, according to Wickes (1953), more interested in children's disease than in infant feeding. However, the famous Moslem physician Avicenna, who flourished in the early eleventh century, laid down the principles of infant feeding and weaning in his Canon of Medicine. The following account of his views on this important subject is based on *A Treatise on the Canon of Medicine of Avicenna* by Gruner (1930).

Avicenna recognized the importance of breast milk in infant feeding and stipulated that whenever possible mother's milk should be given by suckling, for that is the material most suitable and adapted

---

1. M. M. Pickthall, *The Meaning of the Glorious Koran* (New York: New American Library, 1963), p. 54.

Infant Feeding Practices   183

for the infant. According to him it should suffice for the infant to suck the breast twice or thrice in the day at first, and it should not be allowed to take too much. In the case of inability to feed the infant, a wet nurse should be selected.

The normal duration of lactation, according to Avicenna, should be two years (which is in line with the precept of *el Qura'an*). When a supplement is required, addition should be made step by step. Weaning must not be abrupt. After the first two teeth have appeared, a program of stronger aliment is to be considered. To begin, premasticated bread should be given. Things which are hard to chew should not be allowed. Afterwards bread softened with honey water, diluted wine, or milk may be given. In weaning, aliments must consist of articles which can be sucked up. Replacement with bread and sugar should be gradual. Soft meats may be given.

That Avicenna's advice had influenced breast-feeding in the Middle Ages in the European countries as far as England becomes evident from the following passage:

Avicen aviseth to geve the chylde sucke two yeres howe be it amonge us most commenlye they sucke but one yeare. And then ye wyll wene them/then not to do it sodenly but a lytell and lytell and to make for it little pills of bread and sugre to eate and accustom it so/tyll it be able to eate all manner of meate.[2]

Since then the picture has changed beyond recognition as far as Europe and North America are concerned. The modern infant-feeding practices in these regions are based on scientific knowledge and are capable of promoting healthy growth in infants and weanlings.

Phenomenal advances in science and technology and their application have raised, through the industrial and economic development, the standards of life in the western world. The availability of safe cow milk, milk products, infant formulas, and special baby foods has, together with elevation of the general standard of education and spread of knowledge of infant and child care, made it possible for the populations of these regions to adopt satisfactory methods of feeding infants. These changes have passed by the developing countries and have only minimally influenced the standard of life and the ways of living of the large bulk of their populations. This is true of the Arab countries as well. It is small wonder then that the infant-feeding and -weaning practices have changed comparatively little over the past

---

2. Thomas Raynalde, "Byrthe of Mankynde," First Boke, Cap. X, folio Iix, pub. 1540, quoted in Wickes, I. G. (1953).

centuries. If anything, the increasing poverty of the masses may have caused further deterioration because of their inability to buy even the necessities for feeding infants when breast milk supply starts failing.

At the present time, infants are generally breast fed in Egypt and neighboring Arab countries up to two years of age. It is probable that the infant gets milk enough for its needs during the first five months, for its growth during this period is reasonably satisfactory. It is at this stage that supplementary feeding is usually introduced. Social customs, cultural traditions, and economic necessity are the determinants in the actual supplementary feeding practices which prevail. They are not conducive to the healthy growth of the infant. Thus it is the unsatisfactory feeding practices during weaning and immediate post-weaning periods which are largely, if not wholly, responsible for the retardation in growth which sets in in early infancy. These practices lay down the foundations of malnutrition from which children in these countries suffer. It is therefore worth-while to describe in some detail the relevant studies on this subject, if only to point out the current practices and their defects with a view to finding ways and means of improving them.

EGYPT

Abdou, Lebshtein, and Kassim (1965) have studied the weaning practices and supplementary feeding of 1,143 infants up to 24 months in age attending the Maternal and Child Health Centers in Cairo. This was the same sample on which measurements of body weights and lengths were made. The family incomes varied from less than 1£.Eg. to over 5£.Eg. per head per month; 68% of the families had incomes of less than 3 £.Eg. per head per month. Almost all mothers nursed their infants and continued to do so up to the second year of life. Abdou et al. observed that breast-feeding is discontinued, usually abruptly, between 12 and 24 months. In this they may not be entirely correct, for the experience of other workers in Cairo seems to be different. According to Abdou et al. (1965), about 70% of infants were off breast by 18 months. Infants are breast fed exclusively up to 3 months with a few exceptions; supplementary foods are usually introduced after this period. The use of animal milk as supplementary food was limited to comparatively small proportion, starting with 10% of infants before 6 months of age and rising to 22% in infants of 12 to 24 months in age. It was the relatively well-off families in which animal milk was used as a supplementary food. Less than 10% of infants were given rice water, which was introduced in the first three months. Boiled rice, potatoes, biscuits, stewed broad beans, bread, and milk puddings were given as supplementary foods after six months. The proportion of infants receiving these increased in the 9–12 and 12–24 months' periods. In this latter age group 70% of the infants received boiled rice, potatoes, and bread; 47% were given stewed beans, and 37% local cheese and cooked vegetables. Between 20 and 25% of infants in this age group ate biscuits. Eggs and meat as supplementary foods were received by 8 and 14% of infants, respectively, and only after 12 months. These infants, as well as those who received fruit juices, belonged to the families in the higher income groups. Stewed broad beans, or *fool medammès,* seemed to be the only protein-rich food in the list of supplementary foods given to a majority of infants. Rice, bread, and potatoes also contributed their quota of proteins. Less than 3% of infants received orange juice before 9 months; even after 12 months only 22% received it daily. Cooked vegetables, when the children received them, appeared to be the only other and somewhat attenuated source of vitamin C.

It is the practice in Egypt to give to infants infusions of anise or caraway seeds. These can hardly be considered as supplementary foods. These preparations are given in between breast-feedings almost from birth. Their main purpose is to act as carminatives. In the study of Abdou *et al.,* the administration of these infusions was not observed after the infant had reached 9 months in age; in fact it virtually stopped at the age of six months.

Several Egyptian workers interested in the study of protein-calorie-deficiency disease have made reference to the unsatisfactory nature of the current feeding practices, but the only observations which yield some quantitative information are those of Abdou *et al.* described above. Even these, unfortunately, do not take us very far. These authors give the nutrient composition of the various supplementary foods, most of which have been mentioned above. However, they do not indicate the quantities of any of those received by the infants. Furthermore, the breast-milk intakes of infants at different ages have not been studied. In the absence of such information it is difficult to evaluate the calorie and nutrient intake of infants during the supplementary feeding stage. Although the general impression that supplementary feeding is both quantitatively and qualitatively inadequate is borne out by the retardation in growth, the onset of which coincides with the probable diminution in the amount of breast milk secreted in terms of the increasing needs of the infant, one would have liked quantitative information on food intake and the amount of nutrients derived therefrom. The only information about breast milk in Egypt is from an analysis for proximate principles on 40 samples at different stages of lactation from 1 month to 9 months reported by El Soufei (1933). According to him the average composition of breast milk is protein, 1.8%; fat, 3.2%, and lactose, 6.9%.

JORDAN

The ICNND-ICNJ Nutrition Survey on infants and preschool children (ICNND, 1964, and Pharaon et al., 1965) and the WHO study on vitamin A deficiency in Jordan (Patwardhan and Kamel, 1967) are the two principal sources of our information regarding the infant-feeding practices in Jordan. These two studies included observations on 2,843 and 1,297 children, respectively, from birth to 5 or 6 years of age; and the sample was representative of the rural and urban populations of Jordan as well as of the large number of Palestinian refugees in that country awaiting settlement of their problem.

Breast-feeding of infants is universal in Jordan; almost all infants are breast fed till after three months. The proportion of those weaned increases thereafter, but even at 12 months only 25% are weaned, at 16 months 50%. Ten percent of children continue to feed at breast even at 20 months (Pharaon et al., 1965).

Supplementary foods are usually introduced after three months. However, Pharaon et al. found that about 25% of infants of less than three months received some supplementary food. The reasons for this early introduction of supplementary feeding were usually deficient lactation or mother's illness. Under such circumstances the infants generally received animal milk as supplementary food. It was only after three months that other articles of food in addition to or in lieu of animal milk were used as supplements. The progressive increase with age in the use of supplementary foods in addition to breast milk is well illustrated in the figure taken from the publication of Pharaon et al.

The practice of administering infusions of anise, caraway, and other species is observed in Jordan as in Egypt, probably for the same reason. Patwardhan and Kamel (1967) observed, as did Pharaon et al., that commonly food supplementation started with an animal milk (cow, sheep, or goat), usually heavily diluted. They also found tea and rice water being given as beverages in early infancy. As the baby grows older, solid foods, such as bread, boiled rice, biscuits, potatoes, and sometimes soft-cooked portions from the family diet, are gradually introduced. Still later the quantity of bread in infants' diets increases and is supplemented with a variety of other solid foods such

Infant Feeding Practices

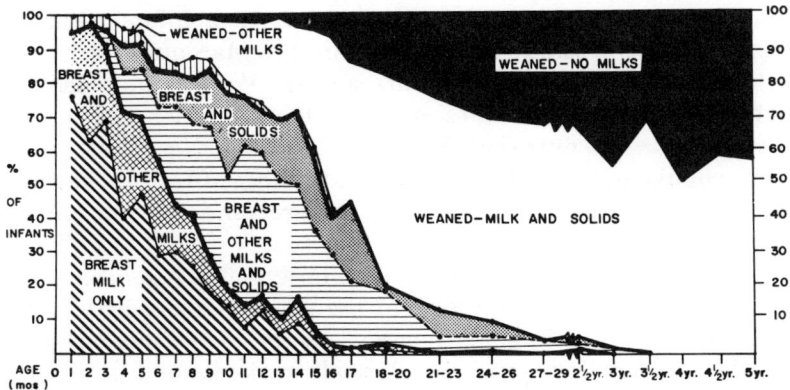

Figure 10.1. Supplementary Foods used in Jordan in infant feeding (ICNND-ICNJ Pediatric Survey Report).

as cooked or stewed beans, cooked vegetables, yoghurt, and local cheese. Eggs, liver, and meat preparations are given even less frequently than animal milks. Patwardhan and Kamel attempted to obtain from mothers at the interview the approximate quantities of food given and their frequency of consumption. On a rough assessment of diets of infants and children which this information provided, the authors concluded that 78% of the infants and children received inadequate amounts of dietary protein, and 38% received an inadequate amount of vitamin A value. Patwardhan and Kamel did not try to assess even roughly the intakes of other nutrients, but the information provided by them is enough to show that the supplementary feeding practices as well as the diets of children between 2 and 6 years of age need to be improved to ensure freedom from nutritional deficiency and appropriate rates of growth.

LEBANON

We have referred in another chapter to the observations of McLaren *et al.* (1964) about the current infant-feeding practices in Lebanon and their effects on the health and growth of infants. A detailed study on 365 mothers and their infants by Harfouche (1965) provides a wealth of information on feeding practices among the Lebanese living in Beirut. The mothers forming the subject of the study were those who had availed themselves of the antenatal services at the American University Hospital, Beirut, and had delivered at full term in the University Hospital. They were followed by periodic home visits for 18 months from the birth of their infants. The self-selected group consisted of 131 Armenian, 120 Maronite (Arab Christian), and 114 Sunni (Arab Muslim) families. We are concerned principally with the Arab families, owing to the limitations set by us in dealing only with nutrition in countries of the Near East almost wholly populated by Arabs. The salient findings of Harfouche among these families are summarized below. For greater details the reader is referred to the original publication.

A large majority of the mothers under observation had been born in Beirut and between 75 and 80% of the Arab mothers had lived in Beirut for more than 5 years. Over 85% belonged to social classes III and IV—i.e., skilled artisans, clerical workers, and semiskilled workers—according to the U.K. Registrar General's classification. The average monthly income per head was estimated at 49 to 52 Lebanese pounds (equivalent to $16–17 U.S.). This represented the earning of the father only, for 94% of the mothers had no occupation other than that of a housewife. Sixty-nine percent of Christian mothers and 84% of Muslim mothers were literate. These details are given to indicate the type of the sample with which Harfouche dealt. It probably is representative of the lower-middle-class urban population in Lebanon.

In the first month after birth 97% of the infants were breast fed; 80% were exclusively breast fed and 17% partially so. Thereafter the proportion of infants fed at breast progressively decreased as shown in Figure 2.

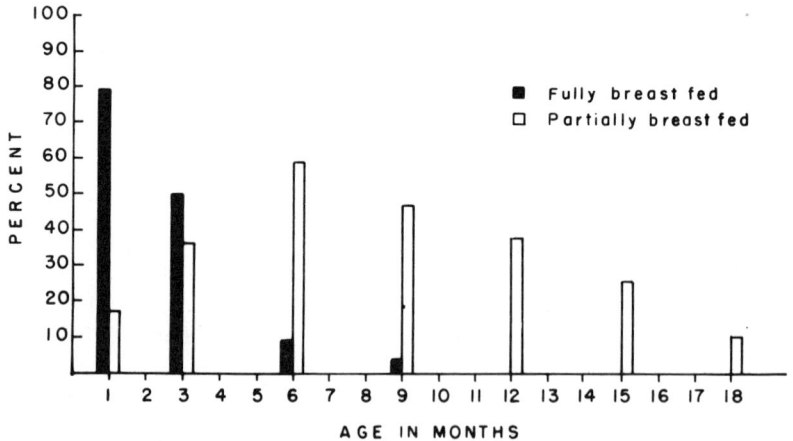

Figure 10.2. Percentage of infants exclusively or partially breast-fed in Beirut, Lebanon (Data of Harfouche 1965 on Maronite and Sunni Infants).

The figure shows that about 4% of infants were, even at 9 months, completely breast fed. Partial breast-feeding continued much longer: about 38% were partially breast fed at 12 months and about 10% at 18 months. In this respect the picture is not dissimilar to that seen in Egypt and Jordan.

In contrast to the assertion of Abdou *et al.* about the prevalent practice of abrupt weaning in Egypt, Harfouche found that among the infants she studied in Beirut, only 8.2% were abruptly weaned. Of these, two thirds were weaned by 1-1/2 months of age. The causes of abrupt weaning were usually emotional or mother's illness. The large majority of infants was weaned gradually, about 90% being completely weaned by 18 months after birth. The remainder probably go on receiving some feeding at breast till about 24 months or even later, as has been shown to occur in Egypt and Jordan.

The commonest cause of complete weaning was pregnancy. The other causes in the order mentioned were spontaneous drying up of the breast or illness of the mother. The refusal of the baby to suckle, the not-infrequent tendency of the infant with erupting teeth to bite the nipple, or the illness of the infant were other important causes for the completion of the weaning process.

Beverages such as tea, coffee, cocoa, and carbonated waters were started, usually three months after birth. Tea was the commonest beverage given and was considered a substitute for milk after six months. The practice of administering a variety of infusions with carminative properties, such as infusions of anise, cumin, orange blossom, or other herbs and flowers, has also been recorded as current in Lebanon.

Soft-cooked cereals such as *burghul* and rice, bread, and biscuits were introduced early, between 4 to 6 months, together with strained soup of lentils. Preparations made from chick-pea were popular among the Lebanese as supplementary food for infants. Other supplementary foods used in the decreasing order of frequency included fruits, vegetables, meat, sweets, dairy products such as yoghurt and white cheese (*leben* and *lebneh*), nuts and roasted chick-peas, eggs, and fish. Fruit juices were more commonly administered to infants by Lebanese mothers than in Jordan or Egypt, reflecting not only the over-all greater availability of a variety of fruit in Lebanon in contrast to the other neighboring countries but also the higher economic status of the families studied by Harfouche.

Harfouche has studied the attitudes of the mothers to breast-feeding and weaning practices. Obviously the cultural background as well as tradition largely influences these attitudes which change only gradually, almost imperceptibly. These attitudes govern the behavior of the mother towards the baby, particularly through the first twelve months of its life. When to put the newborn to the breast, how often to feed it during the day, how long to breast-feed the infant, what supplementary foods to give and when to introduce them, how to control, regulate, and modify infants' feeds during its illness and in convalescence are some of the aspects in which practice is dictated by tradition, tempered by advice from the elderly relations and friends and acquaintances among the neighbors. Physicians, public health nurses, and other maternal- and child-health workers have a minimum influence in the matter. It is therefore only slowly that tradition gives way to the influence of modern scientific knowledge in infant nutrition.

The findings of Puyet, Downs, and Budeir (1963) among the Palestine refugees in UNRWA camps in Lebanon are in general agreement with the Arab practices discussed thus far. They also found that breast-feeding was the rule: 90% of infants were at breast at 6 months, 80% at 12 months, and 40% at 18 months. Supplements were usually started at 4 months. Since the refugees had UNRWA whole milk powder given free, there was much greater use of reconstituted, diluted, and sugared whole milk as a supplement than in other communities. The other supplements were the same as those observed by Harfouche, although meat, fish, and eggs were conspicuous by their absence. This probably reflects the situation among the poor Lebanese as well. The infant starts sampling at one year the food prepared for the family as a whole, and by the end of the second year the majority of children are on the regular family diet.

Puyet *et al.* make one interesting point which is worthy of mention. They found that the earlier a child was taken off breast the slower was its gain in weight. Breast-fed infants with and without supplements gained weight faster than those fed artificially. The findings of Harfouche in Beirut are at variance with this observation. She found that after 6 months and up to 18 months, the partially weaned infants (presumably receiving supplementary foods) showed lower growth increments than those who were completely weaned. It would appear therefore that a fully weaned infant after six months is more likely to get adequate amounts of food as compared to the one who is still at breast. In the latter case the mother probably is unable fully to appreciate the infant's needs, since it partially feeds at breast. Thus there is greater likelihood of its suffering from undernutrition than an artificially fed infant, mostly through ignorance.

REFERENCES

Abdou, I. A., H. E. Ali, and A. K. Lebshtein. 1965. A Study of the Nutritional Status of Mothers, Infants and Young Children Attending Maternity and Child Health Centers in Cairo. Part I—The Nutritional Status of Infants and Young Children. *Bull. Nutr. Inst. U.A.R.* 1: 9.

Gruner, O. C. 1930. *A Treatise on the Canon of Medicine of Avicenna.* London: Luzac and Co.

Harfouche, J. K. 1965. Feeding Practices and Weaning Practices of Lebanese Infants. Beirut, Lebanon: Khayats.

McLaren, D. S., C. Ammoun, and G. Houri. 1964. The Socio-Economic Background of Marasmus in Lebanon. *Leb. Med. J.* 17: 85–96.

Patwardhan, V. N., and W. W. Kamel. 1967. *Studies on Vitamin A Deficiency in Infants and Young Children in Jordan.* Geneva, Switzerland: World Health Organization.

Pharaon, H. M., W. J. Darby, H. A. Shammout, E. B. Bridgforth, and C. S. Wilson. 1965. A Year-Long Study of the Nutriture of Infants and Preschool Children in Jordan. *J. Trop. Pediat.* 11: Monograph 39, No. 3.

Puyet, J. H., E. F. Downs, and R. Budeir. 1963. Nutritional and Growth Characteristics of Arab Refugee Children in Lebanon. *Amer. J. Clin. Nutr.* 13: 147.

Wickes, I. G. 1953. A History of Infant Feeding. Part I—Primitive Peoples: Ancient Works: Renaissance Writers. *Arch. Dis. Child.* 28: 151.

11 GROWTH AND DEVELOPMENT OF CHILDREN

INFANTS

EGYPT. The earliest reported study in Egypt, to our knowledge, of the growth of infants is by Khalik (1929). It comprises his observations at the Kasr-el-Ainy Hospital in Cairo and four Child Welfare Centers in different parts of the city. Khalik has reported his findings on the weights and lengths of the newborn and the growth of infants during the first year of life. These will be referred to in appropriate places in the following discussion. Interest in the important problem of child growth seems to have lain dormant for more than two decades afterward, in spite of the inauguration and development of practical nutrition programs in the country at the beginning of World War II. It is only during the last 10 to 15 years that one finds publications which provide valuable information on infant and child growth.

The average birth weights and lengths of the Egyptian infants seem to be only slightly lower than those of babies in Europe and America. The reported figures from Egypt are given in Table 1.

Little difference appears between the average birth weights reported in 1929 and those reported in more recent years from Cairo and Alexandria. Khalik's (1929) observations were made on infants born in the Midwifery Section of the Kasr-el-Ainy Hospital; so were those of Kamal (1962) in his first series of infants. The figures reported by Sherbini and his colleagues were also from large hospitals in Alexandria. The clientele at these hospitals in Cairo and Alexandria is mostly derived from the comparatively poorer sections of the community, including the lower middle classes.

TABLE 1
THE AVERAGE BODY WEIGHTS AND LENGTHS OF THE EGYPTIAN NEWBORN AT TERM

	Babies M & F No.	Males Weight kg	Males Length cm	Females Weight kg	Females Length cm
Cairo					
Khalik (1929)	802	3.200	50.5	3.030	49.5
Kamal (1962)					
1st series	539	3.300		3.150	
2nd series	300	3.637	49.7	3.403	49.3
Alexandria					
Sherbini and Atallah (1960)	208	3.340		3.230	
Abd and Sherbini (1965)	1790	3.300		3.200	
21 other authors quoted by Kamal (1962) for birth weights in Europe and U.S.A.		3.455		3.306	

Kamal's second series consists of babies who were delivered in a private hospital. Their families were considered to belong to the middle and upper-middle classes, and the mothers did not presumably suffer from malnutrition or from the lack of antenatal care. Although the average birth weights in the second series are higher than those in the first series, the differences are comparatively small. As the table shows, the average birth weights reported by various authors for babies born in some European countries (England, France, Germany) and in U.S.A. fall in between the values given by Kamal for his two series of observations. The findings of Sherbini and Attallah (1960) on the birth weights of 208 infants born in Alexandria University Maternity Hospital were on a sample obtained by weighing every third full-term infant born in the hospital. The average birth weight for girls was 3.230 kg and for boys 3.340. The families of the newborn came from the low, medium, and high income groups in Alexandria, and thus the average birth weights of infants in this series helps to give an average picture of the Egyptian newborn as can be seen by the later report of Abd and Sherbini (1965) on a much larger sample.

The average crown-heel length given in Table 1 shows minor differences between the different sets of observations, which could easily be due to the difference in the techniques of measurement and the quality of the tapes used in measuring the length. The average crown-heel lengths for the male and female newborn, taken together, were as follows:

Khalik (1929) in Cairo	50.1 cm
Kamal (1962) in Cairo, 2nd series	49.5 cm
Abd and Sherbini (1965) in Alexandria	49.88 cm

As Kamal observed, these values are similar to the averages for the European and American babies at birth.

Khalik (1929) measured the weights of 3,064 boys and 2,753 girls of different ages between birth and 12 months at four Child Welfare Centers in Cairo and compared the monthly gains in weight with the then available figures for the English, French, and German infants. Khalik found that after 5 months of age the Egyptian infants showed a fall in the rate of increase in body weight, with the result that their average weight at the end of the year was well below that of the European infants of one year. Thus Khalik anticipated the later observations on the early growth retardation due to malnutrition.

It appears thus that the growth of Egyptian infants occurs at the normal rate up to about 5 months after birth, during which period they double their birth weight. This was also the observation made by Abdou, Ali, and Lebshtein (1965) resulting from a study of 1,143 infants and children up to 24 months of age attending the Well Baby Clinics of four Maternity and Child Health Centers in Cairo. The sample can be considered fairly representative of the urban and suburban population and was chiefly derived from poor and lower-middle socioeconomic strata of the community. Growth seems to start falling off at about five months after birth and continues to deviate from the Iowa means: at 24 months the average weight of the Cairo infants was about 3.2 kg less than that of the Iowa children, and the average height was 14 cm lower. In short, growth was retarded by 16% in length and by 25% in weight. This must have been largely due to the effect of two contributory factors. Abdou *et al.* (1965) found that infants in Cairo suffered during the first year of life from infectious episodes, prominent among which were those involving the gastrointestinal and upper respiratory tracts. According to them the proportion of infants suffering from infection of one kind or the other increased with age, so that by the time the infants had reached 16 months every one of those examined had had one or more bouts of respiratory infections and diarrhea, which must have interrupted the normal rate of growth.

The second contributory factor in growth retardation must have been the unsatisfactory infant-feeding practices, which result in undernutrition and malnutrition of the infant in the weaning period, which presumably starts at about the fifth month of life. This aspect is discussed in detail later.

Wishahi and Khattab (1962) have given figures for "ideal" weights and lengths of Egyptian "full term healthy babies of well-to-do families, well fed, well cared for, regularly weighed and measured from birth up to 2 years by one of the authors." Unfortunately the authors give no more information about the size, composition, and other relevant characteristics of this sample. On the assumption that the figures given by them are based on a fair-sized sample, it would seem that given adequate and appropriate supplementary feeding, medical care, and comparative freedom from infections, the Egyptian infants do nearly as well in growth performance as the U.S. infants during the first 24 months. However as the majority of Egyptian infants from 5 months onwards suffer from malnutrition and are also exposed to frequent episodes of acute infection, it is reasonable to conclude that the curve of growth given by Abdou et al. (1965) would represent the current pattern of infant growth in Egypt. The ideal growth curve constructed from figures given by Wishahi and Khattab and the observations of Abdou et al. on 1,143 infants and children are plotted in the same figure (Figure 1) for comparison.

Singularly enough, the published Egyptian literature does not, so far as we are aware, yield any information on the growth of Egyptian children between the ages of 2 and 5 years. Presumably the children between these age limits are too old to attend the well baby clinics; obviously they are too young for admission to primary schools, the two locations where their heights and weights are likely to be measured and health conditions noted. Thus the preschool child in Egypt seems to have been relatively unstudied. Since at the age of 5 years the average weight of children approximates the 16th percentile of the Iowa values, it is reasonable to conclude that the retardation in growth which set in during the first year of life continues through the preschool age period into the school age.

LEBANON AND JORDAN. The birth weights and lengths of Arab infants in Lebanon and Jordan, as given in Table 2, are comparable with those of the Egyptian newborn. The sample of Pharaon

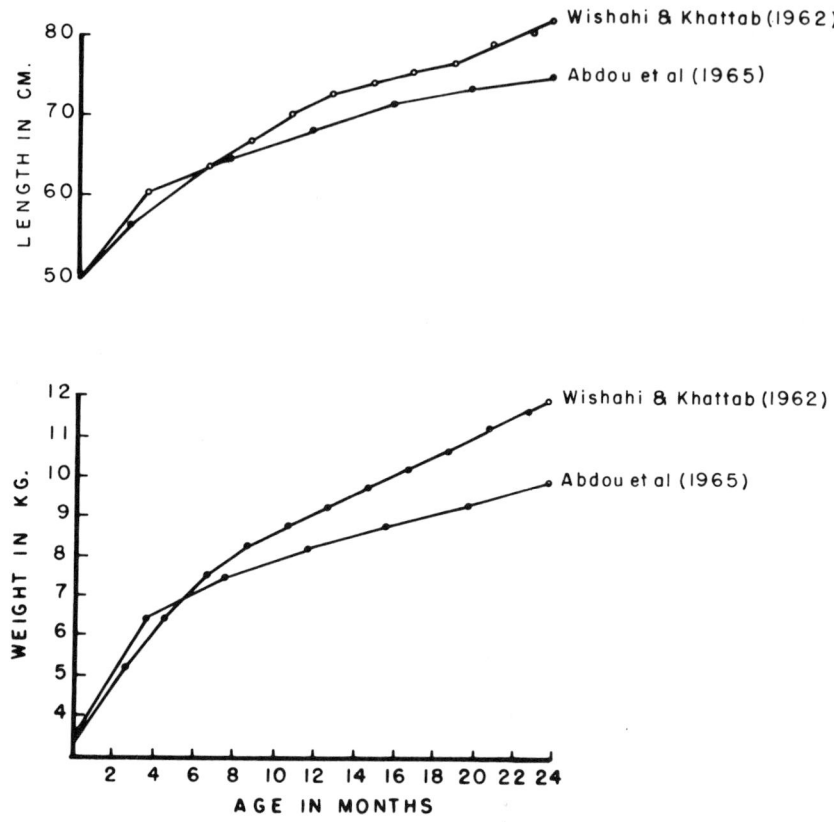

Figure 11.1. Growth Rates of Egyptian infants as average weights and lengths from birth to twenty-four months. For explanation see text.

et al. (1965) is derived from the consecutive deliveries conducted at the Government Maternity Hospital in Amman from June to December 1962. The average birth weights have been calculated on single births only.

The infants observed by Harfouche (1966) were delivered at the American University Hospital, Beirut. They belonged to three communities, namely, Armenian, Maronite (Arab Christians), and Sunni (Arab Muslims). There were slight differences in birth weights within groups, but they were not statistically significant. Harfouche followed these infants by making observations on their growth and health in periodic home visits. The growth chart derived from this study gives a better picture of infant growth in the Lebanese since it was a longitudinal study, and by necessity the group had to be small and manage-

TABLE 2
BIRTH WEIGHTS AND LENGTHS OF FULL-TERM JORDANIAN AND LEBANESE INFANTS

	Birth Weight in kg		Birth Length in cm	
	Male	Female	Male	Female
Jordan	3.300	3.180	49.9	49.7
	(1040)	(912)	(1027)	(898)
Lebanon	3.41	3.33	50.1	49.5
	(198)	(175)	(198)	(175)

able. Harfouche observed slight deviations in increments in weights and lengths which were associated with supplementary feeding and illnesses; however, at the end of 18 months, the situation was much better than expected. The mean weight deficits (from the expected values) were -0.57 kg for males and -0.90 kg for females. In lengths, the average deviation for males was -0.3 cm and for females -1.2 cm. The over-all performance of these infants was satisfactory, as Figure 2, which plots together the growth patterns observed in Jordan by Pharaon et al. and those observed by Harfouche in Lebanon, shows. The growth rate of infants studied by Harfouche is comparable with the "ideal" growth rate of Egyptian infants reported by Wishahi and Khattab (Figure 1). Although the intention of Harfouche in her study was only to obtain information, and not to educate the mothers, the very fact of frequent visits by her team and the health supervision which they offered seemed to have involuntarily produced desirable results in an improved growth pattern. It is however noteworthy that the illness pattern between birth and 18 months was not much different as compared to that in Egypt or Jordan. Almost all children under observation suffered at one time or other from illnesses such as infections of the respiratory tract, diarrheas of varying severity, and infections of the eye, ear, and skin for varying periods. In spite of this, the average growth of these infants was satisfactory. This leads to the inescapable conclusion that better infant-feeding practices in this particular group of infants were probably responsible for a reasonably satisfactory growth pattern.

It will be interesting to compare the results obtained by Harfouche with those of a cross-sectional study in Lebanese infants. If the limited observations of ICNND are any indication, a lower rate of growth in the general Lebanese Arab population, not very much different from that seen in Egypt and Jordan, may be expected. Some light on this aspect is thrown by findings in Palestine refugees in Lebanon mentioned below.

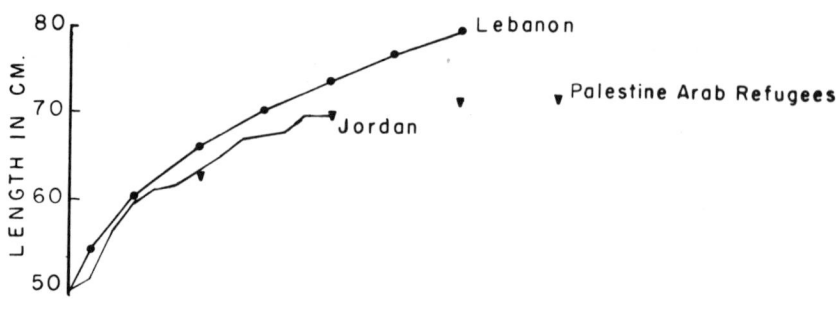
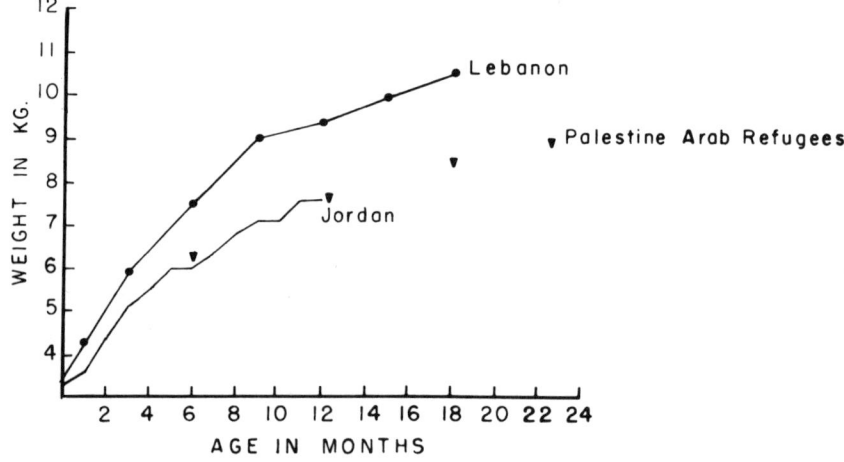

Figure 11.2. Growth rates of Lebanese and Jordanian infants.
•———• Lebanese
———— Jordanian Refugees and Non-refugees Combined.
▼ Jordanian Refugees only.

Puyet, Downs, and Budeir (1963) reported an average birth weight of 3.30 kg in 338 infants born in a year in a small Palestine refugee camp. In a review of about 5,000 infant charts maintained at the Maternal and Child Health Centers of UNRWA in Lebanon, Puyet *et al.* found that the growth of the refugee infants in the first five to six months was fairly satisfactory as compared with the western standards. The growth rate fell off after this period. A further survey of 324 infant charts and follow-up observations on the infants showed that at 24 months the average body weights and lengths of boys and girls were near the 3rd percentile of the Iowa standards. The growth rate continued to be retarded up to 3 years. If observations had continued beyond this period, it is probable that the authors would have found growth retardation to continue in the school age as well.

The findings of Puyet et al. seem to be in general agreement with those made in infants and children among the nonrefugee populations of Egypt and Jordan.

It was found in the Jordan Pediatric Study that the growth of Jordanian infants in the first few months was similar to the average of the Iowa standards. The mean weight curve started falling off between 2 to 3 months. It was followed a month or so later by a fall in length. As a result the average weights and lengths of Jordanian infants at 12 and 24 months were well below the averages of the Iowa standards. The reasons for such growth failure were in general similar to those observed in Egypt. A substantial proportion of infants suffered from single and/or recurrent diarrhea and respiratory infections. The incidence of these infections was two to three times higher in 10% of the 1811 children under 24 months who were considered malnourished.

One can profitably compare the results of the two cross-sectional studies of Abdou et al. in Egypt and Pharaon et al. in Jordan. The sample in Egypt was principally derived from the urban area, whereas the Jordanian sample consisted of the urban and rural populations. The growth curves in the first twelve months of life, constructed from the two sets of observations, seem to run close together. At 12 months the average weight of Jordanian infants was lower than that of the Egyptian infants by 0.7 kg; on the other hand the average length of the Jordanian infants was higher by 1.8 cm. Both the samples had average lengths and body weights lower than the Iowa standards. These observations must lead to the conclusion that the growth of infants in Egypt and Jordan is almost similar in the first year of life and possibly similar also to that in other Arab countries as well. This conclusion is strengthened by the similarity of these growth rates with those observed in many non-Arab developing countries in the tropics and subtropics, in all of which similar contributory factors, namely defective supplementary feeding and frequent infections, operate to the detriment of normal growth.

CHILDREN BETWEEN 2 AND 6 YEARS

We have already deplored the lack of information on the growth rates of Egyptian children between 2 and 5 years of age. Unfortunately we also did not have available to us records of heights and weights of a sufficiently large number of Lebanese and Libyan children of this age as indications of the average growth pattern in these countries. The only reasonably good data are from Jordan, derived principally from the studies of Pharaon et al. (1965) and Patwardhan and Kamel (1967) on a total of a little less than 4,000 infants and children up to 6 years of age. The sample was derived from the urban and rural populations in different parts of Jordan and also included the Palestine refugee population. The growth curves constructed separately for boys and girls based on the observations of Pharaon et al. are illustrated in Figures 3 and 4.

The two studies in Jordan referred to above were done one year apart and for somewhat different purposes, and the sampling was independent. Despite this, the results are close enough, as can be seen from Figures 3 and 4, to justify the conclusion that these curves illustrate the average pattern of growth of the Jordanian children. The average values of weights and heights for boys as well as girls approximate the 3rd percentile of the distribution of heights and weights of American children of comparable age (Nelson, 1959). The figures further show that the retardation in growth which was shown to set in earlier than 6 months during infancy continues throughout the preschool period. The underlying reasons may possibly be the same, that is, continuing malnutrition and frequent infections. This will become clear when we consider at a later stage the nutritional status of preschool children.

The observations of ICNND in Lebanon on 97 boys and 96 girls of 0 to 6 years are in general agreement with those described above for the Jordanian children. Considering the similarity of the growth patterns of infants in Egypt, Jordan, and Lebanon as illustrated earlier, there is no reason to believe that they would be appreciably different in preschool age children in these other countries.

SCHOOL AGE CHILDREN AND ADOLESCENTS

Abboud, Alfi, Hefny, and El Mazny (1957) made an anthropometric survey of Arabian children during which they examined 4,450 boys and 5,300 girls of 5 to 16 years in age from schools in Cairo. Hammoud, Khalil, and Sarhan (1961) measured the heights and weights of 986 boys and 975 girls of 6 to 13 years of age in primary schools of Alexandria as a part of the school health survey in that city. Labib (1964) has reported on the average heights and weights of 910 girls of 5 to 16 years of age from five schools in Alexandria. Abdou

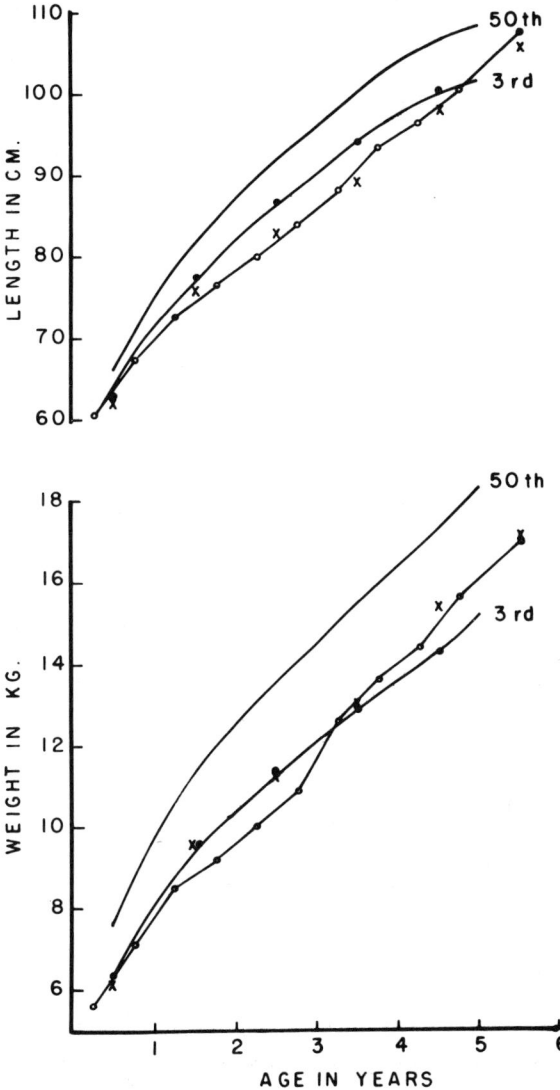

Figure 11.3. Average heights and weights of Jordanian boys 0 to 6 years in age. Third percentile, •———•; Pharaon et al; °———°; Patwardhan and Kamel; x. Both sets of observation include refugee and nonrefugee children from urban and rural areas.

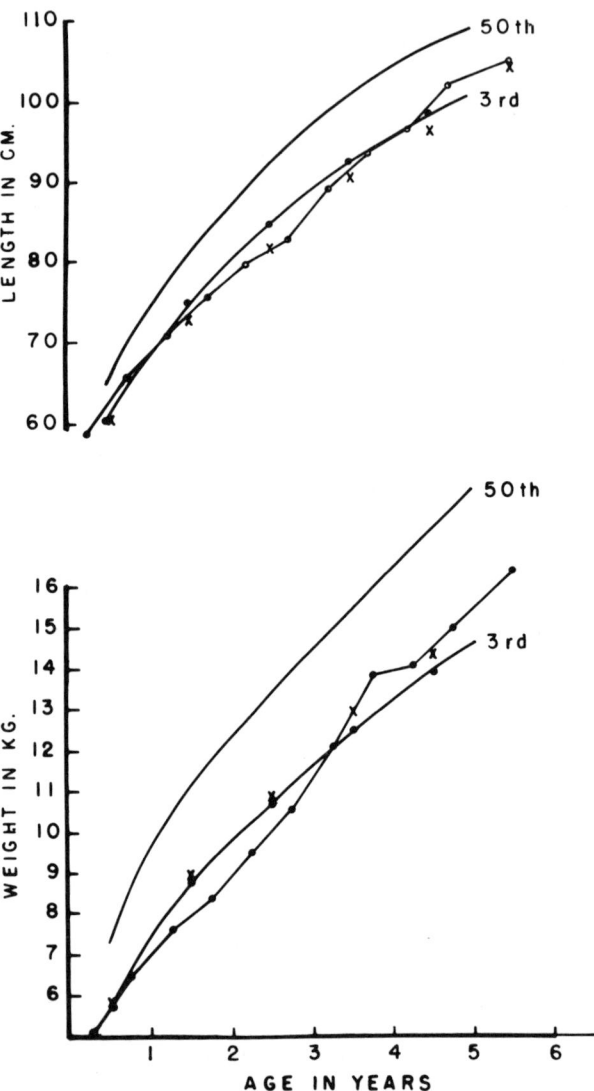

Figure 11.4. Average heights and weights of Jordanian girls 0 to 6 years in age. Third percentile, •———•; Pharaon et al, °———°; Patwardhan and Kamel, x. Both sets of observations include refugee and nonrefugee children from urban and rural areas.

Growth and Development of Children

and Mahfouz (1967) have determined heights and weights in 4,370 boys and 4,560 girls of 7 to 19 years of age. These children were from 252 classes of 64 primary, preparatory, and secondary schools in the north, middle, and south zones of Cairo, selected by the Central Bureau of Statistics of the Egyptian Government; hence they can be considered a representative sample of the population of school children in Cairo.

The values given by Abboud, Alfi, Hefny, and El Mazny (1957) are in percentiles, whereas all other authors give the mean values for heights and weights and standard deviations. The 50th percentile values of Abboud *et al.* (1957) are plotted in Figures 5 to 8 together with the averages reported by other authors.

Boys. The average heights and weights (Figures 5 and 6) of the boys in Cairo schools as reported by Abdou and Mahfouz (1967) are

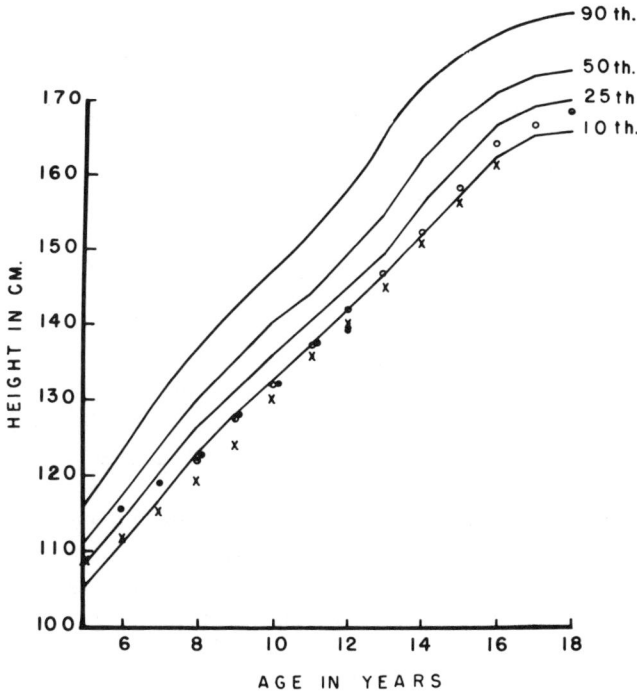

Figure 11.5. Average heights of Egyptian boys 5 to 18 years in age.
° from schools in Cairo, Abdou and Mahfouz.
x from schools in Cairo, Abboud *et al.*
• from schools in Alexandria, Hammoud.

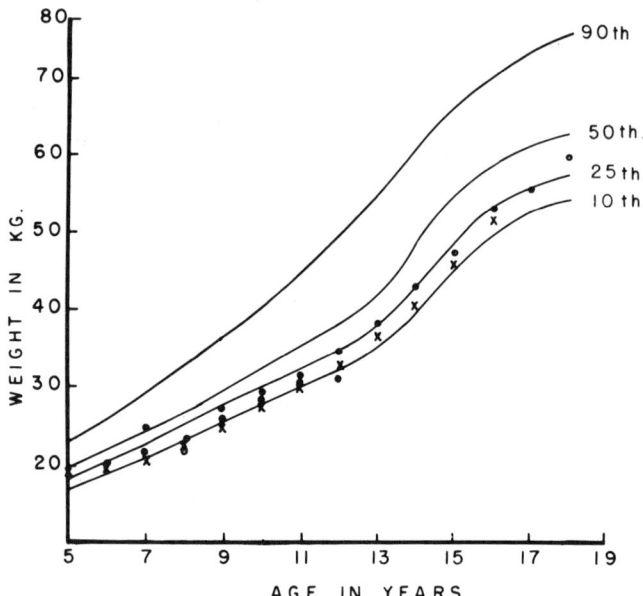

Figure 11.6. Average weights of Egyptian boys 5 to 18 years in age.
° from schools in Cairo, Abdou and Mahfouz.
x from schools in Cairo, Abboud *et al.*
• from schools in Alexandria, Hammoud.

in general higher than those reported by other authors, although the mean values of all observations seem to cluster together, particularly for the age groups of 10 to 15 years. The differences are larger for the earlier age groups, that is, 6 to 9 years. It is difficult to say whether these differences are significant, for the percentile values given by Abboud *et al.* cannot be used for statistical analysis. The height curve of Cairo boys examined by Abdou and Mahfouz lies along the 25th percentile of Iowa standards and the weight curve between the 10th and 25th percentile values of the Iowa standards. This would indicate that there is less retardation in growth in height than one can predict from weights alone. As a result the Egyptian boys are lighter for a given height than their American counterparts. In view of the care taken in the selection of the sample studied by Abdou and Mahfouz, one can conclude that the findings represent the average growth pattern of the urban school children, particularly as there is little difference between the reported mean values from Cairo and Alexandria.

Comparatively little information is available from the rural areas or from Upper Egypt. However Abdou (1965) examined in 1959–1960 a total of 945 boys in the oases of Kharga and Dakhla in the Egyptian Desert, lying between 500 and 600 kilometers southwest of Cairo. He found that the growth of the boys from the oases was at a level lower than that of Cairo school boys. There were minor differences between the oases. The boys from Dakhla had higher average heights and weights than those from Kharga, particularly from ten years on. It is difficult to decide in the absence of the relevant information whether these differences were real. In a recent study on children in a preparatory school in Sindion, a village about 20 kilometers northwest of Cairo, the average heights and weights of 278 school boys of 11 to 17 years were found to be lower than the averages reported by Abdou and Mahfouz for Cairo school children. There is thus reason to believe that in rural areas the growth of school age boys and adolescents will in general be at a lower level than that found in Cairo.

Girls. The growth pattern of Egyptian girls is illustrated in Figures 7 and 8. The findings of Labib (1964) on girls in Alexandria stand out in marked contrast with those of others, in that both heights

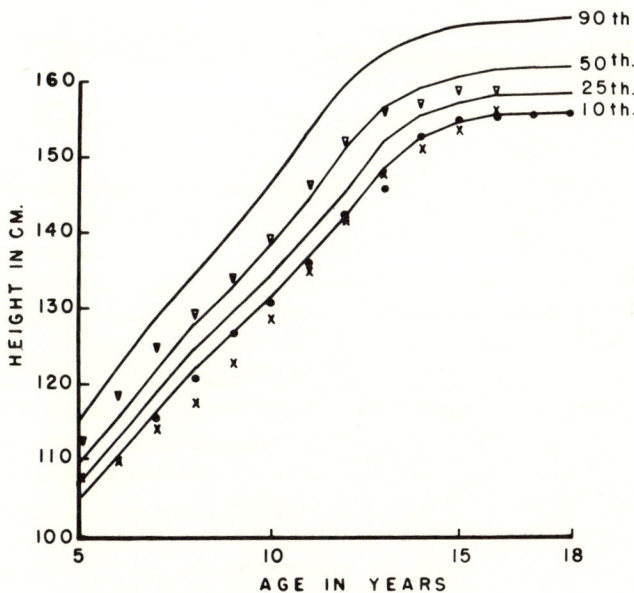

Figure 11.7. Average heights of Egyptian girls 5 to 18 years in age.
° from schools in Cairo, Abdou and Mahfouz.
x from schools in Cairo, Abboud et al.
▽ from schools in Alexandria, Labib.

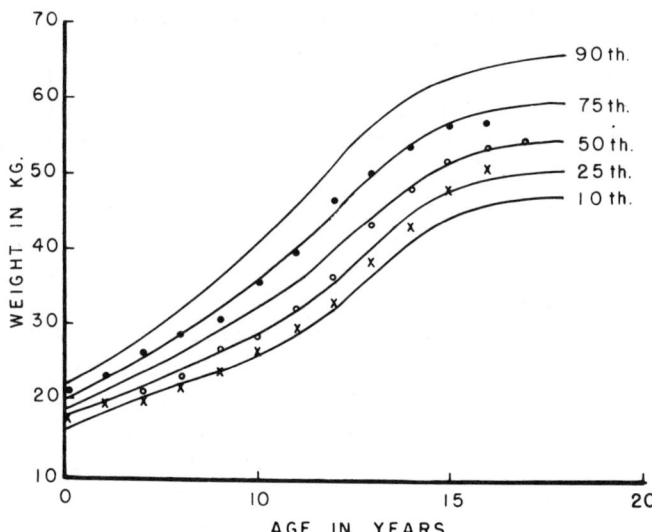

Figure 11.8. Average weight of Egyptian girls 5 to 18 years in age.
○ from schools in Cairo, Abdou and Mahfouz.
x from schools in Cairo, Abboud et al.
• from schools in Alexandria, Labib.

and weights of Labib's subjects are distinctly higher than those reported for school girls in Cairo and also those in Alexandria reported by Hammoud. The five schools in Alexandria in which Labib made his measurements catered to the families of the middle and upper-middle classes of Egyptians. These schools demanded annual tuition fees ranging from 25 to 80 Egyptian pounds for primary education and 45 to 120 Egyptian pounds for secondary education. It stands to reason that families which could afford such fees must be in a position not only to feed their infants and children well but also to take appropriate care of their health. These considerations are reflected in the higher levels of growth achieved by the girls from 5 to 16 years. A reference to the figures will show that whereas the average weights of Cairo school girls lie between the 10th and 50th percentile of the Iowa standards, those reported by Labib are close to the 75th percentile. So far as the average heights of Labib's girls are concerned, they approximate the 50th percentile, whereas the Cairo girls are between the 3rd and 10th percentile of the Iowa standards. Thus Labib's subjects were heavier for a given height as compared with the Iowa curves, whereas the Cairo girls were lighter, as the Cairo boys were found to be. One may be right in suspecting that

Growth and Development of Children

Labib's subjects were probably too well fed. These figures also provide a proof that better nutrition will ensure better growth in Egyptian children population than that currently observed in a majority of school children.

The findings of Abdou on 505 girls from the Kharga and Dakhla oases are consistent with those on boys from these areas in that the growth of the oasis girls was at a lower level than that of the school girls in Cairo.

Other Arab Countries

Our information on the growth of children in the neighboring Arab countries is derived principally from the reports of ICNND surveys in Libya, Lebanon, and Jordan. In addition, the observations on heights and weights reported by Ferro-Luzzi (1958) on school children in Libya and by Abboud et al. (1957) in Kuwait are also available. The number of children between 5 and 18 years of age examined during these studies is given in Table 3.

In Lebanon and Jordan and ICNND surveys included the children from the civilian population as well as those from the Palestine Arab refugees. The latter form a substantial proportion of the total population in these two countries. In fact refugees formed nearly 40% of the Jordanian population at the time of the survey. Since the living conditions of Palestinian refugees are somewhat different from those of the civilian population, it was of interest to see how the health and growth of the refugee children differed from that of their counterparts in the countries concerned.

In Lebanon small differences were apparent between the heights and weights of the civilian and refugee children. In general the refugee children were shorter and weighed less. Considered over the whole range from 5 to 18 years, the differences in favor of nonrefugee chil-

TABLE 3
NUMBER OF CHILDREN IN OTHER ARAB COUNTRIES
EXAMINED FOR HEIGHTS AND WEIGHTS

Country	Source	Boys	Girls	
Libya	Ferro-Luzzi (1958)	4389	651	
Libya	ICNND (1957)	180	262	
Lebanon	ICNND (1962)	492	666	
		489	430	Refugees
Jordan	ICNND (1963)	731	873	
		801	801	Refugees
Kuwait	Abboud et al. (1957)	3800	5667	

dren were as follows: boys, 1.34 cm in height and 1.8 kg in body weight; girls, 1.85 cm in height and 0.8 kg in body weight. On the other hand, in Jordan the differences in the heights and weights between the two groups were negligible. Figures 9 and 10 illustrate the trends in growth of boys and girls in Libya, Lebanon, and Jordan. Although Kuwait lies outside the area of our concern, the data for Kuwait have been included for comparison. Abboud et al. (1957), whose work on Cairo school children has been referred to earlier, also examined a large number of boys and girls in schools in Kuwait, and we found the results sufficiently interesting to include them in the discussion.

The growth of the children and adolescents in other Arab countries follows the general pattern as discussed for Egypt. The growth of Lebanese children is similar to that of Egyptian children. On the other hand, the Jordanian children follow at a lower level. In fact the mean values for their heights and weights are nearest the 3rd percentile of the Iowa standards. It will be recalled that the average growth of the preschool age children in Jordan also followed the 3rd percentile (Boston standards). It is difficult to indicate the reasons for the difference seen between the Lebanese and Jordanian children, since both are from the Arab stock and food habits are not materially different in both countries.

The Libyan sample of school children surveyed by ICNND is too small to permit any meaningful comparison. However, the observations of Ferro-Luzzi (1958) in Libya cover a large number of children of school age examined in Tripolitania, Cyrenaica, and Fezzan, the three important subdivisions of the country. They can therefore be considered fairly representative of the Libyan school child population. Ferro-Luzzi observed that the average heights and weights of children from Fezzan were in general lower than those found in the children of comparable ages from Tripolitania and Cyrenaica. These latter were considerably below the 50th percentile of the U.S. standards but were comparable to the average values found for Italian children. The observations of Ferro-Luzzi on school children from Tripolitania are shown in Figures 9 and 10. It will be clear from these figures that the growth of the Libyan children follows the same pattern as that seen in other Arab countries.

The consistently low averages for heights of Kuwait's boys and girls as compared with the other Arab children is worth noting, particularly in the lower age groups up to 13 years. During the later period the Kuwaiti children seem to catch up with their Jordanian counterparts, although not completely so.

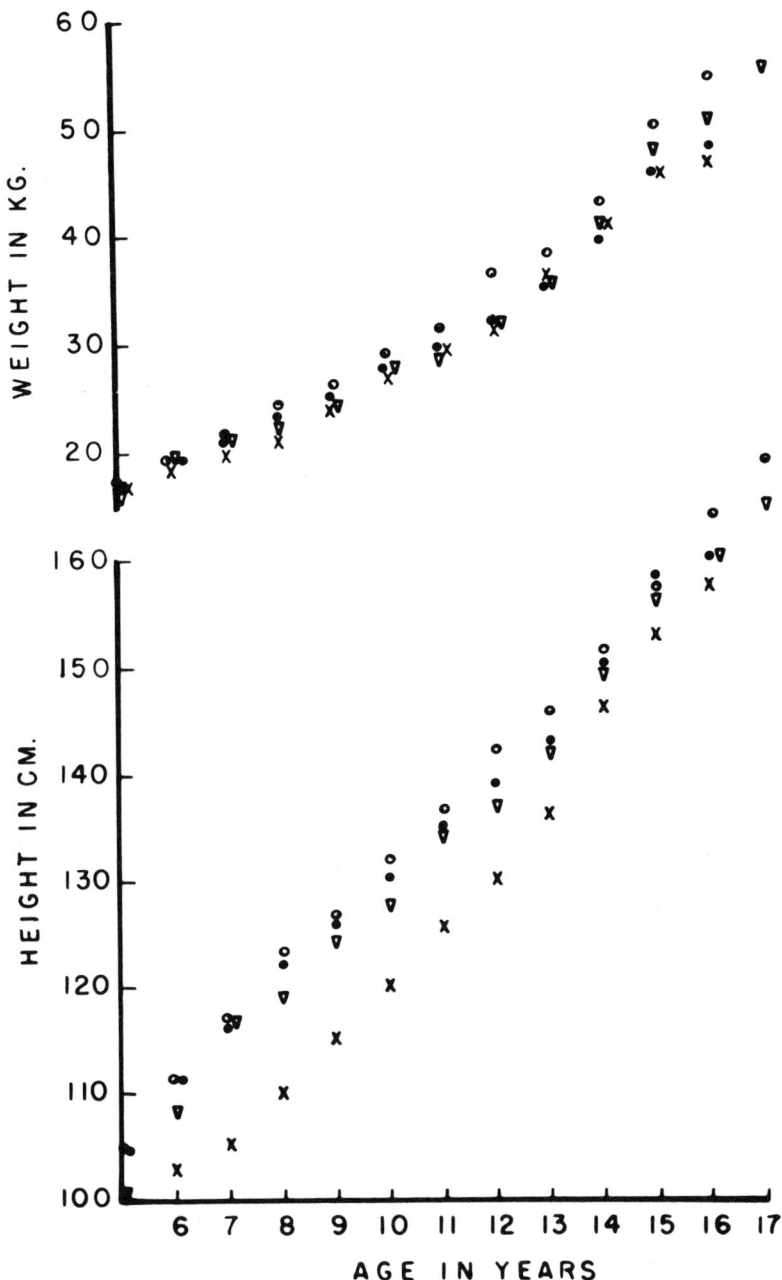

Figure 11.9. Average heights and weights of boys from Libya (•) Lebanon (°) Jordan (▽) and Kuwait (x).

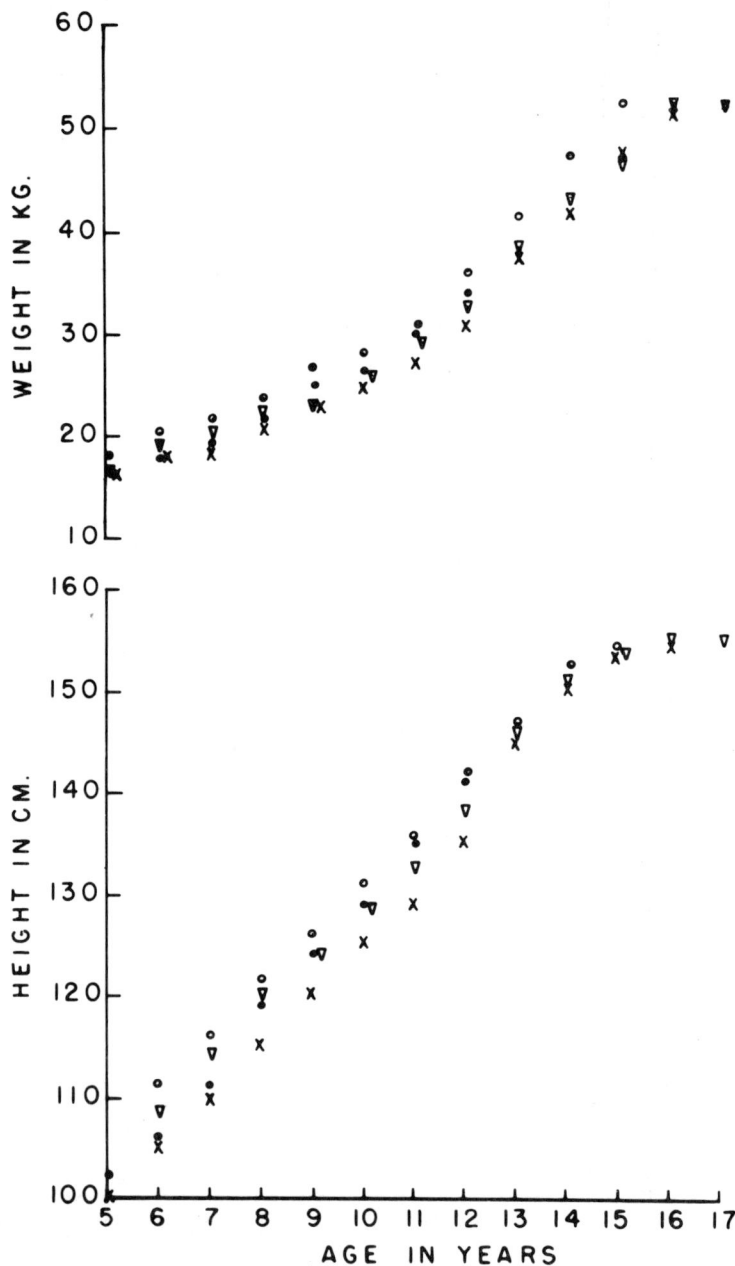

Figure 11.10. Average heights and weights of girls from Libya (•) Lebanon (°) Jordan (▽) and Kuwait (x).

Thus it would appear that probably the best rates of growth are achieved by the Cairo school children. Even these are in the lower percentile values of the Iowa standards. The girls do not achieve better rates of growth. Labib's findings on school girls in Alexandria belonging to the middle- and upper-middle-class families are useful pointers as to the probable causes for the slow growth of Arab children.

It would be appropriate to mention here that one needs to exercise some caution in interpreting the data on heights and weights of school children discussed earlier. It is well known that in most developing countries it is very often difficult to determine correctly the age of children. The older the child, the greater is the uncertainty. The age entered at the school is not necessarily the correct age. Birth registration, although it may be obligatory, is not always feasible or done, and parents' memories are fallible. The investigators who measure heights and weights usually do not take the trouble to check school entries for age against birth registrations where these are available. On the other hand, the data on growth rates of infants up to 2 years are fairly reliable because of the facility with which the age can be checked.

The information so far available shows that in Arab children growth retardation sets in during the first year of life and growth continues at a slower rate throughout childhood. The observations during the latter period are commensurate with those made during infancy. It is therefore legitimate to conclude, in spite of the limitations set by the uncertainty about age, that Arab children show unmistakable evidence of retardation at almost all periods of growth.

The causes underlying the slow growth rate of the majority of Arab children are probably multiple. Undernutrition and malnutrition must be partly responsible. Whereas in infancy and early childhood, diarrheas and respiratory infections are the principal contributory factors together with malnutrition, parasitic infection of different kinds should be considered as another probable cause in the age period 6 to 18 years. The prevalence of parasitism in Egypt and its effects on health are discussed in the chapter on anemia.

REFERENCES

Abboud, M. A., O. Alfi, A. Hefny, and A. R. Mazny. 1957. An Anthropometric Study of Arabian School Children. *Gaz. Egypt. Pediat. Assoc.* 5: 493.

Abd, M., and A. F. Sherbini. 1965. Anthropometric Measures at Birth. I—The Birth Weight. II—The Birth Length. *Alexandria Med. J.* 11: 211 and 217.

Abdou, I. A. 1965. *Nutritional Status in the New Valley* (in Arabic). Cairo, Egypt: National Documentation Center.

Abdou, I. A., and A. H. Mahfouz. 1967. Heights and Weights of School Children in Cairo as Indications of their Nutritional Status. *Egypt. Pub. Hlth. Assoc.* 42: 114.

Abdou, I. A., H. E. Ali, and A. K. Lebshtein. 1965. A Study of the Nutritional Status of Mothers, Infants and Young Children Attending Maternity and Child Health Centers in Cairo. Part I—The Nutritional Status of Infants and Young Children. *Bull. Nutr. Inst., U. A. R.* 1: 9.

Ferro-Luzzi, G. 1958. *Report to the Government of Libya on Nutrition.* FAO Report No. 920. Rome, Italy: Food and Agriculture Organization of the United Nations.

Hammoud, E. T., M. I. Khalil, and A. E. Sarhan. 1961. A School Health Survey in Alexandria, Egypt, U.A.R. Part III—Height, Weight, and Temperature Measurements. *Alexandria Med. J.* 7: 127.

Harfouche, J. K. 1966. *Growth and Illness Patterns of Lebanese Infants (Birth-18 months).* Beirut, Lebanon: Publishers Khayats.

Kamel, I. 1962. Standard Length, Weight, and Cephalic Diameters in Newborn Egyptian Babies. *Gaz. Egypt. Pediat. Assoc.* 10: 1-35.

Khalik, A. K. A. 1929. Standard Development of Egyptian Infants. *Compt. rend. Congr. Internat. Med. Trop. Hyg.* II: 979. Cairo, Egypt: Imprimerie Nationale.

Labib, F. M. 1964. Growth of School Girls in the Kawmiah Schools in Alexandria. *Gaz. Egypt. Pediat. Assoc.* 12: 37.

Patwardhan, V. N., and W. W. Kamel. 1967. *Studies on Vitamin A Deficiency in Infants and Young Children in Jordan.* Geneva, Switzerland: World Health Organization.

Pharaon, H. M., W. J. Darby, H. A. Shammout, E. B. Bridgforth, and C. S. Wilson. 1965. A Year-Long Study of the Nutriture of Infants and Preschool Children in Jordan. *J. Trop. Pediat.* 11: Monograph No. 3, 39.

Puyet, J. H., E. F. Downs, and R. Budeir. 1963. Nutritional and Growth Characteristics of Arab Refugee Children in Lebanon. *Amer. J. Clin. Nutr.* 13: 147.

Sherbini, A. F., and B. F. Atallah. 1960. Some Determinants of Birth Weight. *Gaz. Egypt. Pediat. Assoc.* 8: 867.

Souefi, M. A. 1933. The Average Composition of Breast Milk of Egyptian Mothers. *J. Egypt. Med. Assoc.* 16: 1104.

Wishahi, A., and A. Khattab. 1962. The Effect of Failure of Growth Due to Undernutrition of the Different Parts of the Body in Infancy. *J. Egypt. Med. Assoc.* 45: 1029.

12 | DIETS AND DIETARY HABITS

The foods habitually consumed by the Arabs and hence their diets have undergone comparatively little change over the past eight centuries. Abd Al-Latif Al Baghdadi has described in his book *The Eastern Key,* written in A.D. 1204, many food preparations then used in Egypt, most of which are current and popular today in Arab countries in the Near East. It is true that in the intervening period new foodstuffs such as maize, potato, and tomato were introduced in this region. People learned by experience to make preparations suitable to their taste. Thereafter they were gradually incorporated into the popular diets.

Some features of the Arab diets are common to the Arab countries in the Near East. Bread, largely of the leavened variety, made from wheat, maize, or millet singly or in mixture, is the staple article of the diet. Stewed beans form a useful protein-rich supplement in the diets of the poor people. Many green vegetables are eaten raw as salad. Milk as milk is consumed but little. Much of it is used to make butter, and skim milk is made into cheese. This and the cheese made from whole milk find a place in Arab diets, together with fermented whole and skim milk as yoghurt. Meat is an expensive food item; hence poor people eat it infrequently. Islam forbids the consumption of pig meat. Only the Christians, Maronites in Lebanon and Copts in Egypt, who form a substantial part of the population of Lebanon and Egypt respectively, are not subject to this prohibition. Eggs are valued more for the cash they would bring by sale than for their nutritional value. Hence the poor villagers who keep some poultry more often sell eggs than eat them themselves and give them to their children. Fruit is also a rare article of diet as far as the masses are concerned. Only in times of glut can they afford to eat it.

EGYPT

Dietary habits and food consumption of Arab populations in the Near East have been studied only in recent years. Egypt is one possible exception. The Ministry of Health of the Egyptian government, stimulated by the activity of the Health Organization of the League of Nations, constituted a Permanent Nutrition Committee in 1939. A few nutrition studies were organized between 1939 and 1945 under the auspices of the Permanent Nutrition Committee. Food-consumption surveys were done in some villages in Lower and Upper Egypt and in industrial establishments in Alexandria and near the Red Sea.

The available reports on the results of these surveys are sketchy and lack adequate information on dietary habits and food-consumption patterns. The average calorie and protein intakes recorded in three of these surveys were as follows (*Report of the Permanent Nutrition Committee 1939-1946,* Ministry of Public Health, Cairo, Egypt):

	No. Families	Average Intake per Adult	
		Cal.	Total Protein g
Miniet Shebin, Kaliubieh Province	35	2899	114
El Zahaweien, Kaliubieh Province	45	2511	96
Filiature Nationale in Alexandria	37	3006	—

The average calorie intake in the two villages seemed adequate. However, it is to be noted that nearly 20% of the families surveyed had a calorie intake of 2,000 or less per day. Furthermore, the diets of the villagers were deficient in protective foods, especially milk and milk products and fruits. It was also claimed that diets of workers contained even less milk and milk products but more meat, fish, legumes, and fruit, thus appearing qualitatively better than those of the villagers. This may not be entirely unexpected since the income of an average industrial worker was likely higher than that of an average peasant in the villages.

The Institute of Food and Nutrition, established in 1955, then undertook the responsibility of conducting food-consumption surveys. Among these were surveys done in the oases of Kharga and

Diet and Dietary Habits

Dakhla, among pregnant and nursing women in Cairo, in an orphanage in Cairo, and in villages in Kaliubieh Province about 20 miles from Cairo. A few dietary studies were done by the Nutrition Department of the High Institute of Public Health in Alexandria in and around that city.

A study by FAO (1954) on 23 families in the village of Aghour Soughra in Kaliubieh Province gives a fairly good picture of dietary practices of the people in the villages. These families were selected at random from a total of 280 families constituting the population of the village. Hence the information gained can be considered fairly representative of village life in the Delta area around Cairo.

The families had three meals a day. Breakfast was taken early in the morning before menfolk went off to work; the second meal was at noon and the third just before sunset after return from the field. Little eating was done between meals. Sweetened tea was a popular beverage. Those who could not afford it drank *helba* tea (infusion of fenugreek) instead. The pattern of the meals of a few representative households of different economic status follows.

A fellah who owns a fraction of an acre of land or more has one buffalo and some chickens, hires himself out for labor, and has a family of a wife and two or three children may have the following type of meals:

Breakfast: Maize bread, cheese (skim), *do'a*[1] (a mixture of salt, red pepper, and dried herbs), and tea or *helba* tea.
Luncheon: Maize bread, cheese, *do'a*, chicory.
Supper: Maize bread, broad beans or potatoes and tomatoes cooked in animal fat, cheese, onions, tea.

The above indicates a little variety between meals; there may be none. Among the poor, the same type of food may be consumed at all the three meals. Consumption of meat is usually reserved for feast days.

It is interesting to compare this with the meals taken by an individual who owned 9 acres of land and lived with his brother who owned 8 acres. Their meal pattern was as follows:

Breakfast: Boiled milk and tea, butter, honey, eggs, molasses, wheat and maize bread.

1. The simplest *do'a* is a mixture of salt and ground red pepper or ground cumin seeds. The more elaborate preparations may contain other spices, herbs and ground sesame, peanut or lotus seeds.

Luncheon: Rice, macaroni, meat cooked with vegetables, green salad or pickles, bread, fruit.
Supper: Boiled milk, cheese, bread.

Raw greens, often picked from the fields, were eaten by all families. Those consumed included green beans, green chick-peas, green onions, lettuce, and a variety of wild greens.

This limited study illustrates how economic conditions set the pattern of meals and foods eaten and hence the nutrition derived from such meals.

The FAO Report does not give the actual quantities of food purchased, prepared, or consumed at meals, and hence it is difficult to assess the nutrient and calorie intake of these families. It is probable, however, that the diets of the poorer section of the community may not be adequate nutritionally.

Barakat and Mohamed (1951) conducted a diet survey in the village of Mona el Amir situated 20 miles south of Cairo. Information on food consumption for seven consecutive days was obtained by the questionnaire method. The families surveyed included those of agricultural laborers, land-owners, and industrial workers. Millet bread containing 4% fenugreek formed the staple diet. Cereal and grain legume consumption was the highest in agricultural laborers, whereas the consumption of meat, milk, and milk products was the lowest. This was probably due to the low purchasing power of the agricultural laborer. The results of the survey are summarized in Table 1.

Abdou and Mahfouz (1965) have reported on a diet survey conducted in 1955 in two other villages, Kafr el Hassaa and Mansouriet Namoul in Kaliubieh Province, about 30 kilometers from Cairo. A combination of several methods was used in order to obtain reliable information on actual food consumption. The investigators visited the households at meal times, weighed the food and also obtained samples of foods and composite dishes for chemical analysis. The survey was done in all four seasons of the year and included families with different levels of income, i.e., from less than 1 £.Eg. (Egyptian pound) to over 3 £.Eg. per head per month. The food consumption averaged over the year and the nutrient intake are given in Table 1.

Abdou and Mahfouz compared average daily nutrient intake with the recommendations of the National Research Council (U.S.A.) and concluded that the diets of villagers were deficient in calcium, riboflavin, and ascorbic acid. Certain seasonal trends were noticed. The average intake of calories, protein, vitamin A value, riboflavin, and ascorbic acid was lower in summer and autumn than in winter and

Diet and Dietary Habits

TABLE 1
AVERAGE PER CAPITA DAILY CONSUMPTION OF FOOD AND NUTRIENTS
IN VILLAGES OF KALIUBIEH PROVINCE

Villages Families, Number	Mona el Amir			Kafr el Hasafa and Mansouriet Namoul	
	Indust. Worker 11	Land Owner 15	Agric. 9	160	
				Winter	Summer
Bread, Wheat, g	46	29	22	6	141
Bread, Millet, g	435	521	669		
Bread, Maize, g				436	392
Rice	12	38	9	32	3
Other cereal products	30	66	80		
Legumes (preparations)	152	152	346	7	2
Milk	131	47	—	38	—
Cheese	96	104	110	79	57
Butter	14	12	—		
Cooking Oil	5	2	3	17	14
Eggs	8	6	—	6	2
Meat	76	60	28	26	42
Fish	37	60	28	3	—
Tuber vegetables	105	131	35	66	86
Green vegetables	83	80	41	92	32
Sugar and sweets	14	38	13	—	13
Fresh fruits	21	99	—	30	20
Dried dates	16	35	30		
Calories	2101	2082	2563	2568	2441
Protein g Total	90	77	105	83	76
Protein g Animal	31	21	26	22	19
Fat g	31	34	41		
Ca mg				358	218
Fe mg				12	15
Vitamin A I.U.				5893	2752
Thiamine mg				1.9	1.65
Riboflavin mg				1.48	0.8
Niacin mg				13.2	14.9
Ascorbic Acid mg				54	34

spring. Leafy and other fresh vegetables were consumed less in summer and autumn; so also were milk and milk products, probably because of their low availability in these seasons. The nutritional quality of the diets depended upon the income level of the families. The consumption of such protective foods as meat, milk, grain legumes, vegetables, and fruits was markedly lower in the low income groups. However, the authors concluded that in general food consumption was similar in pattern to that indicated by the country's Food Balance Sheet. Riad (1960) studied the nutrition of young adults attending the army recruiting center in Alexandria. The prospective recruits were from the provinces of Behira and Gharbia. Riad does not give details about food consumption. However, he remarks that the food habits in these two provinces did not differ from those observed in the other parts of the Delta.

That the actual consumption pattern does not vary much in different parts of the country becomes evident from the observations of Abdou (1965) in the oases of Kharga and Dakhla. He describes the typical daily meals as follows:

Breakfast: Majority of people have cooked rice and tea. When rice is not available, wheat bread, skim milk, and/or tea are taken.
Luncheon: This differs according to the occupation. Those who work in fields have skim milk, "sun" bread, greens and tea. Others would eat cooked food such as bread and cooked vegetables, perhaps cooked meat and cooked wheat with tomato sauce.
Supper: Similar to either breakfast or lunch.

The diets in the oases differed from those in the Delta in that grain legumes and skim milk were consumed in much larger quantities in the oases than in the villages in the Delta surveyed earlier by Abdou and Mahfouz. The consumption of green vegetables, fruit, and meat, however, was much lower than in the Delta. These differences were reflected in the estimates of nutrient intakes which are given in Table 2.

A comparison of the nutrient intakes given in Tables 1 and 2 reveals the fact that calcium and iron intakes were higher in the oases than in the Delta villages. On the other hand, the vitamin A value of the oasis diets and their ascorbic acid content were very much lower than in those in the Delta. This is understandable. The large quantities of skim milk consumed in the oases provide a good amount of calcium, but no vitamin A. Comparative lack of green vegetables was responsible for the low levels of vitamin A activity and ascorbic acid in the diet. The only green vegetable consumed in large quantities was Jew's mallow (*Corchorus olitorius*) or *mulukhiyah* in Arabic. This vegetable is popular all over Egypt. When available in season, it is bought in quantity, and the leaf separated from the stalk, dried in the sun, and stored. The dried *mulukhiyah* is soaked in water, cooked with salt and some sour lime juice, and eaten with bread or rice. Those who can afford it cook the vegetable with meat. The ascorbic

Diet and Dietary Habits

TABLE 2
AVERAGE PER CAPITA DAILY INTAKE OF CALORIES AND NUTRIENTS
IN THE VILLAGES OF KHARGA AND DAKHLA OASES

	Kharga Oasis		Dakhla Oasis
	El Mahreek Village	Paris Village	Moot Village
Calories	2653	2714	2770
Protein g Total	86	89	94
Protein g Animal	7.3	7.9	11.3
Calcium mg	600	586	735
Iron mg	21	25	27
Vitamin A value I.U.	87	1098	1408
Thiamine mg	1.2	2.0	1.9
Riboflavin mg	1.2	1.1	1.10
Niacin mg	23	15.7	23
Ascorbic Acid mg	4.3	3.9	14

acid contained in the green leaf is destroyed on drying and storage, as is possibly the vitamin A precursor. Since the practice of drying *mulukhiyah* is common throughout Egypt and the vegetable is frequently eaten, better methods for its preservation ought to be developed.

It must be regretfully admitted that the available information reviewed thus far is still too meager to consider it as representing the dietary habits of millions of people in the Delta and Upper Egypt. The studies described above do not indicate many major defects in the dietary intake. The average energy intake does not appear inadequate except in very poor families. The total protein in the diet is also adequate. Sixty to eighty percent of it is derived from cereals; the animal protein content varies from 10 to 20%. The biological value of dietary protein in terms of NPU is estimated roughly at 65%. The average protein intake must be considered adequate, even allowing for the comparatively low NPU. The vitamin A activity of the diet may be adequate in the Delta, but in the oases and Upper Egypt it is probably insufficient in terms of requirements. The same may be true of ascorbic acid. On the other hand, calcium intake appears to be inadequate in the Delta. Riboflavin intake is probably inadequate in all the diets so far studied, for the observed intakes fall below the level of 0.55 mg/1000 Cal. recommended by the FAO/WHO Report on Vitamin Requirements (1967).

The probability that dietary intakes of certain groups of individuals may be far from satisfactory cannot be discounted, and poverty need not necessarily be the only cause for this. Recently the individual food consumption of school children of Sindion village (20 km. north of Cairo) was studied by Carter et al. (1969). The school had 279 boys, 11 to 17 years of age. Of these, 90 were considered retarded in growth, as they were two standard deviations or more below the Iowa mean. A part of the detailed study on these children was a survey of individual food consumption. Information on food intake was obtained by questionnaire, visits to the homes of children during mealtimes, and weighing the foods consumed. The survey was done in winter and spring of 1966. The composite meal samples were collected a year later, in the spring of 1967. The calorie and nutrient intakes estimated from food tables and calculated from the results of analysis are given in Table 3.

The estimates made from food tables showed that diets were inadequate in calories and marginal in protein. Deficiencies of calcium, riboflavin, niacin, and probably of iron were also indicated. There was little difference between the consumption observed in winter and the spring of 1966.

The analysis of composite meals gives a somewhat different picture as compared to the above. The energy intake was about 300 to 400 calories higher, and protein intake was found to be 23% higher. The difference may have been real, for composite meal samples were collected a year later, as mentioned above. The values for calcium and iron intake obtained on analysis were also considerably higher than those estimated from food tables. The discrepancy in iron can be explained on the assumption that estimates from food tables do not

TABLE 3
AVERAGE CALORIE AND NUTRIENT INTAKE OF SINDION SCHOOL CHILDREN

	Estimated from Food Table		Calculated on Analysis
	Winter 1966	Spring 1966	Spring 1967
Calories	2010	1870	2355
Protein g	56	57	70
Fat g	42	37	35
Calcium mg	260	280	955
Iron mg	12	11	36
Vitamin A value I.U.	3000	2300	981
Thiamine mg	1.30	1.40	—
Riboflavin mg	0.61	0.57	0.87
Niacin mg	9	8	10
Ascorbic Acid mg	61	40	—

include the iron contamination of food due to insufficient cleaning and washing of vegetables and/or cooking in iron utensils. This is an important factor in estimating iron intake which is often missed in diet surveys. Vitamin A value was found to be 33 to 42% of the value estimated from food tables. In spite of these discrepancies between the estimated and analyzed values, it was clear that the diets were deficient in calories, vitamin A, riboflavin, and niacin. It is possible that this multiple deficiency might have been responsible for growth retardation in the boys referred to above. These children were from families which could afford sending them to a preparatory school. Hence dietary inadequacy cannot legitimately be attributed to poverty. Although it is hazardous to generalize, it will be a moot point to consider whether the lower growth rate of Egyptian children is not the result of a possible habitual consumption of defective and inadequate diets.

Three studies relating to diets in pregnancy and lactation are worth discussing in detail. One of these was conducted in Cairo and the two others in Alexandria; thus both were in the urban population.

Abdou and Amer (1965) obtained information on one day's food consumption from 1143 nursing mothers and 763 pregnant women in Cairo. This was achieved partly by questionnaire and home visiting at mealtimes and partly by the analysis of samples of habitual diets. Since the investigation lasted about a year, and as different mothers were being observed at different times of the year, the results were considered representative of the habitual dietary intakes during pregnancy and lactation, particularly as the sample size was fairly large. The women belonged to families with levels of income varying from less than £.Eg. 1 to over £.Eg. 5 per head per month. Abdou and Amer (1965) give no information about the stages of pregnancy in the women studied by them. Since these were women attending the antenatal clinics, it would not be incorrect to assume that they were mostly in the second and third trimesters of pregnancy at the time when their diets were surveyed.

The trends in food consumption in relation to income levels are illustrated with reference to certain foods and well brought out in Figure 1. Even ignoring the values at the two extremes because the number of women was small, some shifts in the foods eaten are apparent with the rising income level. The consumption of bread and of fresh vegetables fell as the income rose. There was not much change in the consumption of legumes, whereas that of all other foods increased with income. In effect the diets of women in higher income groups were richer in protective foods such as meat, fish, eggs, and

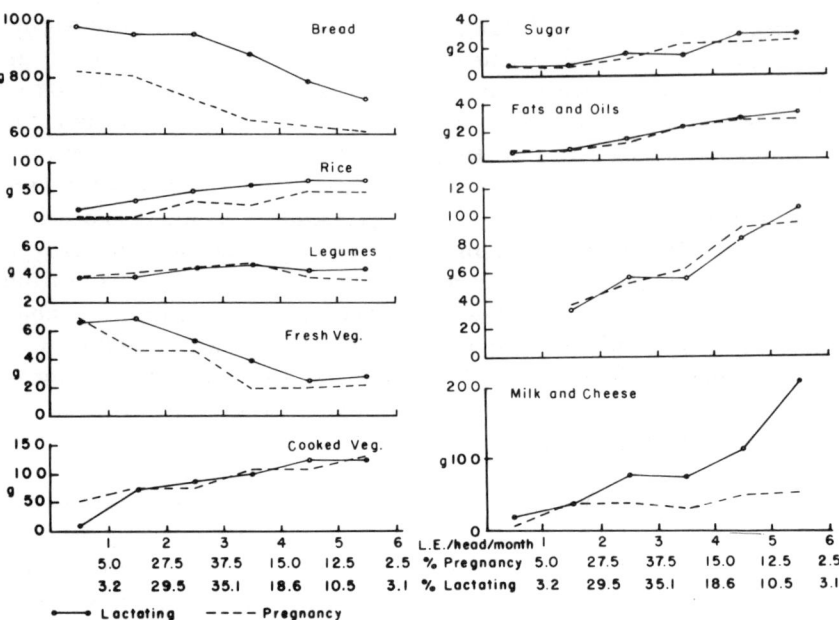

Figure 12.1. Trends in food consumption of pregnant and lactating Egyptian women in Cairo as related to monthly income.

milk and milk products as compared to those of women of the lower income groups.

Differences in food consumption were also found between the diets in pregnancy and in lactation (Table 4). The consumption of bread and rice was uniformly higher in lactation than in pregnancy; so also was that of milk and cheese at three of the five income levels studied. There were no marked differences in the consumption of legumes, cooked vegetables, sugar, fats and oils, and of meat, fish, and eggs. The effect of all these changes considered together is reflected in the estimated energy and nutrient intakes shown in Table 4.

It is clear from the table that the average diet of the lactating woman in Cairo provided more energy, more protein, and slightly larger amounts of all other nutrients than the diet of pregnant women. This placed the lactating woman in an advantageous position to meet the additional needs of milk secretion. However it is not easy to judge whether her total nutritional requirements were actually met. Information on several aspects, such as diets of nonpregnant women, together with information on changes in weight during pregnancy, average milk secretion of mothers, and growth performance of infants would have been invaluable adjuncts to this study.

Of the two studies done in Alexandria, only the details of one by Saleh (1960) were available to the authors. In this study pregnant and lactating women attending the Shatby Hospital were the subjects. Saleh weighed foodstuffs in the homes on seven consecutive days and thus obtained records on food consumption on 142 pregnant women out of 736 attending the antenatal clinic. Thirty-eight of these women were followed after delivery, and information on their food consumption during lactation was collected. The income levels and the distribution of families within these were not dissimilar to those of the group described by Abdou and Amer in Cairo, although there was a slightly higher (10%) representation of families with incomes between 6 and 10 £.Eg. per head per month in the Alexandria sample. A comparison of the average food consumption per day is shown in Table 4.

There are some noticeable differences between the results obtained in the Cairo and Alexandria studies. The average daily intake of bread by pregnant women in Alexandria was less by over 400 g than that observed in Cairo. On the other hand the intake of protective foods in general was higher in Alexandria than in Cairo.

Saleh has not estimated the energy and nutrient intake from the food-consumption data; our own attempts to fill this gap are at best an approximation. However, some information can be gleaned from such an attempt, as shown in Table 4. The results obtained by Sadek in Alexandria are quoted by WHO (1965) merely in terms of average daily intake of energy and certain nutrients. These values have been included in Table 4 for comparison. Sadek observed food consumption in two groups of "poor" women in the eighth month of pregnancy. On the other hand, and for reasons already mentioned, Abdou and Amer and Saleh presumably covered the second and third trimesters, observing women during the period that they attended antenatal clinics. Certain interesting facts emerge from a comparison of these three studies:

(1) The average calorie consumption of pregnant women in Alexandria was lower than that in Cairo. Saleh has recorded the lowest average intake in the smaller group of pregnant women, which he later followed during lactation.

(2) Protein intakes were comparable in all the three groups of pregnant women.

(3) Calcium intake was the lowest in women studied by Sadek in Alexandria, whereas iron intake was lower in both samples from Alexandria than in Cairo. The uncertainty of the estimates of mineral

TABLE 4
DIETS OF EGYPTIAN WOMEN DURING PREGNANCY AND LACTATION (AVERAGE PER CAPITA DAILY INTAKE)

	Cairo			Alexandria			
	(1)		(2)			(3) Pregnant	
	Pregnant 763	Lactating 1143	Pregnant 142	Pregnant 38[1]	Lactating 38	Gr. I—22	Gr. II—23
Bread	725	917	292	305	355		
Cereals other than bread	30	52	62	53	76		
Starchy foods	28	28	64	65	88		
Legumes	43	46	51	45	71		
Fresh vegetables	38	50	42	35	37		
Cooked vegetables	84	86	116	97	154		
Fresh fruit	11	13	75	78	66		
Dried fruit			8	8	7		
Meat	34	38	43	43	52		
Fish	14	13	50	45	53		
Eggs	5	5	10	12	14		
Milk	35	69	103	85	64		
Cheese			26	24	21		
Bean cake	17	18					
Oils and fats	14	16					
Sugar	14	15					

TABLE 4 (Cont'd.)
DIETS OF EGYPTIAN WOMEN DURING PREGNANCY AND LACTATION (AVERAGE PER CAPITA DAILY INTAKE)

	Cairo				Alexandria			
	(1)			(2)			(3)	
	Pregnant 763	Lactating 1143	Pregnant 142	Pregnant 38[1]	Lactating 38	Gr. I—22	Pregnant Gr. I—23
Calories	2200	2761	1680	1620	1980	2046	2124
Protein g Total	77	95	71	68	84	72	78
Protein g Animal	10.7	12.6					
Calcium mg	400	518	612	549	647	300	900
Iron mg	24	30	12	15	15	14	15
Vitamin A value I.U.	3028	3436	4500	3940	5440	2636	2391
Thiamine mg	1.5	1.9					
Riboflavin mg	0.77	0.91					
Niacin mg	24	30					
Ascorbic Acid mg	34	40				23	27

(1) Abdou and Amer, 1965.
(2) Saleh, 1960.
(3) Sadek, 1965.
1. These 38 pregnant women belonging to the larger group of 142 were followed during lactation as shown in column 6.

and vitamin intakes derived from food tables is well known, and hence not much credence should be given to these differences as seen in the table.

(4) In Cairo as well as in Alexandria, the energy and protein intakes of lactating women were higher than those of pregnant women. The relative increases during lactation were larger in Cairo than in Alexandria.

The Egyptian observations are in line with several such made in other countries of the world. Unfortunately, for reasons mentioned already, they fail to indicate the existence, or otherwise, of differences between the diets of pregnant and lactating women on the one hand and those of women of comparable age who are neither pregnant nor lactating. Studies to yield information on this important aspect are obviously needed.

LIBYA

Libya is divided into three large provinces—Tripolitania, Cyrenaica, and Fezzan. The first two border on the Mediterranean and constitute the major areas of food production of the country. The bulk of the population is also concentrated in these two provinces. Fezzan is the interior desert area, interspersed with oases. It contains less than 5% of the total population.

The Interdepartmental Committee on Nutrition for National Defense (ICNND) of USA (1957) conducted a nutrition survey in Libya from 15 June to 15 August 1957. This survey was mainly directed to the study of the food consumption and nutritional status of the Libyan Armed Forces and Constabulary. The sample of civilians included in the survey was comparatively small. The methods used in the study of food consumption of civilians were directed more to gaining general information on food habits and patterns than to obtaining a quantitative appreciation of dietary intakes of the population. They did not, therefore, lend themselves to a quantitative nutritional assessment. Soon after, from 21 August to 23 December 1957, the Food and Agriculture Organization (FAO) sent a consultant, Professor G. Ferro-Luzzi, for a diet and nutrition survey among the civilian population.

The ICNND recommended that nutrition surveys should be conducted periodically by qualified personnel. Ferro-Luzzi (1958) in his recommendations stressed the importance of training local personnel for conducting food-consumption surveys as a part of the nutrition program to be undertaken by the Libyan government. Unfortunately these recommendations did not receive the attention they deserved. In 1962, FAO sent yet another consultant, Dr. Y. H. Yang, to study the problem of nutrition in Libya. Dr. Yang made a few pilot food-consumption surveys in villages not far from Tripoli. Our information on the food habits and nutrient intakes is largely based on the published results of these studies. It must be admitted that in spite of these, our knowledge of the levels of food consumption and nutrient intake of the population in Libya is fragmentary.

According to Ferro-Luzzi, the food habits of the Libyan people in the three provinces do not differ much according to location, but they do so depending upon the economic status. As is to be expected the diets of the poor are limited to a few essential items such as bread made from barley and wheat, dates, figs, onions, tomatoes, green and red pepper, and oil. In rural areas these foods form the mainstay of people's diets. The Italians have influenced to a certain extent, through their long occupation, the food habits principally of the urban population. Pasta and tomato paste are used throughout the country. The consumption of millets, rice, maize, chick-peas, and broad beans is limited. The rare occasions on which the poor consume meat of any kind are similar to those found in Egypt and in most developing countries where meat is relatively scarce and beyond the purchasing power of the bulk of the population. The consumption of milk and milk products is also limited, owing to the same economic considerations.

Ferro-Luzzi found high milk consumption to be common among the pastoral tribes. So far as the majority of the population was concerned, Ferro-Luzzi was of the opinion that only 10% had an adequate level of consumption of milk and milk products. In 1960, the total production of milk was estimated at 45.8 million liters, comprising milk of goats, ewes, cows, and camels in that order. Thus about 3-1/2 ounces of milk per capita per day was produced within the country. This was a very low level of milk production, which has shown only a slight improvement in the intervening years. It is not surprising therefore to learn from Yang's report that in his diet survey he found only 7% of the families consuming milk and milk products. Among the fruits, dried dates and dried figs are available for the best part of the year and form important items in the diet. The consumption of dried dates was high in Fezzan compared with that in Tripolitania and Cyrenaica. In the latter two provinces other fresh fruit, such as grapes, watermelons, melons, and some citrus fruit, is available. The watermelon, being plentiful and comparatively cheap, finds a place in the poor people's diets when in season.

It will appear from the description that the diets of the bulk of the population are simple and the meal patterns more or less what one could call monotonous. Breakfast usually consists of tea, with or without bread. Lunch may consist of one single dish containing several food items cooked together and eaten with tomato and other sauces. Dinner is similar to the midday meal. Tea, highly sweetened, is the beverage used at all the meals.

Ferro-Luzzi studied food consumption in all the three provinces. The number of families covered was, however, small, the total being 145 families in all. Of these 68, or 47% of the total, were from Suk el Djouma, a suburb of Tripoli. Considering that in all locations the families were also divided into two economic classes, middle and low, the number in each category at each location must have been too small to be representative. Ferro-Luzzi obtained information on food consumption by two methods: A questionnaire about quantities of food consumed the day before; and monthly consumption on the basis of food purchased. The results obtained by the two methods agreed in general, although there were a few discrepancies. Cereal consumption varied enormously from 260 g to 700 g per day. It was lowest in Fezzan where the calorie supply seems to have been made up by a large consumption of dried dates amounting to over 350 g per capita per day. There were no other noticeable differences between the three regions, although the diets of the middle income families were better than those of low income families. The estimates of intake of calories, protein, and fats in the three provinces are given in Table

TABLE 5
DAILY PER CAPITA CONSUMPTION OF CALORIES, PROTEINS, AND FAT IN THE THREE PROVINCES OF LIBYA[1]

		Income Group	Cal.	Protein g		Fats g
				Total	Animal	
Tripolitania	Suk-el-Djouma	Middle	1838	55	10.8	38
	Coast	Middle	2898	84	4.4	56
		Low	1960	62	4.5	27
	Djebel	Middle	3088	92	7.9	69
		Low	2090	67	5.2	40
Cyrenaica	Coast	Middle	2877	76	5.3	64
		Low	1920	57	6.1	29
	Djebel	Middle	3130	94	8.0	63
Fezzan		Middle	2344	89	10.8	55
		Low	1720	59	5.9	26

1. Source: Ferro-Luzzi, 1958.

5 and are based on the information obtained on monthly food purchase.

Yang (1963) surveyed food consumption in 43 families selected at random in two villages and a settlement within 50 kilometers of Tripoli. Sixty-seven percent of the families were agriculturists, and 26% were day laborers and others. The economic status of 49% of the families was judged to be poor or very poor; 40% belonged to middle income groups. Yang does not give the average food or nutrient consumption in various classes of families surveyed but gives information on calorie and nutrient intake on one typical family each from the rich and medium economic groups and on three families from the poor group. The levels of intake of the poor families were lower than those of the higher income families. The average values for all the five typical families were as follows: calories 2,030; protein 50.5 g (animal protein 7 g); fat 43.5 g; calcium 131 mg; iron 8.6 mg; vitamin A value 1,450 I.U.; thiamine 0.95 mg; riboflavin 0.42 mg; niacin 8.2 g; ascorbic acid 66.8 mg.

As mentioned before, ICNND surveyed the diets of the Libyan Armed Forces and Constabulary in 1957. The estimates of nutrient intake were made by computation from the official rations issued and by analysis of composite meals collected from the messes. As was to be expected, the army and the police were better fed than the general public. However, some defects were noticed by ICNND, not in the authorized rations, but the actual amounts issued to the units. If the authorized quantities of milk, potatoes, and fresh vegetables were consumed, the army diets would be nutritionally adequate. The computed intake of calories and nutrients in the army and constabulary messes and canteens taken together is given in Table 6.

The composite meal analysis gave different values for several nutrients. Those for calcium, iron, thiamine, riboflavin, and ascorbic acid were higher, and the values for total vitamin A activity were smaller than the computed values. These differences were ascribed partly to the uncertainty about the cooking losses assumed in computation and partly to the fact that computations were based on the average of three days' diets, whereas the composite meal sample was collected on a single day. In view of this, it may be more realistic to assess the adequacy of these diets on computed values. One could conclude that these diets were adequate in calories and proteins but were inadequate in all other nutrients estimated. It might be necessary to make an exception for calcium and iron, however. It is the common experience that values for these nutrients are found to be higher on analysis of composite meals than when computed from food

TABLE 6
AVERAGE CALORIE AND NUTRIENT INTAKE IN LIBYAN ARMY AND THE CONSTABULARY[1]
(AVERAGE PER CAPITA PER DAY)[2]

Location Number Fed	Army More than 6 Months Service		Constabulary Training School	
	Zavia 263	Bengasi 357	Tripolitania 187	Cyrenaica 189
Calories	3229	2911	3276	2884
Protein g	94	88	103	96
Fat g	88	81	62	75
Ca mg	294	318	263	175
P mg	1115	1012	1112	922
Fe mg	12	11	13	10
Vitamin A value I.U.	2023	1888	1271	2390
B_1 mg	0.79	0.71	0.88	0.55
Riboflavin mg	1.09	1.03	0.90	0.81
Niacin mg	15	14	13	16
Vitamin C mg	19	28	17	14

1. Source: ICNND, 1957.
2. These figures are total of mess and canteen consumption, and estimates made allowance for conservative cooking losses.

tables. Whatever the reason, the fact must be accepted, and it may be justifiable to conclude that the diets of the Libyan army and the constabulary may not have been deficient in calcium and iron as judged by the standards of dietary allowances recommended by FAO/WHO Expert Groups (1961, 1968). It is not known what steps the Libyan government took, if any, on the ICNND recommendations to improve the diets of the armed forces.

LEBANON

The standard of living in Lebanon, higher than in other Arab countries of the Near East, has influenced the levels of food consumption in that country. Such foods as milk products and meat are consumed frequently in Lebanon. Furthermore, since large amounts of a variety of fruit are grown in Lebanon for local use as well as for export, the average consumption of fruit by the Lebanese is high (Sabry, 1961).

The foods consumed are generally not dissimilar to those described in an earlier chapter. Wheat is the principal cereal, accounting for 90% of the total cereal consumption. Most of the wheat used in Lebanon is imported as wheat or wheat flour. Although bread made from high extraction wheat flour is common in rural Lebanon, it is the white flour that is used for bread in the urban areas. *Burghul* (boiled wheat) and *kishk* (*burghul* boiled with yoghurt and dried) are also used in Lebanon cooked with lentils, broad beans, and chick-peas or meat.

The average family in the villages eats three meals a day. Bread is consumed with every meal. *Lebneh* (soft sour cheese), jam, pickles, olives, and sweetened tea or Turkish coffee are taken along with bread for breakfast. The midday meal may include yoghurt, pickles, and a hot dish made from *burghul* and lentils. Fresh meat is usually served once or twice a week. When available, raw vegetables are eaten with the meals. The evening meal is simple and may consist of bread and leftovers from the midday meal. Fruit is eaten throughout the day, but not with meals (Cowan *et al.*, 1964).

The entire family is usually present at breakfast and the evening meal. The head of the family and other male "productive" members have the first choice of food prepared for the meal. Women and young children come later. Such a practice leads to an unequal distribution of food within the family, based not on the need of the individual but on considerations of priority. This situation, described by Cowan *et al.* (1964), in rural Lebanon is not unlike that found in many developing countries. It may also prevail in the neighboring Arab countries, although a similar reference to it has not come to our notice.

ICNND (1962) has reported on food-consumption surveys in 129 civilian, nonrefugee and 51 refugee families in Lebanon. The surveys on nonrefugee civilians were done in different parts of the country, and the results may be considered fairly representative of the cross-section of the Lebanese population. The method adopted in the survey was principally that of recall of foods eaten by the family on the day before the interview. Weights of foods prepared and eaten were recorded in a few families as a check on the recall method. Finally composite meal samples were collected and analyzed for principal nutrients. The average amounts and the range of foods consumed and the computed calorie and nutrient intakes are summarized in Table 7.

The average diet of the refugee families was found inadequate in most nutrients. The exceptions were vitamin A value, ascorbic acid, and possibly protein. On the other hand, the average diet of the non-refugee civilian population was considered adequate in calories and other nutrients, with the exception of riboflavin. However, the range of food consumption indicates that in some locations the diets were inadequate in calories and most essential nutrients. Such inadequate intakes were recorded in one village in South Lebanon and also among the Armenian families surveyed in Beirut.

TABLE 7
FOOD AND NUTRIENT INTAKE IN LEBANESE CIVILIANS[1]
(AVERAGE PER CAPITA PER DAY)

	Nonrefugees		Refugees	
	Average	Range	Average	Range
	g	g	g	g
Cereals	477	269–635	422	296–414
Pulses and nuts	30	0–56	33	20–39
Leafy & yellow vegetables	114	42–193	155	80–192
Other vegetables	113	30–177	106	79–133
Fruit	76	1–273	15	6–34
Olives	19	3–43	8	3–19
Milk & Milk products	157	87–275	59	22–87
Eggs	19	4–35	13	9–26
Fats & oils	29	11–48	28	27–36
Sugar & sweets	26	9–47	18	9–31
Meat, poultry, & fish	41	0–78	25	14–33
Miscellaneous[2]	7	0–77	4	
Calories	2312	1679–2667	1955	1775–2630
Protein g	73	58–83	62	58–85
Calcium mg	574	334–913	473	304–638
Iron mg	10.9	7.5–16.0	10.6	8.9–11.6
Vitamin A value I.U.	3843	2116–5889	5374	3122–6556
Thiamine mg	0.79	0.74–0.95	0.44	0.33–0.52
Riboflavin mg	1.11	0.79–1.33	0.88	0.71–1.12
Niacin mg	18.3	13.8–22.8	8.8	8.0–12.4
Ascorbic acid mg	63	23–122	69	53–73

1. Source: ICNND, 1962.
2. This includes *tehina, halaweh,* dried fruit, vinegar, cocoa, etc.

Other studies on food consumption in Lebanese population are those of Cowan and coworkers (1964, 1965) done on 30 families in the northern mountain area of Beqa'a valley in the spring and autumn of 1962 and 25 families in Kfarzubian village on the western slopes of the Lebanon mountain in January, May, and September 1964. The families surveyed in Kfarzubian were of a higher socioeconomic status than those surveyed in Beqa'a. However, Cowan (1965) reported a striking similarity in the meal pattern and foods consumed in the two locations. The fact that the surveys were repeated in different seasons proved useful in elucidating the seasonal variation in food consumption and nutrient intake. The most important change was found in the consumption of fruit, which provided only about 1% of the total daily calorie intake in the spring. On the other hand, in the autumn, fruit consumption accounted for 8.3% and 13.5% of the total calorie intake

Diet and Dietary Habits

in Beqa'a and Kfarzubian respectively. The results of these diet surveys are summarized in Table 8.

The average values recorded in the ICNND surveys and those reported by Cowan et al. are not dissimilar in general. It may be reasonable to conclude therefore that except for the very poor people the diets of the Lebanese are in general adequate. Seasons seem to influence the intake of vitamin A value, ascorbic acid, and riboflavin. It is interesting to see from Table 8 that the intakes of vitamin A value and ascorbic acid seem to move in opposite directions with the season of the year. In spring, the intake of ascorbic acid was the lowest and that of vitamin A value was the highest. The former increased in autumn, and the latter decreased. It is probable that in the season when citrus fruit is in abundance the green and yellow leafy vegetables are consumed less. Fresh vegetables and fruits are available throughout the year. It is possible, however, that their relative abundance varies in different seasons of the year. The changes in the intake of other nutrients with season as judged from the results of these surveys do not indicate any specific trend.

ICNND surveyed the food consumption of Lebanese armed forces in four locations. Information was collected on authorized rations and food as served in the messes; an additional check was made by analysis of composite meals. The results of the estimates of calorie and nutrient intake based on food tables and those calculated from analysis of the composite meals are summarized in Table 9.

TABLE 8
CALORIE AND NUTRIENT INTAKE IN LEBANESE RURAL POPULATION
(AVERAGE PER CAPITA PER DAY)

	Beqa'a Valley[1]		Kfarzubian[2]		
	Spring 1962	Autumn 1962	May 1964	September 1964	January 1964
Calories	2304	2454	2323	2438	1986
Protein					
Total g	75	74	84	86	70
Calcium mg	552	544	680	794	722
Iron mg	10.2	15.0	19.5	20.8	16.8
Vitamin A value I.U.	3374	2520	2566	2854	1679
Thiamine mg	1.6	1.6	1.9	2.0	1.9
Riboflavin mg	1.8	1.0	1.3	1.5	1.1
Niacin mg	15.5	10.6	19.3	20.0	16.2
Ascorbic acid mg	50.0	85.0	49.2	85.4	106.8

1. Source: Cowan, J. W., et al., 1964.
2. Source: Cowan, J. W., 1965.

TABLE 9
CALORIE AND NUTRIENT INTAKE IN LEBANESE ARMED FORCES[1]
(AVERAGE PER CAPITA PER DAY)

	Planned Menu[2]	Recipe Method[3]	Food Composite Analysis[3]
Calories	3808	3238	2778
Protein g	122	103	85
Fat g	114	96	52
Calcium mg	661	547	560
Iron mg	24	21	50
Vitamin A value I.U.	7169	5247	2000
Thiamine mg	1.64	1.45	0.84
Riboflavin mg	1.49	1.19	0.81
Niacin mg	21	19	17
Ascorbic Acid mg	194	140	36

1. Source: ICNND, 1962.
2. Four locations, month of March 1961.
3. 1254 rations in 4 two-day surveys.

There were marked differences between the three methods of assessment of the daily diets. The differences between the planned menu and recipe methods were ascribed to the losses as food waste and not to the differences in the rations issued. On the other hand the differences between recipe and composite meal-analysis methods were ascribed to excessive cooking losses, except for the differences in protein and fat, which were considered to be due possibly to sampling errors. Whereas the recipe method indicated that the diets were nutritionally adequate, the analysis showed that the diet actually eaten was deficient in thiamine and riboflavin and vitamin A activity. The ICNND recommended that proper cooking methods be adopted to reduce the cooking losses of labile vitamins.

JORDAN

The only source of information on food consumption and dietary habits in Jordan is the ICNND report of the nutrition survey carried out in 1962. As mentioned elsewhere, Jordan has large numbers of Palestine Arab refugees who constitute roughly 40% of the total population of the country. Many of them are housed in camps, others live in border villages, and some live among the urban and rural population of the country. The survey included representative samples from different locations of the refugee as well as the nonrefugee population. Their dietary habits are similar. Wheat bread forms the staple. Other cereal products may include *burghul, kishk,* rice, and pasta. The protein-rich grain legumes are consumed in appreciable quantities. The consumption of meat, eggs, and milk and milk products is subject to economic considerations as in the neighboring countries. Jordan has a negligible coastline, and hence fish consumption is practically nil.

The results of diet surveys by the twenty-four-hour-recall method on the 61 nonrefugee and 39 refugee families in different areas of Jordan are given in Table 10.

Foods available and consumed on the east and west banks of the

TABLE 10
FOOD CONSUMPTION AND NUTRIENT INTAKE[1] OF NONREFUGEE AND REFUGEE FAMILIES IN JORDAN (PER CAPITA PER DAY)

	Nonrefugees—9 Locations		Refugees—5 Locations	
	Average	Range	Average	Range
	g	g	g	g
Bread	371	290–540	397	340–506
Other cereals	77	6–142	44	22–88
Milk and *leben*	96	36–250	31	0–49
Cheese	25	0–57	16	6–41
Eggs	15	0–32	14	3–27
Meat	38	4–80	25	0–74
Legumes	19	0–60	49	27–100
Fats and oil	17	5–31	13	9–17
Green & yellow leafy vegetables	64	10–160	72	20–123
Other vegetables	162	15–310	172	81–429
Citrus fruit	35	0–100	23	8–42
Other fruit	44	0–100	15	0–30
Sugar	35	10–58	22	8–33
Miscellaneous	2	—	2	—
Calories	2063	1794–2443	2041	1600–2857
Protein g	64	53–80	68	51–88
Fat g	45	24–70	37	25–52
Calcium mg	429	291–595	363	258–456
Iron mg	8	4–12	10	7–14
Vitamin A value I.U.	2889	1102–6184	2524	1275–3939
Thiamine mg	1.19	1.07–1.39	1.36	1.02–1.71
Riboflavin mg	1.01	0.75–1.35	0.90[2]	0.63–1.03
Niacin mg	13	10–15	13	10–15
Ascorbic acid mg	66	5–147	48	14–74

1. Cooking losses are not considered.
2. These estimates are lower for the actual users of UNRWA ration flour, which is of enriched variety.

Jordan and in the Jordan valley itself were similar in variety. In the South, however, less vegetables and fresh fruit were available; e.g., the diets in the village of Ras en Naqb in Ma'an district consisted mainly of bread and other cereals, milk and *leben* (yoghurt). Other foods such as grain legumes, meat, eggs, and green and yellow leafy vegetables were consumed in very small quantities. As a result the diet in this village was inadequate in most respects. As mentioned before, the dietary patterns of the nonrefugee and refugee families were not dissimilar. However, in the refugee families the consumption of milk and milk products, meat, fruit, and sugar was less than in the nonrefugee families. This could have been due to the fact that the per capita income of refugees was probably less than that of the ordinary civilian population of Jordan.

The intake of calories and nutrients derived from the above-mentioned diets as calculated by reference to food tables and given in Table 10 indicates a very wide range of consumption levels. Some of the diets were totally inadequate. There is no indication in the ICNND report of the economic status of the families surveyed. It may, however, be reasonable to conclude on the basis of experience elsewhere that families with the lowest incomes must possibly have been living on inadequate and defective dietaries. Among other things, the iron intake appears to be very low. However the values calculated from composite meal analysis in a few families in each of the three locations gave intakes of 44, 26, and 28 mg per day when the intakes estimated from food tables were 8, 11, and 9 mg respectively for the same families. This again shows that at least so far as iron is concerned, estimates from food tables usually give low values for intake.

The rations planned for Jordanian armed forces and their food consumption in the messes and canteens were studied by ICNND as in Libya and Lebanon. The Jordanian ration, as compared to that in Lebanon, contained more bread, sugar, and rice and less grain legumes, fresh fruit, fresh vegetables, and meat. The calorie and nutrient intakes estimated from food tables and from analysis of composite meals in 11 units of the armed forces are given in Table 11.

The differences between the values obtained by calculation and analysis could not be explained particularly for protein and fat. The analysis of one day's composite meal will most likely give different figures from those obtained by averaging the intakes by recipe or recall method. Such discrepancies have repeatedly been observed in ICNND studies in Libya and Lebanon as have been mentioned earlier in this chapter.

Diet and Dietary Habits

TABLE 11
CALORIE AND NUTRIENT INTAKE OF JORDANIAN ARMED FORCES IN 11 UNITS
(AVERAGE PER CAPITA PER DAY)

	Calculated	Analyzed[1]
Calories	3280	3219
Protein g	93	123
Fat g	82	30
Calcium mg	1184	954
Iron mg	15	29
Vitamin A value I.U.	1560	—
Thiamine mg	1.52	1.55
Riboflavin mg	1.07	0.85
Niacin mg	16	14
Ascorbic acid mg	41	35

1. From composite food samples.

ICNND considered that the diets of the Jordanian armed forces were inadequate in vitamin A and riboflavin. It recommended greater use of leafy green and yellow vegetables, and the fortification of hydrogenated oil with vitamin A and carotene and of white flour with riboflavin.

GENERAL COMMENTS ON ARAB DIETS IN THE NEAR EAST

A reference has been made earlier to the basic similarity of diets in different Arab countries in the Near East. This is reflected so far as can be ascertained from the published data, in some common features in nutrient intakes and their sources in diet. These are summarized below:

1. Cereals, of which wheat is the most important, provide between 54 to 79% of the total calories ingested. This proportion is greater in the diets of the poor people and becomes less in higher income groups when the diets attain greater variety.

2. Cereals also provide between 52 to 82% of the total protein intake, and the extent of this contribution is subject to the same considerations as the calorie intake.

3. Animal-protein intake shows great variation; recorded figures show a range of 2 to 31% of the total protein ingested in Libya, Egypt, Lebanon, and Jordan taken together. The relative unavailability and high cost of animal products determine the level of their consumption.

4. The intake of calcium and iron "appears" to be low. However, analysis of the composite meal samples has almost always shown

higher levels of intake than the estimates from food tables and within the realm of adequacy. The reason for iron-deficiency anemia prevailing in certain of these communities must lie elsewhere.

5. Inadequacy in thiamine intake seems to be comparatively rare. In most diet surveys an intake higher than 400 mcg/1000 Cal has been recorded. However inadequacy of riboflavin intake appears far more common as judged from the FAO/WHO recommendation of 550 mcg/1000 Cal. Very few of the published data exceed the recommended level, and the estimated deficit has been as much as 50%.

6. The intake of ascorbic acid is considered adequate in spite of a few low recorded values. The Arab practice of eating salads and raw vegetables, as mentioned earlier, protects them against the deficiency of this vitamin.

Several of these features are also common to other developing countries. Insufficient food production, the high cost of protective foods, and the low purchasing power of the masses make it inevitable that bulk of the population must depend to a large extent on the consumption of the cheapest foods, sacrificing quality for quantity in order to satisfy their hunger.

REFERENCES

Abdou, I. A. 1965. *Nutritional Status in the New Valley* (in Arabic). Cairo, Egypt: National Documentation Center.

Abdou, I. A., and A. K. Amer. 1965. A Study of the Nutritional Status of Mothers, Infants, and Young Children Attending Maternity and Child Health Centers in Cairo. Part II—Dietary Intake and Nutritional Status of Pregnant and Nursing Mothers. *Bull. Nutr. Inst., U.A.R.* 1: 21.

Abdou, I. A., and A. H. Mahfouz. 1965. A Survey of the Diet in the Egyptian Village and Its Seasonal Variation. *Bull. Nutr. Inst., U.A.R.* 1: 51.

Barakat, M. R., and G. Mohamed. 1951. A Comparison of Food Consumption of Industrial and Agricultural Labourers in Rural Egypt. *J. Egypt. Med. Assoc.* 34: 462.

Calcium Requirements. 1962. Report of an FAO/WHO Expert Group, Wld. Hlth. Tech. Rep. Ser. Geneva, Switzerland: World Health Organization.

Carter, J. P., L. E. Grivetti, J. T. Davis, S. Nassif, A. Mansour, W. A. Mousa, A. Atta, V. N. Patwardhan, M. A. Moneim, I. A. Abdou, and W. J. Darby. 1969. Growth and Sexual Development of Adolescent Egyptian Village Boys: Effects of Zinc, Iron, and Placebo Supplementation. *Amer. J. Clin. Nutr.* 22: 59.

Cowan, J. W. 1965. Dietary Survey in Rural Lebanon, Part II. *J. Amer. Dietet. Assoc.* 47: 466.

Cowan, J. W., S. Chopra, and G. Houry. 1964. Dietary Survey in Rural Lebanon. *J. Amer. Dietet. Assoc.* 45: 130.
Ferro-Luzzi, G. 1958. *Report to the Government of Libya on Nutrition.* Rome, Italy: Food and Agriculture Organization of the United Nations.
Hafuth, K., J. A. Videan, and I. E. Videan, trans. 1964. *The Eastern Key.* (Abd el-Latif Baghdadi, *Kitab al-Ifadah wal I'tibar,* Cairo: 1204). London: George Allen and Unwin Ltd.
Interdepartmental Committee on Nutrition for National Defense. *Reports of Nutrition Surveys in Libya 1957; Lebanon 1962; and Jordan 1963.* Bethesda, Md.: National Institutes of Health.
Report of the Permanent Nutrition Committee. 1939–1946. Cairo: Ministry of Public Health.
FAO/WHO Expert Group. 1967. *Requirements of Vitamin A, Thiamine, Riboflavin, and Niacin.* Wld. Hlth. Org. Tech. Rep. Ser. Geneva, Switzerland: World Health Organization.
Riad, H. 1960. A Nutriture Survey of Young Adults Attending the Army Recruiting Center of Alexandria. Thesis (M.P.H.), High Institute of Public Health, Alexandria, Egypt, U.A.R.
Ross, M., M. Khoury-Schmitz, and Z. Hefnawy. 1954. *Preliminary Report on Visits to 23 Families in Aghour Soughra.* Rome, Italy: Food and Agriculture Organization of the United Nations.
Sabry, Z. I. 1961. *Protein Foods in Middle Eastern Diets in Meeting Protein Needs of Infants and Children.* Publ. 843. National Academy of Sciences. Washington, D.C.: National Research Council.
Sadek, 1960. Unpublished thesis. Quoted from Nutrition in Pregnancy and Lactation. Report of a WHO Expert Committee. Wld. Hlth. Org. Tech. Rep. Series 1965, 302, p. 47.
Saleh, A. 1960. A Study of the Food Habits of Pregnant and Lactating Mothers Attending Shatby Hospital. Thesis (M. P. H.), High Institute of Public Health, Alexandria, Egypt, U.A.R.
Yang, Y. H. 1963. Food and Nutrition Policy-Report to the Government of Libya. Rome, Italy: Food and Agriculture Organization of the United Nations.

13 NUTRITIONAL STATUS OF POPULATION GROUPS IN EGYPT, JORDAN, LIBYA, AND LEBANON

EGYPT

The permanent Nutrition Committee of Egypt, established in 1939 by the Ministry of Public Health, had as one of its functions the evaluation of the nutritional status of population groups in the country. However, it was only in 1944 that the Committee could arrange for nutrition surveys and dietary studies in different areas in Upper and Lower Egypt. In 1952 a Nutrition Division was formed in the Ministry of Public Health which took over the work connected with nutrition surveys. Three years later, with the establishment of the Nutrition Institute of Egypt, the responsibility concerning dietary and nutritional studies devolved on the latter. Despite this apparent continuity, there are not many publications reporting on the nutritional status of the different segments of the Egyptian population. It is possible that the reports of most surveys carried out under the auspices of the Ministry of Health might be found in the archives of the Ministry. At infrequent intervals, consolidated and abridged reports were prepared by the Ministry for presentation at the international meetings such as those arranged by FAO and WHO. Furthermore, the results of such nutrition surveys as have been published have not been very informative. Consequently not much published information is available in detail on the nutritional status of the Egyptian population.

The growth patterns of the Egyptian infants, children, and adolescents, which have been reviewed in another chapter, provide the only reliable information on the nutritional status of the young growing population groups. The general conclusion one reaches after the study of growth patterns is that growth is retarded in a majority of Egyptian children. However, the interpretation of growth data is difficult, for one is not in a position to decide whether the retarded growth is the result of general undernutrition or whether specific nutritional deficiencies also take their toll. Besides, studies on growth have not in many instances provided information on nonnutritional factors such as parasitic infections, which should influence growth. An attempt will, however, be made in the following pages to review such information, published and unpublished, as is available, meager though it proves to be.

Two villages in Shebin el Kanater District were surveyed in 1944. Growth of children in general was reported to be retarded; however, differences between socioeconomic groups were noticed. Children from the higher socioeconomic groups of population showed a higher growth rate than those from the poorer classes. The average hemoglobin levels were lower than normal. A few cases of rickets in infants were found. Serum ascorbic acid was less than 0.4 mg/100 ml in 17 of the 100 subjects examined, but no scurvy was found. Although no figures are given, the survey team reported that there was less pellagra in this area than was prevalent in 1939.

Also in 1944 a nutrition survey was done in Quena and Aswan provinces of Upper Egypt. This followed an epidemic of malaria with high mortality in an area where malaria was endemic. The physique of the people in general was poor. The growth of children showed unmistakable evidence of retardation. The average weights of school children of 7 to 15 years of age were lower by 3 to 8 kg at different ages than those of the school children in Cairo; similarly the Quena and Aswan school children were shorter by 5 to 12 cm than their Cairo counterparts of comparable age. The heights and weights of adults from Upper Egypt were also lower than those of adults from Cairo. Angular stomatitis, rough and dry skin, and nutritional edema were common, especially among school children. A few cases of night blindness were also encountered. It was concluded that the population from these provinces was generally under- and malnourished. The fact that its economic status was also very bad may be one of the principal reasons for their poor nutritional status.

The nutritional status of industrial workers was also studied in 1944. Among these were the workers and their families in a textile yarn mill in Alexandria and in mines, quarries, and oil fields near the Red Sea. No clinical evidence of specific nutritional deficiency was found in the workers and their families from Alexandria. However, the heights and weights of children and the adult population were lower than those of their Cairo counterparts, and hemoglobin levels were also low, indicating a generally low level of nutritional status.

On the other hand the survey reported finding clinical signs of nutritional deficiency in varying degrees among the workers and their families in the Red Sea area. Unfortunately no details in support of this statement are vouched in the report. The detailed reports of individual surveys, which must have been made to the Ministry, were not available to the authors.

It may be mentioned here that these surveys were done during the latter part of World War II, when the economy of the country must have been disturbed. Food production suffered; imports were limited; demands of the Allied Armed Forces, which were stationed in the country in increasingly large numbers through a large part of the war years, must have affected the availability and prices of food; an increase in the general price level made the lot of the bulk of the population difficult so far as its dietary intake was concerned. As a result, the general level of nutrition in Egypt could have been expected to be adversely affected.

There must have been a few more surveys done after the formation of the Nutrition Division as mentioned before. Unfortunately no information about the results is available except such as appears in a report prepared for the FAO Regional Nutrition Committee in 1953, which does not add much to the information on nutritional status given above.

During 1956–1957 Abdou, Ali, and Lebshtein examined 1143 infants of up to 24 months attending four Maternal and Child Health Centers in Cairo. The authors found low hemoglobin values: the average was 9.1 g/100 ml below 3 months and 8.6 g/100 ml between 12 and 24 months. As a matter of fact, between 40 and 70% of the infants up to 12 months could be considered anemic, and the proportion of anemic infants increased progressively with age from 0 to 12 months. Other evidence of malnutrition was the occurrence of clinically diagnosed rickets in 13% of the infants. The authors believe that the actual prevalence of rickets would have been found to be higher if radiological and biochemical methods of diagnosis had been used. Delayed dentition was observed in 22% of the infants, and delayed sitting and standing in 18%. No other signs of malnutrition are mentioned.

Not many observations are on record so far as the nutritional status of children of preschool age children is concerned. Abdou *et al.* (1967) report on the clinical examination of 1,637 boys and 1,219 girls of 7 to 19 years from Cairo schools. This was a subsample of the group on

TABLE 1
CLINICAL FINDINGS IN CAIRO SCHOOL CHILDREN[1]

	Boys 1637 %	Girls 1219 %
Cheilosis	16.3	15.6
Angular stomatitis	9.2	3.8
Tongue atrophy (papillary)	1.8	5.0
Tongue hypertrophy (papillary)	1.5	4.4
Scorbutic gums	2.7	5.1
Dry skin	7.4	6.9
Hyperkeratosis follicularis	3.2	3.6
Enlarged Thyroid	1.7	17.8

1. Source: Abdou, Ali, and Lebshtein (1965).

which heights and weights had been reported earlier. Their findings on the prevalence of nutritional deficiency signs are given in Table 1.

The table shows that among the Cairo school children a certain proportion showed overt signs of malnutrition, which could probably be ascribed to dietary deficiencies of the vitamin B complex and possibly of vitamin A.

The average hemoglobin levels were below 12 g per 100 ml in boys and girls of 6 to 10 years; they rose gradually, but the average was around 13 g in the 14-to-19-years group. These values are indicative of the existence of anemia in a certain proportion of Cairo school children.

In a recent study of 279 boys aged 11 to 17 years of a high school in Sindion about 20 km from Cairo, Carter *et al.* (1969) also noted the occurrence of clinical signs of nutritional deficiencies. They examined the boys once in October 1965 and then again in October 1966. Their observations are summarized in Table 2.

It is of interest to compare the findings of Abdou *et al.* in Cairo and of Carter *et al.* made in a rural community. Although the findings in Cairo were published in 1967, the actual study was done in 1959–60. Thus, apart from the fact that one sample is urban and the other rural, there is also a time interval of 5 to 6 years between the two studies. Yet there are some similarities in the findings. For example, the relatively high prevalence of angular lesions of the lips and cheilosis was observed in both studies; so also were the lesions of the tongue, although a very much higher figure for papillary atrophy is recorded by Carter *et al.* Dryness of the skin was observed by both the groups. Carter *et al.* found no hyperkeratosis follicularis, although the age group studied by them is most prone to developing this deficiency

TABLE 2
CLINICAL FINDINGS IN 279 BOYS IN SINDION HIGH SCHOOL[1]

		October 1965 %	October 1966 %
Skin:	Dry or scaling (xerosis)	9	2
Hair:	Dyspigmented	1	0
Lips:	Angular lesions	21	44
	Cheilosis	21	35
Tongue:	Papillary atrophy	19	21
	Red beefy: glossitis	3	0
	Magenta	4	1
Eyes:	Bitot's spots	4	5
	Circumcorneal injection	0	2
	Corneal scars	2	1
Glands:	Parotid enlarged	4	1
	Thyroid enlarged Grade I	4	12
Abdomen:	Hepatomegaly	29	17
	Splenomegaly	15	8

1. Source: Carter et al. (1969).

sign. The significance of Bitot's spots in the age groups 11 to 17 as a sign of vitamin A deficiency is questionable (McLaren, Oomen, and Escapini, 1966). Also, the observations of Carter *et al.* do not make clear whether the rather high prevalence of hepatomegaly had any nutritional significance.

In the study reported by Carter *et al.* is to be found a tentative estimate of nutrient intake based on the result of a diet survey carried out in the families of the school children. The results indicate that the diets of the boys were limited in calories, calcium, iron, vitamin A, riboflavin, and ascorbic acid. An appreciable proportion of boys showed low excretion of riboflavin as expressed per gm of creatinine. Thus it is possible that the high prevalence of the lesions of the tongue and the lips may be an expression of riboflavin deficiency.

Abdou (1965) reports a phenomenally high prevalence of certain clinical signs of nutritional deficiency in school children in the oases of Kharga and Dakhla as is shown in Table 3.

Since Abdou was involved in the clinical examination of school children in Cairo as well as in the oases, one can only conclude that the reported figures for the children in Dakhla and Kharga represented the correct state of affairs, which, if true, should be considered indicative of an unusually high prevalence of some nutritional deficiencies. Commenting on the skin manifestation, Abdou describes

TABLE 3
CLINICAL FINDINGS IN CHILDREN FROM KHARGA AND DAKHLA OASES, EGYPT[1]

		Kharga (1102) %	Dakhla (249) %
Lips:	Angular lesions	52	41
	Cheilosis	67	59
Tongue:	Inflamed	13	3.2
	Red margins only	60	43
Gums:	Inflamed	73	68
Skin:	Rough	45	29
	Scaly dermatosis	51	36

1. Source: Abdou (1965).

rough skin as similar to that seen in hyperkeratosis follicularis both as regards its description as well as distribution on arms, legs, and the trunk. He also described scaly dermatosis as characterized by roughness and peeling of the skin, leaving hypopigmented areas confined to the dorsum of the hand extending up the forearm and found covering the exposed areas of joints such as elbows and knees and around the mouth. Abdou distinguishes it from the pellagrous type of dermatitis. Vilter, Darby, and Glazer (1954) in their report on pellagra in Egypt also describe a similar dermatosis as distinct from that of pellagrous origin. They felt that this type of dermatosis may connote malnutrition of a nonspecific type. Its nutritional significance must, however, remain uncertain until some positive proof is forthcoming. Inflamed gums could easily be a manifestation of the wide prevalence of periodontal disease which in fact has been found to occur in Egypt.

Riad and Barakat (1964) make a report without relevant details on a nutrition survey of 958 males of 19 to 20 years of age in Beheira and Gharbia provinces. They find the lesions of lips, tongue, gums, and the skin present in a proportion of the sample examined but give no figures of prevalence.

OTHER COUNTRIES

The information on the nutritional status of population groups in the neighboring countries has been derived mainly from the surveys carried out in Libya, Lebanon, and Jordan by the ICNND. The dates of the surveys and the population sample examined are given in Table 4.

Apart from the armed forces personnel, which included males only,

TABLE 4
POPULATION GROUPS SURVEYED BY ICNND

	Libya	Lebanon	Jordan
Date of Survey	June–August 1957	February–April 1961	April–June 1962
Population groups surveyed			
Armed Forces	2,199[1]	2,284	1,528
Civilians	1,629	4,857	3,663
Palestine Arab Refugees	—	1,485	2,583

1. Included personnel from the police force.

the civilian sample comprised males and females of all age groups. The civilian sample was selected from different regions in each country, so that within the limits of feasibility a fair cross-section of the population in all geographic areas of the country was included in the survey.

In Lebanon and Jordan, the Palestine Arab refugees were surveyed as a separate group. Some explanation about them is necessary. When Israel was established in 1948, a large number of Arabs either migrated willingly or were driven out from the areas where they had been living for generations. Political unrest and armed clashes with the neighboring Arab states subsequent to the partition of Palestine added to the number of Arab refugees who were separated into four countries, namely, Egypt, Jordan, Syria, and Lebanon. In Egypt the refugees were confined to an isolated area bordering on Israel known as the Gaza Strip and had little communication with the rest of the country. In Jordan, Syria, and Lebanon, the bulk of them was settled in organized camps in different parts of the country and in border villages. A certain number lives in villages and towns among the local inhabitants. The number of refugees in relation to the total populations of Lebanon, Syria, and Jordan was much larger than in Egypt. The largest concentration of Arab refugees is in Jordan, where they formed in 1965 about 40% or more of the total population of the Hashemite Kingdom of Jordan.

A special United Nations Agency known as the United Nations Relief and Works Agency (UNRWA) looks after the health and welfare of the refugees in all of the four countries where they have been settled. UNRWA provides dry basic rations equivalent to 1500–1600 calories per day to all refugees registered with the agency. Infants, children, and pregnant and nursing women get special supplements as well. UNRWA also provides medical and health services for the refugees. It was therefore naturally of special interest to compare

Nutritional Status of Population Groups

the nutritional status of refugees with the local civilian population, and this was the reason for including them as a special group in the ICNND surveys in Jordan and Lebanon.

The ICNND nutrition surveys included the examination of the food situation within the countries visited and the patterns and levels of the food consumption. The determination of nutritional status was based on anthropometric measurements, clinical examination for the overt signs of malnutrition, and biochemical examination of a subsample of the population group under study. The clinical examination itself was in an abbreviated form for the whole sample and more detailed on a subsample. In general the results of the detailed examination confirmed the findings of those made in the abbreviated examination. The biochemical examination consisted of determinations of hemoglobin and hematocrit on whole blood and total protein, vitamin C, vitamin A, and carotenoids in serum. The excretions of thiamine, riboflavin, and N-methyl nicotinamide were determined in random samples of urine and the results expressed in terms of per gram of creatinine in urine. The suggested guide for the interpretation of data on vitamin concentrations in blood and in urine are given in Table 5. The table has been adapted from the ICNND *Manual for Nutrition Surveys* (1963). This guide is used in the following discussion of the results of vitamin determinations in blood and urine reported in surveys in Libya, Lebanon, and Jordan.

Libya

The civilian sample in Libya comprised 1,029 men, 364 women (61 pregnant), 135 children 5 to 15 years, and 103 children 1 to 2 years of age. There were only 13 girls in the age group 5 to 15 years; hence findings on them have been ignored in the discussion that follows.

The findings of clinical examination by survey groups are summarized in Table 6.

The interpretation of the clinical findings alone for evaluating the nutritional status is often beset with difficulties. A certain amount of assistance is provided by biochemical determinations such as concentrations in blood or excretion in urine of nutrients or their metabolites. Even then the results are seldom conclusive. Hence the conclusions reached on the basis of clinical and biochemical examinations should be viewed with certain caution, the more so if the available evidence is restricted to clinical observations alone.

The results of the clinical (Table 6) and biochemical examinations (Table 7) in Libya showed that in general the nutritional status of the police and defense forces personnel was satisfactory, although there

TABLE 5
SUGGESTED GUIDE TO INTERPRETATION OF BIOCHEMICAL DATA[1]

	Deficient	Low	Acceptable	High
Blood				
Adults and children				
Plasma ascorbic acid mg/100 ml	< 0.10	0.10–0.19	0.20–0.39	> 0.40
Plasma retinol µg/100 ml	< 10	10–19	20–49	> 50
Plasma carotenoids µg/100 ml		20–39	40–99	> 100
Urine				
Adults				
Thiamine µg/g creatinine	< 27	27–65	66–129	> 130
Riboflavin µg/g creatinine	< 27	27–79	80–269	> 270
N'-methylnicotinamide mg/g creatinine	< 0.5	0.5–1.59	1.6–4.29	> 4.3
Children				
Thiamine µg/g creatinine				
1–3 yrs.	< 120	120–175	176–600	> 600
4–6 yrs.	< 85	85–120	121–400	> 400
Riboflavin µg/g creatinine				
1–3 yrs.	< 150	150–499	500–900	> 900
4–6 yrs.	< 100	100–299	300–600	> 600
Pregnant women				
Thiamine µg/g creatinine				
1st trimester	< 27	27–65	66–129	> 130
2nd trimester	< 23	23–54	55–109	> 110
3rd trimester	< 21	21–49	50–99	> 100
Riboflavin µg/g creatinine				
1st trimester	< 27	27–79	80–269	> 270
2nd trimester	< 39	39–119	120–399	> 400
3rd trimester	< 30	30–89	90–299	> 300
N'-methylnicotinamide mg/g creatinine				
1st trimester	< 0.5	0.5–1.59	1.60–4.29	> 4.3
2nd trimester	< 0.6	0.6–1.99	2.00–4.99	> 5.0
3rd trimester	< 0.8	0.8–2.49	2.50–6.49	> 6.5

1. Source: Adapted from ICNND Manual for Nutrition Surveys, 1963.

TABLE 6
LIBYA: PHYSICAL FINDINGS IN ABBREVIATED EXAMINATIONS, BY SURVEY GROUPS[1]

	Men			Boys	Women	Women
	Police	Army	Civilian	5–15 yrs.	Nonpregnant	Pregnant
Number Examined	808	941	865	120	228	61
	%	%	%	%	%	%
Thyroid enlarged	0.1	0	0.2	0	1.3	4.9
Nasolabial seborrhea	9.7	12.1	15.3	0.8	10.5	14.8
Follicular keratosis	1.6	1.4	1.8	4.2	2.6	18.0
Scrotal dermatitis	2.8	2.8	0	0		
Pellagrous lesions	0.1	0	0.1	0	0	0
Bitot's spots	0	0.6	0	0	0.9	1.6
Lips, angular lesions	6.6	3.7	5.1	5.0	4.8	9.8
Lips, angular scars only	2.7	4.7	3.6	2.5	7.5	27.9
Lips, cheilosis	0.7	0.6	0.5	0.8	0.9	0
Tongue:						
Filiform pap. atrophy, Mod., sev.	0.5	0.5	1.5	0.8	5.3	14.8
Glossitis	1.0	0.6	2.0	0.8	1.3	4.9
Magenta-colored tongue	0	0	0.5	0	0.9	1.6
Lower Extremities:						
Bilateral edema	0	0	0	0	5.3	0
Calf tenderness, slight	0	0	0.9	0.8	0.9	0
Loss of ankle jerk	1.0	1.0	2.1	1.7	24.6	1.6

1. Source: Adapted from ICNND *Report on Nutrition Survey in Libya*, 1957.

TABLE 7
THE RESULTS OF BIOCHEMICAL EXAMINATION IN LIBYAN SURVEY[1]

	Police and Defense Forces		Army		Civilian Men		Women			
							Nonpregnant		Pregnant	
	No.	%	No.	%	No.	%	No.	%	No.	%
Hemoglobin g/100 ml	77	14.8	67	14.7	97	14.96	37	12.88	35	11.09
Hematocrit %	77	47.6	67	46.9	97	47.1	37	41.9	35	35.8
MCHC %	77	31.1	67	31.3	97	31.7	37	31.0	35	30.8
Total Protein g/100 ml serum	77	7.93	67	8.01	97	7.97	37	8.29	35	7.55
Vitamin C mg/100 ml serum	77	0.07	67	0.10	97	0.26	37	0.16	35	0.33
Vitamin A µg/100 ml serum	77	38.2	67	26.9	97	32.4	37	27.0	35	8.0
Carotenoids µg/100 ml serum	77	143	67	164	97	138	37	168	35	162
Urine (Median values)										
Thiamine µg/g Creatinine	76	80	66	71	103	98	35	80	33	306
Riboflavin µg/g Creatinine	76	190	66	170	103	230	35	260	33	280
N-Me-Nicotinamide mg/g Creatinine	76	0.65	66	0.56	103	0.75	35	0.78	33	1.60

1. Source: Adapted from ICNND Report on Nutrition Survey in Libya, 1957.

were indications of deficiencies of vitamins of the B complex. These were more common in the civilian population groups, particularly among the women. A study of the urinary excretion of thiamine, riboflavin, and N-methyl nicotinamide throws some light, but not enough to prove satisfactory. For example, between 30 and 40% of the subsample of the police, military, and civilian men and nonpregnant women excreted thiamine in the deficient or low range. Thiamine excretion in pregnant women was in the acceptable and high range. Twenty-five percent of the nonpregnant women examined showed loss of ankle jerk as against 1 to 2% found in all other groups. This sign was also present among pregnant women in spite of the acceptable to high thiamine excretion in this group. The distribution of riboflavin excretion pattern is even more discordant. Not more than 4% of the subsample was in the category of deficient or low, and yet as Table 6 indicates, the signs attributable to riboflavin deficiency (WHO Rep. TRS 258, 1963) were fairly common.

However, from the evidence obtained during the survey, it can be concluded that certain signs of malnutrition, such as those attributable to deficiencies of vitamins of the B complex and possibly that of vitamin A as well, existed in the Libyan population. The serum concentrations of ascorbic acid were in general low; those of vitamin A ranged from deficient to low levels. In general the pregnant women exhibited physical signs of malnutrition with greater frequency than nonpregnant women, with the exception of the loss of ankle jerk which was exhibited by 24.6% of nonpregnant women as compared with only 1.6% in those who were pregnant. Urinary thiamine excretions in the two groups do not provide a satisfactory answer for this discrepancy.

Lebanon

The sample of population surveyed in Lebanon consisted of 2,284 individuals from the armed forces, 4,857 local civilian population, and 1,485 refugees. Both sexes and all ages were represented in the latter two groups; 65.2% of the armed forces sample was made up of male adolescents and young adults between the ages of 15 and 24 years, and 33.8 were between 25 and 44 years.

Among the signs of nutritional deficiencies seen in the population groups examined, follicular hyperkeratosis and angular lesions of the lips, together with angular scars and cheilosis, were encountered most frequently. Their prevalence among infants and children up to 4 years was less than in later age groups. Furthermore these signs were more frequent in refugee children of 0–4 years than in nonrefugees.

Thereafter such differences were not noticeable. A comparison of clinical findings in women who were not pregnant with those who were pregnant or lactating showed almost similar frequency of the occurrence of nutritional deficiency signs in both the groups. It is for these reasons that clinical findings are presented in a composite form in Table 8, prepared from the data contained in the ICNND report on Lebanon.

The biochemical findings given in Table 9 are more informative. The hemoglobin, hematocrit, and MCHC values indicate the existence of anemia, much of which could probably be of the iron-deficiency type, in about 40% of the population. Among the military personnel, length of service did not seem to make any difference in this regard. The average serum total protein levels were normal in all

TABLE 8
LEBANON: CLINICAL FINDINGS IN MILITARY AND CIVILIAN POPULATION GROUPS[1]

	Military 1938 %	Civilian[2] Nonrefugees 1871 %	Refugees 1286 %
Eyes:			
Bitot's spot	0.6	0.4	0.3
Face and Neck:			
Nasolabial seborrhea	3.2	1.5	1.1
Lips:			
Angular lesions	12.5	12.8	16.9
Angular scars	3.2	7.0	6.4
Cheilosis	20.9	23.6	44.2
Gums:			
Swollen red papillae diffuse	2.7	0.4	2.3
Tongue:			
Filiform papillary atrophy	0.6	1.0	0.4
Glossitis	0.2	0.5	1.0
Magenta	1.8	1.5	1.2
Glands:			
Thyroid enlarged	49.1	45.8	39.6
Skin:			
Follicular hyperkeratosis			
Arms	9.0	21.4	26.2
Thighs	14.8	18.3	28.0
Lower Extremities:			
Bilateral edema	0.0	0.1	0.2
Bilateral loss of ankle jerks	0.6	0.2	0.1

1. Source: Adapted from ICNND *Report on Nutrition Survey in Lebanon,* 1962.
2. The civilian sample consisted of males and females of all ages.

TABLE 9
LEBANON: BIOCHEMICAL FINDINGS IN LEBANON MILITARY AND CIVILIAN (NONREFUGEE) POPULATIONS[1]

	Children 5–9 yrs.		Male 10–14 yrs		Female 10–14 yrs		Male 15–44 yrs.		Female 15+ yrs.		Military	
	No.	%	No.	%	No.	%	No.	%	No.	%	No.	%
Hemoglobin g/100 ml	43	11.8	22	12.4	31	12.4	45	14.1	32	12.0	231	14.3
Hematocrit %	47	30.0[2]	23	40.0	31	41.6	45	46.6	32	40.3	231	46.3
MCHC %	43	30.0	22	31.1	31	30.0	45	30.2	32	29.4	231	30.8
Total Protein g/100 ml serum	47	8.1	22	8.2	32	8.6	44	8.6	33	8.7	226	8.5
Vitamin A μg/100 ml serum	33	22.9	20	26.3	25	25.8	39	42.3	24	34.8	225	43.9
Vitamin C mg/100 ml serum	40	0.95	18	0.83	21	1.18	30	0.52	22	0.74	206	0.61
Carotenoids μg/100 ml serum	34	88	20	109	26	115	40	103	24	118	229	98
Urine[3]												
Thiamine μg/g Creatinine	37	684	17	575	17	425	6	249	7	550	168	150
Riboflavin μg/g Creatinine	45	105	24	71	26	77	48	68	36	77	231	41
N-Me-Nicotinamide mg/g Creatinine	39	4.6	15	2.30	24	3.93	40	3.87	24	2.97	225	2.7

1. Source: Adapted from ICNND Report on Nutrition Survey in Lebanon, 1962.
2. Figure is wrong; it is probably nearer 40.
3. Median values.

the groups. The average vitamin C concentrations in serum showed a tendency to decrease with age. On the other hand serum vitamin A tended to increase with age, although the values were on the low side. In pregnancy and lactation all the biochemical values tended to be lower. Since their number was very small, the data have not been included in the table.

The urinary excretion figures for thiamine were considered satisfactory. On the other hand, 40 to 60% values for urinary riboflavin per gram creatinine were either in the "deficient" or "low" range. This percentage showed an increase in pregnancy and lactation.

The average urinary excretion of riboflavin in military personnel was lower than in nonrefugee civilian males: 88% of the values were in the low and deficient ranges. The daily average intake of riboflavin in military messes was estimated at 0.37 mg per 1,000 Cal. as against 0.477 per 1,000 Cal. in civilians. Both these values indicated a marginal intake of riboflavin, that of the military being lower of the two. The low excretion of riboflavin, together with the lesions of the lips and tongue, indicate widespread deficiency of riboflavin in the Lebanon population groups examined by ICNND.

Commenting on the nutritional status of infants and children up to 5 years, the ICNND report suggests that the clinical and biochemical findings indicate limitation of calories as well as several nutrients such as protein, iron, iodine, ascorbic acid, and vitamin A. Clinical evidence of rickets was seen in refugee infants, namely, cranial bossing in approximately 40% and costochondral beading in 4 to 10 per cent.

Jordan

The ICNND survey of 1962 in Jordan was followed a year later by a detailed nutrition survey of infants and children of 0 to 6 years, undertaken jointly by ICNND and the Interdepartmental Committee of Nutrition in Jordan. In this survey, more than 2,800 infants and children from different parts of Jordan were examined; 23% of the sample was made up of the Arab refugee children. The findings of this survey are illustrated in Table 10 and summarized below.

The signs of frank protein-calorie deficiency were found in an appreciable number of children. In general, marasmus was twice as common in girls as in boys. One does not know what significance should be attached to this except to suggest that girls are more likely to be neglected by their mothers than boys. This is true in some communities in developing countries, and it may be true in this case as well. Pharaon *et al.* (1965) distinguish a category of pre-kwas-

TABLE 10
CLINICAL FINDINGS IN A PEDIATRIC SURVEY IN JORDAN[1]

	Refugees		Nonrefugees	
	Male 0–6	Female 0–6	Male 0–6	Female 0–6
Age Group Number	360 %	299 %	1200 %	978 %
Hair:				
Dyspigmented	6.9	12.4	5.0	5.9
Thin	8.3	17.1	7.5	10.5
Easily pluckable	3.9	6.4	2.7	3.4
Eyes:				
Dry conjunctiva	0.3	0.3	0.3	0.3
Bitot's spot	0.3	—	0.2	0.3
Xerophthalmia	0.3	—	0.1	—
Lips:				
Angular lesions	6.7	7.4	5.2	8.5
Cheilosis	1.4	1.3	0.6	1.5
Gums:				
Swollen red papillae	—	0.3	0.2	0.3
Tongue:				
Atrophic filiform papillae	1.9	4.3	1.0	1.9
Glossitis	4.2	2.7	4.0	3.2
Glands:				
Thyroid enlarged	0.6	—	0.1	0.1
Skin:				
Inelastic	1.4	1.7	1.2	1.4
Petechiae	—	—	0.1	0.2
Dermatitis	1.9	0.3	0.9	1.6
Follicular hyperkeratosis	—	—	—	—
Abdomen:				
Hepatomegaly	36.1	43.8	37.7	38.1
Splenomegaly	4.2	4.3	3.9	4.5
Pot belly	3.1	6.7	3.1	3.0
Lower Extremities:				
Bilateral edema	0.6	1.7	0.8	0.8
Calf tenderness	—	—	—	0.1
Skeletal:				
Craniotabes	—	—	0.1	—
Cranial bossing	1.2	—	0.1	0.3
Beading of ribs	—	—	0.1	—
Enlarged joints	0.3	—	0.1	—
Muscle wasting	16.4	21.7	13.2	16.9

1. Source: Adapted from ICNND-ICNJ *Report on Nutrition Survey on Infants and Preschool Children in Jordan,* 1964.

shiorkor which according to the ICNND *Manual* (1963) includes children who are underweight, undersized, and underdeveloped, with poor muscle tone and with or without dyspigmented hair. It should represent a stage which could later develop into marasmus or kwashiorkor. This term can therefore be taken to include such mild to moderate cases of protein-calorie deficiency as can be classified neither as marasmus nor as kwashiorkor. According to Pharaon *et al.* about 6.5% of the boys and 10.7% of the girls of 0–6 years of age were found to show overt signs of moderate to severe protein-calorie deficiency. In this respect there was no difference between the refugee and nonrefugee children.

Among the other signs of malnutrition seen in the children, angular lesions of lips and cheilosis and lesions of the tongue, such as atrophy of the filiform papillae and glossitis, were found in an appreciable number of children.

The estimates of Pharaon *et al.* on the occurrence of the ocular signs of vitamin A deficiency are probably an underestimate. A careful survey on vitamin A deficiency in infants and preschool children undertaken a year later by Patwardhan and Kamel (1967) under WHO auspices revealed its prevalence to the extent of about 8% in a randomly selected population principally from Amman and Jerusalem districts. Among 1,180 children examined, they detected 95 cases of xerophthalmia and its sequelae with the following signs: xerosis conjunctivae, 77; Bitot's spots, 7; pigmented conjunctiva, 15; xerosis cornea, 1; corneal ulcer,1; and leukoma, 2.

The observations of Pharaon *et al.* and Patwardhan and Kamel on serum vitamin A levels, on the other hand, have yielded almost identical values, namely, 21.9 $\mu g/100$ ml and 20.3 $\mu g/100$ ml, respectively. In over 43% of children out of 303 in Pharaon's series in whom vitamin A in serum was determined, and in 50% of 283 in the series of Patwardhan and Kamel, the serum vitamin A was less than 20 $\mu g/100$ ml, indicating a deficient and low range. Thus in spite of a reasonably good agreement in biochemical findings, the clinical assessment in the two investigations is at variance. All that can be said is that the results of serum vitamin A determinations would be more in keeping with a higher prevalence of clinical vitamin A deficiency than indicated by the observations of Pharaon *et al.*

The hemoglobin and hematocrit values indicate mild to moderate anemia more common in infants below 2 years. Hypoalbuminemia was also more common in the first two years of life and least in children of 5 years and over. On the other hand, vitamin C in serum indicated a satisfactory status up to 5 years. The urinary excretion of thiamine was low in 6.7% of the children studied, whereas that of riboflavin was low in nearly 40%. This may have a bearing on the occurrence of the oral manifestations attributable to riboflavin deficiency.

The ICNND Survey Team examined 898 refugee children and 796 nonrefugee children of both sexes, 5 to 9 years of age. Angular lesions of the lips, swollen red papillae of the gums, and hyperkeratosis follicularis were encountered more frequently than in the younger age groups examined by Pharaon *et al.* Between the refugee and nonrefugee children there were few differences, with the exception of angular scars of the lips in the refugee children. The interpretation of this difference is difficult because, as the ICNND report admits, some examiners were inclined to overreport this sign.

In the next age group, 10 to 14 years of age, consisting of 1,300 children of both sexes, there were no marked differences in the prevalence of nutritional deficiency signs between the refugees and nonrefugees. In the latter group, angular lesions of the lips, swollen red papillae of gums, and follicular hyperkeratosis occurred more frequently in boys than in girls.

The biochemical findings in blood in age groups 5 to 14 in the refugee and nonrefugee groups were similar. Anemia of moderate degree in a certain proportion and low vitamin A in serum were found in both the groups. High urinary excretion of thiamine was found in both the groups. A higher percentage of nonrefugee children excreted riboflavin in amounts which were considered to be in the deficient and low ranges than the refugee children.

A comparison of clinical findings in adults, i.e., 15 years and over, for the military personnel, nonrefugee, and refugee population groups is illustrated in Tables 11 and 12. Various signs of nutritional deficiency were found in all the groups. Apart from the fact that angular lesions of the lips and swollen red papillae of the gums were found more frequently among the civilian population—both refugees and nonrefugees—there were no appreciable differences between the three groups. Follicular hyperkeratosis was observed less frequently in age groups beyond 45 years than in younger people. The older age group also showed the prevalence of bilateral edema in the lower extremity (4.4%) and bilateral loss of ankle jerk (5.3%).

Among the biochemical findings (Tables 13 and 14) was a decrease in serum ascorbic acid values with age in both males and females, refugees and nonrefugees. This trend was less marked in females than

TABLE 11
CLINICAL FINDINGS IN JORDAN—MALES[1]

				Civilians	
		Military	Refugees	Nonrefugees	
	Age Group	15–44	45+	15–44	45+
	Number	1528	199	128	271	225
		%	%	%	%	%
Eyes:						
Bitot's spot		0.8	0.5	—	1.5	0.4
Face and Neck:						
Nasolabial seborrhea		9.0	5.5	5.5	11.4	5.3
Lips:						
Angular lesions		1.8	8.5	10.2	8.1	6.7
Angular scars		30.9	25.1	28.9	24.7	36.4
Cheilosis		6.3	5.0	3.9	6.3	2.7
Gums:						
Swollen red papillae		1.9	13.1	15.6	30.3	29.8
Tongue:						
Atrophic filiform papillae		0.6	1.5	3.9	1.5	1.3
Glossitis		0.4	—	—	—	0.4
Magenta					—	0.9
Enlarged Thyroid:						
Grade I		4.3	5.0	1.6	5.2	2.2
Grade II		0.2		0.8	0.7[2]	—
Skin—General:						
Follicular hyperkeratosis		10.3	8.0	4.7	9.2	4.4
Lower Extremities:						
Bilateral edema						4.4
Loss of ankle jerk					0.7	5.3
Calf tenderness					—	—
Teeth:						
Fluorosis		22.7	14.1	12.5	18.1	7.6

1. Source: Adapted from ICNND *Report on Nutrition Survey in Jordan,* 1963.
2. Grades II and III.

in males. The average vitamin A level in serum showed a tendency to increase with age but less so than was observed in the Lebanon survey. These changes are depicted in Figures 1 and 2.

Pregnancy and lactation did not seem to make much difference with respect to vitamin A in serum. On the other hand vitamin C levels in serum were appreciably lower in pregnant than in nonpregnant women. Serum ascorbic acid levels were even lower in lactating women than in pregnant women.

The average urinary excretion of thiamine in terms of creatinine was high, and there were hardly any subjects up to 15 years of age who were either in the deficient or low levels of excretion. On the

TABLE 12
CLINICAL FINDINGS IN JORDAN—FEMALES[1]

	Refugees				Nonrefugees			
Age Group	15–44	45+	Pregnant	Lactating	15–44	45+	Pregnant	Lactating
Number	235	74	65	136	340	247	131	273
	%	%	%	%	%	%	%	%
Eyes:								
Bitot's spot	0.8	—	—	1.5	0.9	—	0.8	0.7
Face and Neck:								
Nasolabial seborrhea	3.0	1.1	1.5	2.9	2.6	0.8	2.3	0.4
Lips:								
Angular lesions	2.6	6.4	3.1	14.7	7.9	8.1	6.9	7.3
Angular scars	31.1	45.7	36.9	30.9	26.5	36.4	25.2	18.7
Cheilosis	5.5	3.2	3.1	3.7	5.9	4.0	3.8	1.8
Gums:								
Swollen red papillae	10.2	10.6	18.5	10.3	25.6	27.5	34.3	27.8
Tongue:								
Atrophic filiform papillae	2.1	1.1	—	2.2	1.8	4.0	1.5	2.6
Glossitis					0.9	0.8	—	1.1
Magenta					0.3	0.4	—	—
Enlarged Thyroid:								
Grade I	31.9	9.6	43.1	32.4	19.4	6.9	21.4	20.1
Grade II	1.7	2.1	6.2	4.4	7.4[2]	2.4[2]	5.3[2]	7.3[2]
Skin—General:								
Follicular hyperkeratosis	14.4	6.4	10.8	8.1	12.6	4.8	4.6	5.9
Lower Extremities:								
Bilateral edema					0.9	2.4	1.5	—
Loss of ankle jerk					0.3	3.6	—	0.4
Calf tenderness					0.3	0.4	—	0.4
Teeth:								
Fluorosis	21.3	17.0	13.8	22.0	19.7	7.3	18.3	26.4

1. Source: Adapted from ICNND Report on Nutrition Survey in Jordan, 1963.
2. Grades II and III.

TABLE 13
BIOCHEMICAL FINDINGS IN JORDAN CIVILIAN (NONREFUGEE) POPULATION—MALES[1]

Age Group in Years	5–9		10–14		15–44		45+	
	No.	%	No.	%	No.	%	No.	%
Hemoglobin g/100 ml	29	12.3	26	12.9	41	14.2	29	13.8
Hematocrit %	30	39.7	26	42.5	41	44.7	29	43.0
MCHC %	29	31.2	26	30.8	41	32.0	29	32.0
Total Protein g/100 ml serum	28	7.0	25	6.9	39	7.4	28	7.5
Vitamin C mg/100 ml serum	21	0.72	23	0.79	31	0.43	22	0.33
Vitamin A µg/100 ml serum	22	23.2	22	25.1	36	32.7	23	28.7
Carotenoids µg/100 ml serum	22	89	22	94	36	94	23	94

1. Source: Adapted from ICNND *Report on Nutrition Survey in Jordan,* 1963.

other hand, the average urinary riboflavin excretion in children was high; but at the same time 22 to 32% of children excreted riboflavin within "deficient" and "low" ranges. This could probably account for the occurrence of oral signs of riboflavin deficiency seen in a certain proportion of children.

In general the refugee children excreted more thiamine and riboflavin in urine than nonrefugee children. This was attributed to the consumption of bread made from the imported enriched wheat flour issued to the refugees by UNRWA as a component of dry rations. The nonrefugees on the other hand had to depend largely on the locally produced flour, which was not enriched.

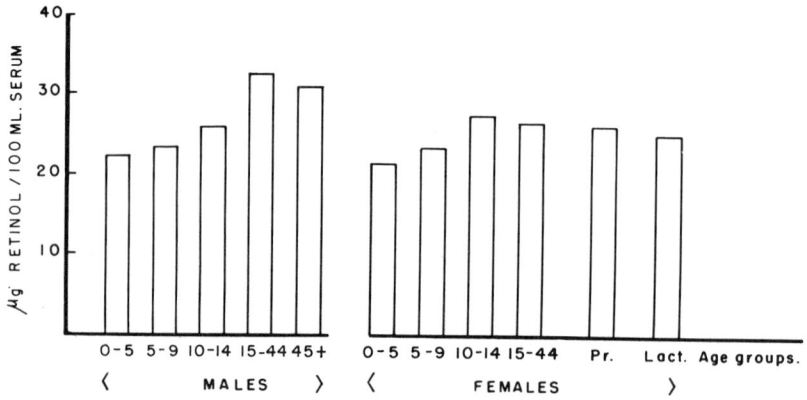

Figure 13.1. Average serum retinol levels in Jordanian males and females according to age.

TABLE 14
BIOCHEMICAL FINDINGS IN JORDAN CIVILIAN (NONREFUGEE) POPULATION—FEMALES[1]

| | Age Group in Years |||||||| | Pregnant || Lactating ||
| | 5-9 || 10-14 || 15-44 |||| | | | | |
	No.	%	No.	%	No.	%	No.	%	No.	%
Hemoglobin g/100 ml	24	12.5	35	12.4	41	12.4	16	11.7	30	12.4
Hematocrit %	24	40.3	34	40.9	41	39.7	17	37.1	30	39.6
MCHC %	22	31.2	34	31.0	41	31.2	16	31.0	30	31.4
Total Protein g/100 ml serum	22	7.1	35	7.2	41	7.5	16	7.2	29	7.4
Vitamin C mg/100 ml serum	19	0.80	33	0.82	38	0.63	16	0.46	27	0.37
Vitamin A µg/100 ml serum	20	24.0	34	26.6	39	30.7	15	23.3	30	22.0
Carotenoids µg/100 ml serum	20	110	34	91	39	97	15	116	30	86

1. Source: Adapted from ICNND *Report on Nutrition Survey in Jordan*, 1963.

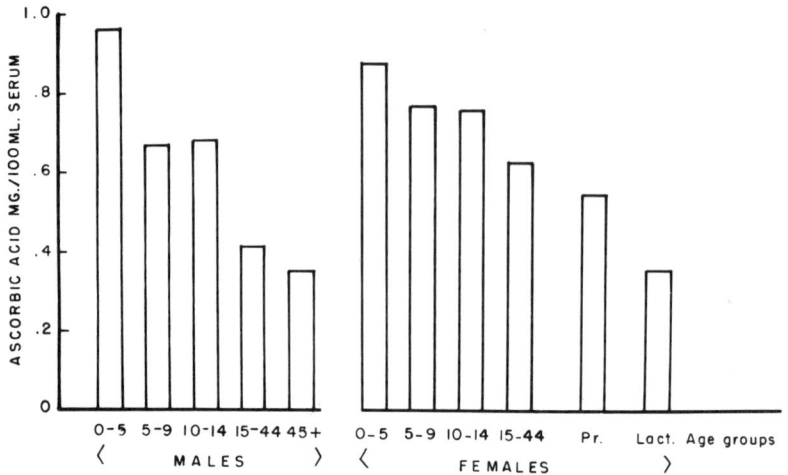

Figure 13.2. Average levels of serum ascorbic acid in Jordanian males and females according to age.

The urinary excretion of thiamine and riboflavin both showed a decrease with age as shown in Figures 3 and 4. Similar findings were recorded in the Lebanon survey. Their significance will be discussed later in relation to nutrient intakes.

The preceding account of the studies on nutritional status of population in Egypt, Jordan, Libya, and Lebanon will have made it clear that malnutrition exists to an appreciable extent in these countries. Growth retardation in infants and young children, continued low rate of growth in late childhood and adolescence, presence of signs of protein-calorie malnutrition in infants and young children, low blood concentrations of vitamin A at all ages, low urinary excretions of thiamine and riboflavin, and finally the occurrence of a variety of clinical signs of nutritional deficiency are the manifestations of the poor nutritional status of the populations.

The reasons for this state of affairs are many and varied, and they are inseparable from the stage of economic development, organization of public services, social customs, and cultural traditions which determine the standard of life and ways of living in a country.

A low level of food production within the country and inability to import food to make up the deficit result in relative unavailability of food and high food prices. The low purchasing power of the masses limits the purchase of foodstuffs, particularly the protective food-

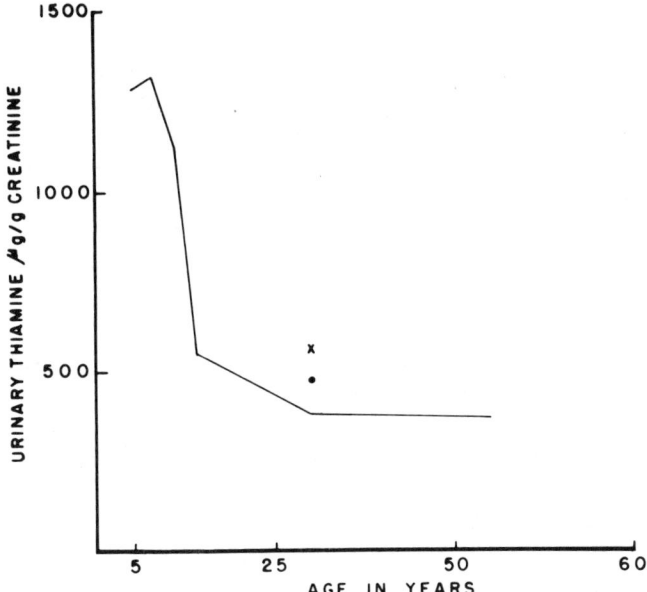

Figure 13.3. Urinary excretion of thiamine in Jordanians. Data on males and females combined. •Pregnant women and ˣLactating women.

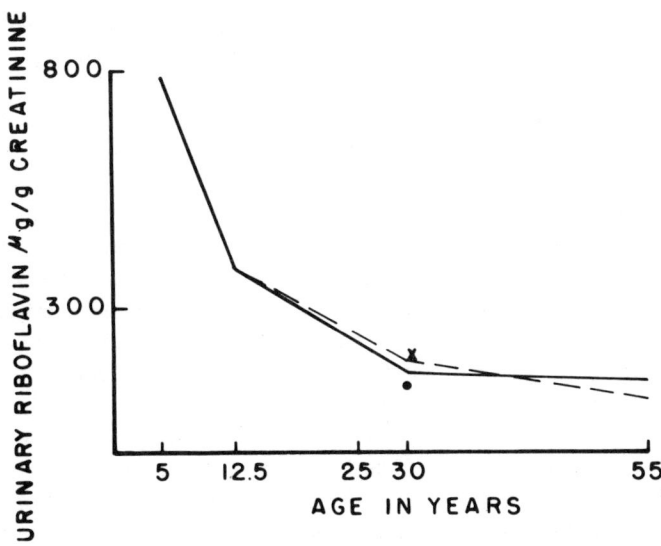

Figure 13.4. Urinary excretion of riboflavin in Jordanian males (———) and females (- - -); •Pregnant women and ˣLactating women.

stuffs, leading to inadequate food consumption and hence to undernutrition and malnutrition. The social habits, customs, and taboos which govern the feeding of infants and young children, coupled with the inability of the poor people to purchase appropriate foods for them, introduces malnutrition at the most important stage in life, that is, when the infant is rapidly growing and its demand for nutrients is great. As the child grows older, the difference between its needs and the food that it gets gradually diminishes; but in general the deficit still continues, if not in calories, in many of the essential nutrients that the child needs. Such a situation may continue even in adult life.

The level of medical and health care and environmental sanitation also plays an important role in determining the nutritional status of the population. For example, appropriate antenatal care would be effective in preventing malnutrition in pregnancy, thereby giving a good start to the infant to be born. A network of Maternal and Child Health Centers would provide health services and advice to mothers in problems such as breast-feeding and weaning, supplementary feeding, and child care in general. Besides, they would, by providing facilities for immunization, for teaching elementary hygiene to mothers, and for early treatment, reduce the incidence and the ill effects of gastrointestinal and respiratory infections from which a majority of infants and young children suffer in most developing countries. The provision of community water supply and control of the housefly and other pests can minimize the hazard of infections in the community as a whole.

There is not the least doubt that infection in association with malnutrition adversely influences the status of nutritional health of a population. Malnutrition may lower the resistance to infection. It may also modify the effects of infection in that the resulting disease follows a more severe course, and the outcome is not infrequently fatal. Infection on the other hand may itself cause secondary malnutrition or exacerbate the existing malnutrition through reduction of appetite, consumption of carbohydrate-rich, bland diets of inferior nutritional quality, impaired absorption of the food eaten, and increased metabolic wastage because of fever which usually accompanies infection. When infection and malnutrition both are present together, the synergistic effect is far more damaging to the body than when either of them is present alone. High morbidity and mortality among infants and children from gastroenteritis, bronchopneumonia, and measles, for example, found in malnourished populations, illustrate these points very well. Those infants and children who survive, since they continue to live in the same environment, seldom attain the full potential of growth and continue to suffer from mild to moderate degrees of malnutrition in adolescence and adult life (Reports of WHO Expert Committees: *Medical Assessment of Nutritional Status,* 1963; *Nutrition and Infection,* 1965).

Finally, the illiteracy of the masses which one commonly finds in developing countries also contributes to the present state of affairs. The level of education of the population determines its attitude and response to a situation. Education, and through it the understanding of the problem involved, permit the adoption of rational attitudes and tend to lessen the grip of tradition and taboos which are known to be harmful. In the field of nutrition and health and within the economic limitations, one can expect from educated persons an intelligent purchase of food items, better dietary habits, improved child-feeding and care, avoidance of unhygienic personal and social habits, and appropriate use of medical and health-care facilities provided for the community.

This discussion is intended to convey the impression that the improvement of nutritional status of populations is a complex problem. It cannot be solved by merely making more food available. Advance on all fronts which will raise the standard of life is essential for success. There is no simple solution. However, the problem is not insurmountable. The administrators must plan a concerted attack on the problem of improving the nutritional status of the populations.

REFERENCES

Abdou, I. A. 1965. *Nutritional Status in the New Valley* (in Arabic). Cairo, Egypt: National Documentation Center.

Abdou, I. A., H. E. Ali, and A. K. Lebshtein. 1965. A Study of the Nutritional Status of Mothers, Infants, and Young Children Attending Maternity and Child Health Centers in Cairo. Part I-The Nutritional Status of Infants and Young Children. *Bull. Nutr. Inst., U.A.R.* 1: 9.

Abdou, I. A., H. E. Ali, A. K. Said, W. A. Mousa, H. G. Demian, A. M. Soliman, and L. H. Hawary. 1967. Incidence of Nutritional Deficiencies, Goiter and Dental Caries Among School Children in Cairo. *J. Egypt. Publ. Hlth. Assoc.* 42: 175.

Carter, J. P., L. E. Grivetti, J. T. Davis, S. Nasiff, A. Mansour, W. A. Mousa, Alaa-El-Din Atta, V. N. Patwardhan, M. Abdel Moneim, I. A. Abdou, and W. J. Darby. 1969. Growth and Sexual Development of Adolescent Egyptian Village Boys: Effects of Zinc, Iron, and Placebo Supplement. *Amer. J. Clin. Nutr.* 22: 59–78.

Interdepartmental Committee on Nutrition for National Defense and Interdepartmental Committee on Nutrition for Jordan. 1964. *Report of a Nutrition Survey on Infants and Preschool Children in Jordan.* Bethesda, Md.: National Institutes of Health.

Interdepartmental Committee on Nutrition for National Defense. *Nutrition Surveys in Libya 1957; Lebanon 1962; and Jordan 1963.* Bethesda, Md.: National Institutes of Health.

———. 1963. *Manual for Nutrition Surveys.* 2nd ed. Bethesda, Md.: National Institutes of Health.

McLaren, D. S., H. A. P. C. Oomen, and H. Escapini. 1966. Ocular Manifestations of Vitamin A Deficiency in Man. *Bull. Wld. Hlth. Org.* 34: 357.

Patwardhan, V. N., and W. W. Kamel. 1967. *Studies on Vitamin A Deficiency in Infants and Young Children in Jordan.* Geneva, Switzerland: World Health Organization.

Pharaon, H. M., W. J. Darby, H. A. Shammout, E. B. Bridgforth, and C. S. Wilson. 1965. A Year-Long Study of the Nutriture of Infants and Preschool Children in Jordan. *J. Trop. Pediat.* 11: 1–39.

Report of the Permanent Nutrition Committee, Ministry of Health. 1948. Cairo, Egypt: Government Press.

Riad, H., and M. R. Barakat. 1964. Nutriture Survey of Young Male Adults of Behera and Gharbia Provinces. *J. Egypt. Med. Assoc.* 47: 272.

Vilter, R. W., W. J. Darby, and H. S. Glazer. 1954. A Study of Pellagra and Nutritional Anemia in Egypt. Geneva, Switzerland: World Health Organization.

WHO Expert Committee on Medical Assessment of Nutritional Status. 1963. Technical Report Series No. 258, pp. 12–13. Geneva, Switzerland: World Health Organization.

WHO Expert Committee on Nutrition and Infection. 1965. Technical Report Series No. 314, pp. 1–30. Geneva, Switzerland: World Health Organization.

14 THE NUTRITIONAL SITUATION IN IRAQ

The principal cereal crops in Iraq are barley, wheat, and rice, in that order. Appreciable amounts of millet and maize are also produced. Between 30 to 50% of the barley production is for export, about 20% is put to nonfood uses, and the remainder of the crop is available for consumption as food within the country. The staple in the Iraqi diet is bread made from barley, wheat, millet, or maize or from a mixture of more than one cereal. With the expanding production of wheat, bread made from wheat has become increasingly popular.

Lentils, cowpeas, chick-peas, and beans are not cultivated in sufficient quantities; thus grain legumes of any kind form a comparatively minor component of dietaries in Iraq.

Many kinds of vegetables and fruits are grown, such as tomatoes, eggplant, okra, marrow, green beans, spinach, cabbage, potatoes, carrots, and onions. Among the fruits, watermelon, melon, citrus varieties, pomegranate, apples, peaches, and apricots deserve mention. Dates are an important crop in Iraq, for this country is the largest producer of dates in the world, and a considerable proportion of the produce is exported.

The production of animal foods is comparatively low. The FAO estimates for 1954–56 gave the available supplies for human consumption per day as follows: Meat (of all kinds) 42 g; fish 9 g; milk 420 g (not all of it available as fluid milk); eggs 6 g. These animal foods are expected to provide about 24 g animal protein per day. In this respect Iraq seems to be nearer to Lebanon than its sister countries in the region. The situation with regard to food production per capita has not improved much in Iraq. Hence it may be reasonable to assume that animal foods available for human consumption remain at the same level as in 1954–55; they may even have registered a decrease.

An attempt to study the state of food and nutrition in the comparatively young state of Iraq was made as early as 1937 with the formation of a Nutrition Committee in that year. A survey of the food situation in terms of the needs of the population was made and the potential for food production assessed. Since about 20% of the total area of Iraq is cultivable, the estimated cultivable land area of over 5 acres per capita was considered sufficient to provide a liberal diet for the Iraqis on the assumption that even half of the cultivable land could be utilized for food production. Although the proportion of cultivable land per capita must have decreased substantially since 1937, owing to a rapid increase in population (the estimate for 1963 was 6,974,000), there still exists sufficient potential for finding adequate food for the population of Iraq.

The Nutrition Committee also promoted studies of dietary habits of population groups and of the nutrient composition of Iraqi foods. The outbreak of World War II must have interrupted these activities, and their resumption after the termination of hostilities was slow and uncertain. However, with the stimulus provided by FAO and on advice and assistance from this agency and also partly from WHO, the government of Iraq established a National Institute of Nutrition in Baghdad. The functions of the Institute were to interest itself in the study of food and nutrition problems, to foster activities contributing to the spread of nutrition education, to organize and participate in applied nutrition programs, and to act as adviser in nutrition to the national government.

The Institute has done some valuable work during the comparatively short period of its existence, but its activities have been limited, largely because of the inability or unwillingness of the government to provide adequate funds for it to function properly. Occasional visits by FAO and WHO staff from headquarters and regional offices and of consultants appointed by them may have helped barely to maintain the interest of the government in nutrition and to keep the Institute alive. It is not too much to hope that the authorities that be will remedy the situation soon.

We shall review in the following pages such information as is available from the published reports of nutritional studies in Iraq, most of which were done at the Nutrition Institute.

Diets

The levels and patterns of food consumption vary in different parts of Iraq. Two main patterns can be considered, one rural and the other urban. In urban areas the economic status would seem to determine the composition of the dietaries, as is usual in most countries. The pattern of the rural dietaries would depend largely on the types of food locally produced. Since the majority of village population is poor, the diets usually contain few foodstuffs beside bread. Three meals are the rule, dinner being the main meal. Bread with tea serves for breakfast. Raw vegetables such as onions, lettuce, and carrots may accompany bread at the midday meal. Cooked vegetables, grain legumes, and meat when it is available are eaten with bread at dinner. Fruit in season is consumed when it is in glut and the prices are low. Dates form a substantial portion of the poor man's diet, particularly in the south.

Abdul Nabi and coworkers (1959, 1961, 1962) have analyzed a large variety of Iraqi foodstuffs for their nutrient composition. Among the foodstuffs investigated were cereals and cereal products, vegetables, fruits, meat, milk and milk products, including varieties of Arab and Kurdish cheeses. Abdul Nabi and Dhia (1964) also determined phytate content of cereals, legumes, and nuts. A knowledge of phytate content is important in diets which contain a large proportion of foods made from cereals and their products, for phytate is known to interfere with the absorption from the intestinal tract of nutrients such as calcium, iron, and zinc. As was to be expected, 44 to 63% of total phosphorus in cereals and their products was in the form of phytate. The results of this food analysis proved helpful in the evaluation of nutrient intakes from Iraqi diets discussed below.

Jalili, Georges, and Fadhil (1950) surveyed the diets of 55 families. Of these, 39 families were from Baghdad and Mosul with incomes varying from 200 to over 1,000 Iraq dinars (1 Iraqi dinar = 1 £ sterling) per year. Two other low-income groups, one urban and the other of poor peasants from villages near a big city, were included in the survey. The study was based on the records of food as purchased. Jalili *et al.* stated that they attempted to cover the period of one whole year; however, they failed to mention how they accomplished the difficult task of keeping records over such a prolonged period. It is probable that the survey covered a few days at a time during different seasons of the year. The authors concluded that the diets of the families with incomes of over 200 dinars were satisfactory. It appears from the table of nutrient intake contained in the paper that the diets of the low-income urban group were also not unsatisfactory. On the other hand, the diets of the peasants were inadequate in calories, iron, and vitamin A. A more recent study of rural dietaries in Baghdad province by DeMarchi et al. (1962) provides a slightly better picture. A sample made up of ten families each was randomly selected in villages from five administrative districts of Baghdad province. The families were those of peasants who lived in mud huts, the men working on the farms. During the survey foods were weighed on three consecutive days, and the survey was repeated in different seasons of the year. The findings expressed by the authors as the average for the year are given in Table 1.

The diets appeared to be adequate in calories, proteins, calcium, iron, and thiamine. The probable deficiencies were those of vitamin A, riboflavin, and ascorbic acid.

The findings of DeMarchi et al. indicate a much better level of food consumption in rural areas than that suggested in the report of Jalili et al. in 1950. It is probable that in rural areas, as in the urban, the extremely poor represented by the landless laborers subsist on a totally inadequate diet, whereas the small farmers and their families consume diets which are adequate in calories and proteins but marginal or inadequate in certain essential nutrients. Although there is not much information to substantiate such a statement, experience in other countries would probably support it.

DeMarchi et al. (1963) surveyed food consumption in 105 families of brick workers who form over 20% of the total industrial labor in Baghdad. The average wage was about 429 fils (1 dinar = 1000 fils) per day. Workers' families lived in mud houses in the neighborhood of Baghdad with no communal protected water supply. Water was carried by women from irrigation canals nearby or in certain seasons purchased from tankers at the rate of 10 fils per 4 gallons. The average composition of the diet and its nutrient content are given in Table 1. The diets showed the same characteristics in respective adequacy and insufficiency as those of the small farmer.

One other diet survey, also in Baghdad, done by DeMarchi and coworkers (1966) deserves particular mention. The subjects were 157 pregnant women randomly chosen from those attending the Sheikh Omar Maternal and Child Health Center. Of these, 97 women were between 2 and 5 months and 60 between 5 and 8 months pregnant. Information on food consumption was obtained by the questionnaire method over 7 consecutive days. Since there are comparatively few studies on the dietary intake of pregnant women, the findings of DeMarchi et al. (1966) as given in Table 2 should prove of interest.

TABLE 1
THE AVERAGE FOOD CONSUMPTION OF SMALL FARMERS IN BAGHDAD PROVINCE AND OF WORKERS IN BRICK INDUSTRY NEAR BAGHDAD

	Small Farmers (50 Families) Food in g/Capita/Day	Brick Workers (105 Families) Food in g/Capita/Day
Whole wheat flour	380	468
Barley flour	104	35
Rice	71	50
Grain legumes	5	2
Meat, fish, chicken	20	33
Eggs	4	2
Milk	41	7
Diluted sour milk	139	83
Cheese	—[1]	—
Butter, ghee	17	5
Vegetable fat	7	9
Potatoes	2[2]	3
Other vegetables (winter)	30	39
(summer)	114	141
Fruits	82	51
Dates and date syrup	74	27
Sugar	61	83
Calories	2758	2545
Protein Total g	79	82
Animal g	7.6	7.3
Calcium mg	530	410
Iron mg	20	18
Vitamin A I.U. total	2011	2583
Vitamin I.U. Preformed	478	—
Thiamine mg	1.8	2.0
Riboflavin mg	1.1	1.0
Niacin mg	21	20
Ascorbic Acid mg	17	22

1. No assessment of cheese intake could be made since the records were incomplete.
2. For the same reason the figure for potatoes is tentative.

It is worthy of note that apart from a difference of 180 calories between the two groups, the average nutrient intake was surprisingly similar. The diets were deficient in calcium, iron, and riboflavin and marginal in vitamin A, thiamine, and possibly niacin. In general they were not very much different from the dietaries of pregnant women in Cairo and Alexandria except in calorie intake. The average body weight for almost identical average height was higher in the latter half of pregnancy, as was to be expected. The average hemoglobin

TABLE 2
ENERGY AND NUTRIENT INTAKE OF PREGNANT WOMEN IN BAGHDAD

Particulars	Pregnancy 2–5 Months	Pregnancy 5–8 Months
No. examined	97	60
Av. Height cm.	154.6	153.8
Av. Weight kg.	55.5	58.2
Calories	1815	1996
Protein Total g	57.6	57.4
Protein Animal g	15.8	15.9
Calcium mg	364	325
Iron mg	10.3	11.8
Vitamin A I.U.	2579	3569
Thiamine mg	0.76	0.73
Riboflavin mg	0.84	0.78
Niacin mg	8.9	9.5
Ascorbic Acid mg	33.3	38.7

determined in 200 pregnant women was between 10 and 11 g/100 ml with no significant difference between the three trimesters of pregnancy.

Gounelle *et al.* (1956) have studied the diets of young Iraqi male adults serving with the army and police forces. The average intake of calories was over 3500 and that of protein over 100 g per day. The average daily calcium intake was 407 mg in the police force and 327 mg in the army. These figures are indicative of a low calcium intake; the figures quoted for vitamin A activity of the diet, namely, 1620 I.U. in police and 2769 I.U. in the army, indicate that vitamin A intake was also low in the former. The young men examined were often below the standard weight for height, and mild anemia was frequent, as was nutritional glossitis. The ration scales were apparently adequate, according to the authors. However, the duration of service of the recruits was not long enough for the diets based on these rations to have shown a beneficial effect on their nutritional status.

The above account should indicate that dietary studies have been concentrated in and around Baghdad, whereas for the remainder of the country not much information is available. This is true for studies on nutritional status as well, which are described below. However, the picture revealed by the published studies is not dissimilar to that seen in other Arab countries which we have described earlier. Hence it is

Nutritional Status of Population Groups

unlikely that it would be very much different in other parts of Iraq except perhaps with some minor local features.

DeMarchi et al. (1965) have studied the growth and nutritional status of infants and young children in Baghdad. They quote from a personal series of observations of a Dr. Chaderchi that the average birth weight of the newborn Iraqi infant is 3.63 kg for males and 3.46 kg for females. These averages are slightly higher than those given earlier for Jordan and Egypt and are comparable with the birth weights reported from West Europe and North America.

DeMarchi et al. (1965) observed 2,501 infants and children between 1 month and 5 years of age at three MCH. Centers. These centers, situated in three different areas of Baghdad, served populations with different economic status. One was attended by women and children of the low socioeconomic group, the second by those mostly of low economic status but slightly better than the last, and the third center served a population which was "comparatively better off." The increase in body weight of infants up to 4 months of age was satisfactory and comparable with that reported for European infants. Growth retardation set in during the fifth month and was quite marked by the seventh month. The growth deficit continued up to 5 years of age. The observations of DeMarchi et al. on the prevalence of second and third degree of malnutrition in children from 1 to 18 months are shown in Figure 1.

The figure unmistakably points to the association of poverty with malnutrition in infants. The proportion of infants showing the second and third degree of malnutrition increased in the 7–12-month period, and it was still higher in the 13–18-month period. The increase in the third degree of malnutrition, which is a fairly severe condition in a growing infant, was not quite so marked, but it was noticeable in the 13–18-month age group. The figure also shows that 2 to 5% of infants in the "comparatively better off" families suffered from this severe form of malnutrition. Obviously there must be some factor other than poverty for this comparatively high prevalence of protein-calorie-deficiency disease, possibly ignorance of proper child-feeding and frequency of infections. Other signs of malnutrition were also found in the total sample of 2,501 children. Frequency varied with the degree of malnutrition, as Table 3 will show.

Surprisingly enough, the authors make no mention of rickets. Considering the experience in the neighboring Arab countries, it seems unlikely that rickets was absent.

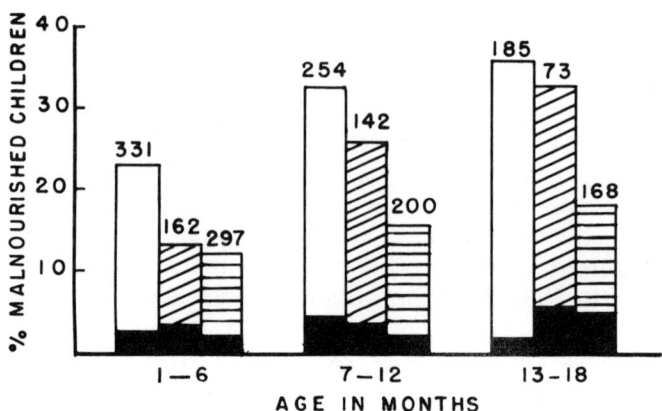

Figure 14.1. Percentage of infants between 1 and 18 months of age from three income groups with second and third degree of malnutrition.

☐ low income   ▨ middle income   ☰ "comparatively better off"

Shaded area indicates 3rd degree of malnutrition.

TABLE 3

SIGNS OF NUTRITIONAL DEFICIENCY ASSOCIATED WITH THIRD DEGREE MALNUTRITION IN IRAQI INFANTS AND YOUNG CHILDREN AS COMPARED TO APPARENTLY HEALTHY CHILDREN OF SAME AGE

Physical Sign	In Apparently Healthy Children %	In Malnourished Children %
Enlarged liver	1.1	5.4
Xerosis conjunctivae	0.08	0.2
Angular stomatitis	0.20	2.7
Angular scars of mouth	0.04	0.2
Cheilosis	0.60	1.6
Tongue—Papillary atrophy	0.91	8.1
Tongue—Papillary hypertrophy	1.20	3.8
Nasolabial seborrhea	0.20	1.35
Redness and swelling of gums	3.43	9.46
Edema of lower extremities	0.10	2.7
Mosaic skin	0.60	1.81

It will be clear from the above that, in general, the pattern of growth in infants and young children in Baghdad was not very much different from the patterns seen in Lebanon, Jordan, and Egypt. The causes for early growth failure were almost similar, namely, inadequate and inappropriate supplementary feeding and frequency of gastrointestinal infections.

DeMarchi et al. (1967) have reported on the nutritional status of 1,142 boys and 358 girls, 6 to 9 years in age, belonging to the first grade in schools in Baghdad, with a comparison of the various nutritional indices derived from children in families with high and low income. They did not find any significant difference in heights and weights between the two groups. The children of the high income groups had a higher skin-fold thickness (measured on triceps and subscapular region) than the children of the low income groups. Physical signs of malnutrition, such as lesions of the lips and tongue and follicular hyperkeratosis, were much more frequent in the low income group. The average hemoglobin values ranged between 12.05 to 13.00 g/100 ml, and according to the authors no hemoglobin value was less than 11.5 g/100 ml, which represents a reasonably satisfactory situation. This finding is particularly significant since the sample included 201 children of low income groups of families from the rural area as well.

Parasitism and Iron Deficiency Anemia

It is known that parasitic infections involving hookworm and bilharzia among others are prevalent in the rural areas of Iraq, mostly along the two great rivers, Euphrates and Tigris, and the irrigation systems emanating from them (Simmons et al., 1954). The species of hookworm found in Iraq is *Ankylostoma duodenale*. The infection rate of 10 to 20% has been recorded in the northern provinces, with about 40% in the south. *Schistosoma hematobium* is the principal infecting parasite responsible for the endemicity of schistosomiasis in Iraq. The rate of infection varies between 0 and 80%, with an average of 18 to 25% in the irrigated regions of the Delta. A survey in 1950 showed the following prevalence rates for schistosomiasis in four provinces: Amarah, 67%; Basra, 23%; Baghdad, 35%; and Kut, 48%. The situation with regard to parasitism is thus not dissimilar to that existing in Lower Egypt. There must therefore be a great deal of iron deficiency anemia in Iraq, particularly in adults. Unfortunately we have little information about its prevalence in that country.

Some evidence for this exists, however, as can be seen from the results of a nutrition survey of young army recruits reported by

DeMarchi and coworkers (1966). They examined 1,622 recruits, mostly 18 years in age, who had been in service from 2 to 12 weeks. The recruits came from different parts of Iraq, 70% being from the urban communities. Their average hemoglobin values ranged from 12.4 to 13.8 g/100 ml according to location. The lowest average value was recorded among the recruits from the central rural area of Iraq; 26% of these had hemoglobin less than 12 g per 100 ml. Furthermore the average MCHC values for all the groups were less than 30%. MCHC values above 32% were found in 0 to 11.1% of the entire group of recruits. The anemia was probably mild; nevertheless its presence has to be accepted. Urinary schistosomiasis and ankylostomiasis were found in the recruits from the central and southern areas demonstrating the role of parasitism in the anemia. These and other findings indicative of malnutrition in recruits are summarized in Tables 4 and 5.

It will be clear from Table 5 that lesions of the lip and tongue were fairly common among the recruits and were suggestive of ariboflavinosis. Commenting on the urinary riboflavin excretion in the light of the ICNND guidelines for interpretation, the authors state that 11%

TABLE 4
RESULTS OF A BIOCHEMICAL AND PARASITOLOGICAL EXAMINATION OF ARMY RECRUITS FROM NORTHERN, CENTRAL, AND SOUTHERN REGIONS OF IRAQ[1]

		Urban			Rural		
		North	Center	South	North	Center	South
Hemoglobin g/100 ml	No.	44	176	58	15	64	35
	Av.	13.4	13.8	13.3	13.4	12.4	13.1
MCHC %	No.	21	18	34	8	22	12
	Av.	29.6	29.6	29.6	28.6	28.6	29.8
Serum retinol	No.	20	38	36	6	27	11
µg/100 ml	Av.	21	24	21	18	26	23
Urine							
Thiamine µg/g Cr.	No.	28	40	42	10	25	12
	Med.	486	364	325	455	410	307
Riboflavin µg/g Cr.	No.	28	40	42	10	27	13
	Med.	241	117	163	189	149	172
N-Me-Nicotinamide	No.	28	40	41	10	27	13
mg/g Cr.	Med.	4.6	2.4	3.0	4.3	2.9	3.1
Parasitic Infection							
S. hematobium	No.	40	153	59	15	34	37
	%	0	5.2	25.4	0	8.8	16.2
A. duodenale	No.	31	145	43	11	38	27
	%	0	6.2	6.9	0	18.4	14.8

1. Source: DeMarchi et al. (1966).

TABLE 5
RESULTS OF A NUTRITION SURVEY OF ARMY RECRUITS[1]

	Urban			Rural		
	North	Center	South	North	Center	South
No. examined	186	734	222	102	219	159
Height cm Average	166.4	164.5	166.4	165.7	165.6	167.4
Weight Kg. Average	57.6	60.7	60.3	58.3	58.2	60.7
	%	%	%	%	%	%
Eyes: Bitot's spots	—	—	—	—	—	1.3
Lips: Angular Scars	1.6	5.3	0.9	2.0	1.4	1.3
Angular lesions	0.5	1.1	0.9	3.9	0.4	0.6
Cheilosis	4.8	1.5	4.0	4.9	5.0	2.5
Tongue: Filiform Pap. atrophy	8.1	13.8	2.7	12.7	13.2	6.3
Pap. hypertrophy	7.5	8.2	13.1	2.9	13.2	6.9
Glossitis	5.9	1.1	31.6	3.9	2.7	3.1
Gums: swollen	11.3	5.2	14.4	16.7	13.6	18.9
red	5.4	10.1	10.8	5.9	6.4	5.0
Skin: Follicular hyperkeratosis	6.4	4.2	9.5	18.6	4.6	11.3
Lower limbs: Loss of ankle jerk	2.1	2.7	2.2	2.0	5.0	1.3
Calf tenderness	—	1.4	0.4	—	2.3	—
Spleen: enlarged	—	0.3	—	—	0.4	0.6
Liver: enlarged	—	0.4	0.4	1	0.9	—

1. Source: DeMarchi et al. (1966).

of the sample examined excreted riboflavin in the low and deficient ranges. This supports the suggestion made above regarding the relation of riboflavin deficiency to the observed frequency of the oral lesions. There is, however, a discrepancy between the results of urinary thiamine excretion and clinical findings suggestive of thiamine deficiency. According to the authors, none of the subjects excreted thiamine in urine in the low and deficient ranges. And yet loss of ankle jerk and calf tenderness were found in 1 to 5% of the recruits examined. Unless some other reason can be postulated for the occurrence of these signs, the two findings cannot be reconciled.

The over-all picture emerging from the survey clearly indicates that malnutrition is not infrequent among adolescents in Iraq. In this the situation is similar to that in the neighboring countries.

Goiter

The occurrence of endemic goiter in Iraq was first described by Caughey and Follis (1965). The account of this was published for a second time by Caughey (1966) and contained essentially the same information. Caughey had earlier been impressed by the high prevalence of goiter in hospital patients in Mosul in the North of Iraq. Caughey and Follis found 55% of 273 adult hospital patients with thyroid enlargement. The majority of the patients were Arabs or Kurds. The authors also surveyed over 900 school children of both sexes, 11 to 18 years of age, in Mosul and 228 girls of the same age in the neighboring rural region. They recorded the occurrence of goiter in 98% of girls and 64% of boys examined in Mosul and 72 to 95% of girls in the neighborhood. The majority of enlargements was made up, according to the authors, of (1) glands just visible at the isthmus and a palpation felt as a thickened band across the isthmus and (2) glands which caused slight alteration of the contour of the neck. Caughey and Follis combined these two categories and considered them equivalent to Group 1 of WHO classification. Ghalioungui (1967), who made later a more detailed survey in Mosul Province, was not satisfied with this grouping and felt that an unusually high level of goiter prevalence had been recorded by Caughey and Follis.

Ghalioungui examined 1,632 male and 1,619 female subjects comprising school children, school teachers, industrial workers, and a few unselected persons. Of these more than half were from the city of Mosul. Ghalioungui followed the WHO classification and found the figures shown in Table 6 for goiter prevalence in different parts of Mosul Province.

Northern Iraq is partly mountainous, and hence endemicity of goiter was to be expected. Goiter in areas in Turkey bordering on Iraq to the north had been reported. On the other hand the occurrence of goiter in Baghdad, which is in the plains, was not to be expected. However, Ghalioungui reported it in 18% of the school girls he examined in Baghdad. This would suggest the need for a more detailed survey of endemic goiter in other regions of Iraq.

TABLE 6
GOITER IN MOSUL PROVINCE

Town	% Prevalence in	
	Males	Females
Mosul	26	49
Dohuk	41	54
Tell Afar	34	50
Amadia	80	87
Baghdad (school children only)	6.4	18

That goiter in Mosul Province is due to iodine deficiency is not to be doubted. The results of analysis of iodine in water supplies reported by Caughey and Follis and of urinary iodine excretion reported by them as well as Ghalioungui support this assumption. Obviously iodization of salt could be the appropriate preventive measure in this situation. The nutritional status concerning goiter and iodine are separately treated in the chapter on goiter.

The account given in the preceding pages should indicate that malnutrition exists in Iraq and that, as in the other Arab countries, infants and young children are the most affected. The findings of DeMarchi et al. and Gounelle et al. suggest that malnutrition also exists in school children and adolescents. The prevalence of endemic goiter in northern Iraq revealed by recent studies presents a challenge, as do the other forms of malnutrition whose prevalence we need to study further so as to plan for their prevention. Thus there is plenty of scope for work in nutrition. The Nutrition Institute has indeed done valuable work in spite of the limitations of funds and personnel. It is all the more necessary and urgent that its organization be strengthened and adequate funds placed at its disposal.

REFERENCES

Abdul Nabi, M., and L. Y. Dhiya. 1962. Vitamin B_{12} Content of Some Iraqi Foodstuffs. *J. Fac. Med. Baghdad* 4: 153.

———. 1964. Phytic Acid Content of Some Iraqi Foodstuffs. *J. Fac. Med. Baghdad* 6: 109.

Abdul Nabi, M., S. Shukri, and L. Y. Dhiya. 1962. The Nutritional Value of Some Iraqi Foodstuffs. *J. Fac. Med. Baghdad* 4: 22.

Abdul Nabi, M., N. Abutrab, L. Y. Dhiya, F. Kamil, S. Shukri, and A. Yahya. 1959, 1961. The Nutritional Value of Some Iraqi Foodstuffs. *J. Fac. Med. Baghdad* 1: 173 and 3: 10.

Caughey, J. E. 1966. Endemic Goiter in Iraq. *J. Fac. Med. Baghdad* 8: 7.

Caughey, J. E., and R. H. Follis. 1965. Endemic Goiter and Iodine Malnutrition in Iraq. *Lancet* i: 1032.

DeMarchi, M., M. Mohanty, M. Ali, M. Azzawee, and S. Saidi. 1962. A Dietary Survey in Rural Areas in Baghdad. *J. Fac. Med. Baghdad* 4: 140.

DeMarchi, M., I. S. Saidi, M. Azzawee, M. Ali, and N. Elmilli. 1966. Food Consumption and Nutrition Status of Pregnant Women Attending A Maternal and Child Health Center in Baghdad. *J. Fac. Med. Baghdad* 8: 20.

DeMarchi, M., M. Mohanty, M. Ali, M. Azzawee, S. Saidi, and A. Isa. 1963. Family Food Consumption Survey of Workers Belonging to the Brick Industry. *J. Fac. Med. Baghdad* 5: 173.

DeMarchi, M., R. Haider, M. Mohanty, M. Ali, M. Azzawee, S. Saidi, and M. Isa. 1965. Nutritional and Growth Status of Infants and Young Children Attending Maternal and Child Health Centers in Baghdad. *J. Fac. Med. Baghdad* 7: 36.

DeMarchi, M., M. Abdul Nabi, N. Elmilli, U. Hiti, H. Taj el-Din, L. Y. Dhiya, S. Shafik, and H. Askari. 1967. A Nutrition Study of School Children. *J. Fac. Med. Baghdad* 9: 151.

DeMarchi, M., M. Abdul Nabi, N. Elmilli, U. Hiti, H. Taj el-Din, A. Ubaidy, Z. Nejjar, L. Y. Dhiya, S. Shafik, and A. Yahya. 1966. Nutritional Status of New Army Recruits in Iraq. *J. Iraq. Army Med. Ser.* 2: 13.

Ghalioungui, P. 1967. Endemic Goiter in Mosul Area, Iraq. Report to World Health Organization. Alexandria, Egypt: Regional Office for the Eastern Mediterranean.

Gounelle, H., M. DeMarchi, H. Rabii, R. Rashid, S. Findalky, H. F. Selloumi, and S. Cofmann. 1956. Enquete de nutrition en Moyen-Orient sur des jeunes adultes. *Bull. Soc. Sci., d'Hyg. Alimentaire* 44: 269.

Jalili, M. A., F. Georges, and A. Fadhil. 1950. The State of Nutrition in Iraq. *J. Fac. Med. Iraq., Baghdad* 14: 73.

May, J. M. 1961. *The Ecology of Malnutrition in the Far and Near East.* New York: Hafner Publ. Co., Inc.

Simmons, J. S., T. F. Whayne, G. W. Anderson, and H. M. Horack. 1954. *Global Epidemiology: A Geography of Disease and Sanitation.* Vol. 3. Philadelphia: J. B. Lippincott Company.

15 | PREVENTION

The account given in the preceding chapters of the state of nutrition in the Arab countries of the Near East makes it abundantly clear that dietary deficiencies, nutritional disorders, and malnutrition in general are common among the population of these countries. Continuation of this situation can but lead to further deterioration in health with damaging effects on productive capacity and on the economic development of the countries concerned. It is essential, therefore, to combat malnutrition, to control its spread, to prevent and eradicate it.

Malnutrition cannot be considered as a problem in isolation; it results from the interaction of a variety of factors. Even when "simple" dietary deficiencies are the immediate cause of malnutrition, they result from the interplay of such factors as the purchasing capacity of the people, the availability of food, and knowledge of how best to use it. Illnesses due to microbial and parasitic infections and the lack of medical and health-care facilities in the community further aggravate malnutrition. Malnutrition is as much an economic, social, and health problem as it is one of food supplies and food consumption levels. It stands to reason, therefore, that attempts to control malnutrition should be directed to the solution of many problems which severally and collectively contribute to its existence, rather than concentrating merely on augmenting food supplies.

In economically underdeveloped countries the majority of people are generally poor, and there is a high rate of population growth. The total food production is low, largely because agricultural practices vary from primitive to medieval. In those developing countries where improved techniques are being used in agriculture and animal husbandry, their effectiveness is reduced to a large extent by considerations such as those briefly mentioned in Chapter 2. The result is seen in the uncertain success of the efforts to increase food production either in absolute terms or as related to the growing population.

The meager economic resources of developing countries and the relative lack of expert knowledge not only limit food production but also hamper the progress of industrial and economic development. Through such development alone, improvements in education, housing, sanitation, environmental hygiene, and medical and health care can be accomplished.

The approach to the control and prevention of malnutrition must therefore be broad based. Measures to improve the nutritional status can be considered under two heads: general and specific. General measures encompass a range of national and governmental activities which are beyond the scope of this book. Most developing countries have adopted the concept of national planning for economic development. Plans usually are made for specific periods varying from three to seven years. External aid for their implementation is usually forthcoming from the developed countries on a bilateral basis or from the specialized agencies of the United Nations. Assistance provided is in the form of advice in planning and finance to supplement national resources for the fulfillment of these plans. The national plan often includes provisions for increased food production, its processing, distribution, and marketing among other equally important aspects of industrial, social, and economic development. It is with respect to development in the field of food that we shall draw attention to some specific aspects as part of the general measures for the control and prevention of malnutrition.

Food Production. There must be an improvement in total food production of all kinds,—the staple cereals, grain legumes, livestock yielding meat and meat products, milk and dairy products, fish, vegetables, and fruit. Often great effort is concentrated on the increase in the production of such staple foods as cereals or starchy tubers and secondary attention given to such protective foods as vegetables, fruit, meat and fish; and milk and its products. Such a policy is self defeating, for without an adequate supply of protective foods proper nutrition of the population can never be assured. Although the production of protective foods is comparatively costly and yields in terms of calories are lower than from the staples, neglect in planning for production of them will not improve the nutritional status of the population.

Control of Pests. Efforts to increase the production of food must be accompanied by greater attention to its preservation. Natural phenomena like drought, excessive rain, and floods often limit food production. On the other hand, insect and fungus pests of the standing crops also cause appreciable losses. Then again fungus, and insect and rodent pests cause a great loss during the storage of the harvest. Of these, fungal spoilage of foodstuffs is of special significance. It not only causes loss of food by making it unsuitable for human consumption, but it also presents a danger to the health of man and domestic animals. Several examples of toxic effects in animals resulting from the consumption of contaminated feed are on record (Wilson; 1966). Only two need be mentioned here as being of topical interest.

Since 1949, seasonal epizootics, mainly in the autumn and involving the equine species, have been reported in Egypt. Donkeys in the farm lands of the Nile Delta were mostly affected, and the mortality was high, with great economic loss. Two major outbreaks occurred in 1965 and 1966. Loss of appetite, impairment of vision, stupor, unco-ordinated gait, inability to stand, and recumbency accompanied by convulsions were the signs of the disease, which often proved fatal. Careful studies of the latest epizootic followed by experimental work showed that the disease was due to the consumption of moldy maize (Badiali et al., 1968). Maize is harvested in the autumn and is indifferently stored with the result that mold infection of partly damaged grains sets in and spreads to undamaged maize in favorable conditions of temperature and humidity. The uninfected maize is taken for human consumption, leaving the infected maize ears for the donkey. On occasions camels, horses, and water buffalo also are known to suffer from the disease if they consume mold-infested maize.

The second example is that of the fungal infection of peanuts. In 1960, a disease outbreak involving a large number of turkey poults, ducklings, pigs, and calves was reported in England. Mortality was high among turkey poults and ducklings. Brazilian peanut meal was a common constituent of the feed given to all these animals. Subsequent investigations led to the isolation of the toxic substances from peanuts infected with *Aspergillus flavus*. They were given the name of aflatoxins. Aflatoxins were later found to occur in varying quantities in samples of peanut and its press cake obtained from crops grown in different countries. Thus all these were potentially toxic. The manifestation of toxic effect depends upon the concentration of the toxin contained in the feed, the amount consumed, and the animal species involved. The loss of appetite, failure to gain weight in young animals, unthriftiness, and profound liver damage are some of the common effects. Laboratory investigations demonstrated that aflatoxins were also carcinogenic in certain species of animals.

Peanut is universally consumed, and the low-fat and fat-free meals are widely used as protein concentrates in feeds for domestic animals. One can imagine the extent of the harm which fungus infection of indifferently stored peanut harvest can do the consumer. The scare caused by the ubiquitous presence of aflatoxin in peanut and its products from almost all over the world had an adverse influence for a time on the FAO/WHO/UNICEF-sponsored protein-rich food program based on the use of fat-free peanut flour in formulations of weaning foods.

There is no evidence yet that fungus-infected maize or peanut causes toxic effects in man. However, one need not go to the length of demonstrating its harmfulness. If not in his own interests, at least in the interests of the animals who serve him, it is the duty of man to take steps to prevent fungus pests from attacking foodstuffs.

If losses in the field and during storage caused by various pests are reduced to a minimum, considerably more food will become available for human consumption in developing countries than exists now, even at the present rate of production. Reliable estimates of these losses are, however, not available.

Food-Processing. The processing of foods has three main purposes, all of them of significance in extending food supplies. One is to conserve supplies of perishable foods such as milk, meat, fish, vegetables, and fruits. Some of these, especially fruits, vegetables, and some fish and seafoods, are seasonal; when they are in season there is a glut. Food preservation achieved through appropriate processing eliminates losses through spoilage and ensures their availability throughout the year. The second object of processing is to refine coarse foods, remove undesirable materials, and add others designed to improve the nutritional quality of the resulting product. Milling of wheat followed by enrichment of the flour can be cited as the best example. The third purpose of food-processing is to convert perishable and nonperishable foods as well into products acceptable to the people as ingredients of their daily diets. Fruit juices and preserves; yoghurt, cheese, and butter from milk; refined and hydrogenated vegetable oils; soya sauce and other soya products; sugar from sugar cane or beet; syrup from maize; and a variety of products made from staple cereals are only a few examples which indicate how important food-processing can be and how successful it is in achieving its major objectives.

Food-processing may cause the loss or diminution of some essential nutrients contained in the food. Thiamine is lost during milling of rice, and this loss is an important factor in the prevalence of beriberi in the Southeast Asian countries. Vitamins of the B-complex and iron are lost during milling of wheat. Vitamin C may be lost in the processing of fruits and vegetables unless care is taken to maintain conditions of processing that reduce or minimize such losses. The preparation of protein concentrates from defatted oil seeds or fish may cause a loss of various vitamins, minerals, or nutritional value of the protein. Modern technology can minimize losses through improved methods of processing, and, where this is not possible, the nutrients removed during processing can often be restored. The choice of methods of food-processing is of great importance in developing countries where new food industries are being established.

A variety of traditional food-processing methods exists in the countries of the Near East. Preparation of butter, *ghee,* and cheese is common in villages and towns; drying of such fruits as dates, grapes, figs, and apricots is a traditional way of preserving fruit; pressing of oil from oil seeds and milling of wheat and rice in small mills are time-honored small industries. So also are baking bread and confectionary. However, large-scale food-processing plants are gradually increasing and expanding in their scope. Large flour and rice mills; sugar factories; confectionary factories; canneries of fruit, vegetables, and meat; breweries; wineries; distilleries; and factories for soft carbonated drinks and other food industries have been established and are contributing in an increasing measure to the food economy of this region. But much remains to be done in order that full benefit is derived from the food produced within the countries either for local consumption or for export.

Enrichment and Fortification of Foods. Enrichment is the addition of nutrients to a foodstuff during processing. This term often means restoration to original levels of nutrients lost during processing. Enrichment is now an accepted concept in developed countries; for example, almost all white flour produced and marketed in the United States is enriched with thiamine, riboflavin, niacin, and iron; iodine is added to salt and vitamin A to margarine.

Fortification of food makes possible the addition of one or more nutrients to a food product in quantities more than are found in the foodstuff in its unprocessed state. An essential nutrient may be incorporated in a food where it did not exist at all. The specific purpose of fortification is to meet nutritional needs and thereby prevent nutritional deficiencies.

Food Standards and Food Laws. One of the major responsibilities of a government is to ensure safe and wholesome food for the population. Unfortunately, however, this responsibility is not being discharged in an appropriate manner in most developing countries. The ICNND nutrition survey teams in Lebanon and Jordan specifically recommended that appropriate food laws be enacted and enforced. In fact the ICNND recommendations for Jordan were very specific and detailed, for the probable reason that at the time the survey was done a draft law was before the Jordanian Parliament.

Food in the countries of the Near East is produced by numerous small producers and is also processed on a small, almost domestic, scale in villages and towns. The quality of the products offered to the consumer varies enormously, and furthermore there is always a possibility that spoiled and damaged food, food products, or preparations are marketed. Adulteration of food is not uncommon. The lack of food standards, appropriate food laws, and mechanism for their enforcement make for an unsatisfactory, often harmful, situation against which the consumer has little redress. Even in situations where food laws exist, their enforcement leaves much to be desired. Enforcement requires trained personnel and adequate laboratory facilities. Unless these are properly provided for, mere enactment of food laws will have little success in ensuring wholesome food for the public.

In 1962 an Agricultural Marketing Bureau was established in Jordan with the responsibility for developing market standards and food regulations. A central laboratory for analytical purposes was equipped and staffed; provision for inspection was also made. The Central Laboratory in Amman in the Ministry of Health and the Army Laboratory for tasting of foods are operative in their respective spheres.

In Lebanon, a central public health laboratory functions in the Ministry of Health and is charged with the analysis of imported foods, alcoholic beverages, milk and milk samples, and water. The lack of enforcement of existing regulations, however, would seem to nullify much of the effort involved, a situation also commented upon by the ICNND survey team in 1962.

In Egypt food control is administered by the Ministry of Public Health. The administration is charged with: (a) planning of laws, rules, and regulations for the protection of the public against food-poisoning; (b) preparation of food standards; (c) inspection of food for spoilage, contamination, and adulteration; and (d) educating food-handlers in appropriate methods of food-handling and storage. Both the imported food and food for export are subjected to inspection according to the standards formulated by the government for a

Prevention

large variety of foods and beverages produced within the country. The slaughter of animals for food is regulated, and ground rules for slaughterhouses laid down. Thus it would appear that Egypt is the most advanced within the region in respect to food laws. It is difficult to determine, however, the efficiency with which food laws are enforced. It is not unlikely that in large towns and cities their enforcement may be reasonably good and that manufactured foods must satisfy the standards. On the other hand, the rural population, which forms the majority and which does not usually consume manufactured or processed foods, may probably be less well protected.

FAO and WHO (1967) jointly established a Codex Alimentarius Commission with a Food Standards Program. Among the main objectives of this program are the protection of consumers' health, the assurance of fair practice in the food trade, and furtherance of food-standards work in developing countries. The work of the Codex Alimentarius Commission is therefore of immediate interest and benefit to the developing countries. However, among the six countries covered by this book, only Jordan and Syria were members of the Codex and participating in its food-standards program. It is hoped that other countries will join the Codex before long and derive the fullest benefit from this international effort.

SPECIFIC MEASURES

The measures discussed above for the prevention of malnutrition will require time to implement. Much more time will be required after implementation for them to affect the nourishment of the people. More food and a better standard of living will undoubtedly contribute to improvement in the nutritional status of the people. However, one should not believe that nothing can be done until more food becomes available and the standard of living is raised. Effective measures which are within the means of the governments concerned can be instituted immediately to control malnutrition and its increasingly ill effects.

A readily applicable series of specific measures utilizes the techniques of food enrichment and fortification. The intelligent use of these measures can control certain nutritional deficiencies and reduce the prevalence of certain specific diseases. Both enrichment and fortification can be effective if foods or food adjuncts most commonly used by the majority of the people in daily dietaries are selected as vehicles for the nutrients to be added.

Fortification of common salt with iodide or iodate is one example of proved efficacy in countries with endemic goiter. There is ample evidence that this deficiency disease exists over much of the region with which we are concerned. It is disappointing to see that a country with a high rate of endemicity, where iodization of salt has been recommended, has not yet seen fit to introduce it as a control measure. One does not know what considerations operated against the adoption of iodization; whatever they were, one must say that the country was ill advised not to adopt this wholesome measure. The result is that even though seven to eight years have passed since the goiter survey, little reduction in the prevalence of endemic goiter seems to have occurred.

The fortification and enrichment of wheat flour is another useful measure. Ariboflavinosis and iron-deficiency anemia are common in this region. The enrichment or fortification of flour with riboflavin and iron can readily reduce the prevalence of these two conditions. Since anemia in Egypt is in part a reflection of the parasitic burden, it is true that fortification of flour by itself, without measures to reduce the parasitism, cannot completely control the anemia. Parasitism itself is more difficult of solution. Nevertheless, an assured increment in the daily intake of available iron from fortified flour would do much to alleviate the ill effects of the widespread anemia in the population. The doubt on the efficacy of the current practice of iron-enrichment of flour resulting from the recent investigations in England (Elwood, 1963) in no wise should be interpreted as discrediting the process and its effectiveness. Many forms of iron suitable for use and readily available from food are known.

Investigations in Jordan showed a relatively high rate of vitamin A deficiency in infants and preschool children. Even in adults comparatively low average levels of vitamin A in serum were found, suggesting a marginal deficiency of this vitamin in the population. Considering that the majority of the people find it difficult to consume foods rich in vitamin A in adequate quantities, the obvious immediate solution was to fortify a commonly used food with vitamin A or its precursor β-carotene. The fortification of olive oil and hydrogenated vegetable oil was considered and judged unsuitable because vitamin A was likely to be destroyed while food was being cooked in the fortified oil. Fortification of *ghee* with vitamin A was initiated. However, it was concluded that the poorer people could not be expected to consume *ghee* in adequate quantities to provide enough vitamin A for protection against deficiency.

Modern technology, however, had found a solution to this problem.

Prevention

A stable, solid vitamin A preparation (containing vitamin A palmitate) was available. It was suitable for fortification of wheat flour, a foodstuff used in the form of bread by everyone, rich or poor. Preliminary trials demonstrated that the vitamin A could be evenly distributed in the fortified flour, that the latter had satisfactory shelf life, and that no more than 20% of the added vitamin was destroyed during the baking of bread. A project was thereupon planned jointly by the Jordanian government and U.S. AID in 1966 for the fortification of wheat flour with vitamin A in Jordan. The cost of fortification at the level of 3,250 I.U. vitamin A per pound was estimated to be between 250 to 300 fils per ton (1,000 fils = 1 dinar = 1 £ sterling). The pilot trial in one large flour mill in Amman was to be followed by further expansion to include all such large mills in Jordan. The pilot stage started in December 1966, and the expansion of the project was set for the middle of 1967. Unfortunately the Arab-Israeli war put a stop to all such developments and even the pilot project was discontinued. What would have been a beneficial measure for the people, the controlling of vitamin A deficiency and the demonstration of one of the easier and cheaper ways of achieving it was frustrated by the exigencies of the political situation.

Pellagra is peculiar to Egypt among the Arab countries in the Near East and is largely associated with maize-based diets. Fortification of maize flour with nicotinic acid should be one appropriate and far-reaching measure for the prevention of pellagra. Such was recommended in 1954 by an expert team from WHO requested by the Egyptian government, but the measure has not yet been instituted. The arguments advanced earlier for fortifying wheat flour with riboflavin and iron should apply to maize flour as well and hence should deserve serious consideration.

Fortification of foodstuffs can only succeed if it can be applied on a nation-wide scale. Under the present circumstances this seems limited because methods of production, distribution, and marketing range from the small-producer effort, which predominates, to large undertakings. Attempts should, however, be made to introduce fortification procedures in all the large flour mills. This step will ensure that at least the consumers who use that flour or bread made from it will benefit nutritionally. As more and more large mills are established, possibly at the cost of the small units, the benefits of fortification can be extended to a larger population than at present. Even for the small producers, methods adaptable for small units are available and should be used where pellagra and anemia are endemic. This may require encouragement from the government, possibly in the form of a subsidy, followed by supervision to ensure proper functioning of the equipment.

Nutrition in Public Health

Medical and public health services have an important role to perform in the control and prevention of malnutrition. In any country, infants, young children of preschool age, and women of child-bearing age are among those most vulnerable to malnutrition. They can be reached through the maternal- and child-health (MCH) services which now form an integral part of the basic health services in most countries. In theory, these services are expected to look after the nutrition of mothers and children. In practice, this is only indifferently achieved. The staff, including the medical officer-in-charge of the center, know comparatively little about practical nutrition, and, they usually have had no training in how to deal with problems of malnutrition found commonly to occur in pregnant women and infants who attend the MCH centers. Their understanding of the interrelation between infection and malnutrition is elementary, particularly where infants are concerned. Besides, the MCH centers usually care only for infants of up to one year of age, whereas the most serious problems of malnutrition, which are accompanied with and often triggered by the recurring respiratory and gastrointestinal infections, are likely to arise between six months to two years of age. The experience of Abdou et al. (1965) has shown that in MCH centers in Cairo almost all infants examined had suffered from repeated episodes of infections by the time they reached one year of age and most of them were malnourished. The situation in the villages must be the same or possibly worse.

It is the common practice in many developing countries, including the Arab countries of the Near East, to withhold food from the infant during attacks of diarrhea or fevers or to give thin cereal or starchy gruel and to continue the restricted diets during convalescence as well. In this malnourished state the infant falls an easy prey to the next bout of gastroenteritis, the danger of which is always present because of the unhygienic manner in which infant's food is prepared and handled by the ignorant mother. Thus a vicious circle of malnutrition and infection is set up which can only be broken by proper advice and health education at MCH centers. We believe that the role of MCH centers in combating malnutrition in mothers and children is of the utmost importance. Its functions as they pertain to nutrition can be briefly described as follows:

1. To advise and to educate pregnant and nursing women regarding their own food and diet and the appropriate methods of feeding their infants in health and during minor illnesses. Emphasis on breast feeding as the best way of providing nourishment to the infant is essential.

2. To provide nutrient supplements to pregnant women, especially iron supplements, for anemia in pregnancy is common.

3. To provide and demonstrate the use of nutrient supplements intended for infants, such as protein-rich foods and vitamin preparations.

4. To provide nutrition-rehabilitation service which should consist of: (a) detection and treatment of early malnutrition; (b) treatment of cases of malnutrition discharged from hospitals since continued hospitalization is considered unnecessary after the cure has been initiated; (c) rehydration of cases suffering from diarrhea and dehydration; (d) education of mothers concerning the preparation of meals for infants, methods of appropriate feeding, and elements of hygiene, including food-handling.

MCH services should be extended to cover not only infants but also children of preschool age. Under the present conditions care of infants up to one year of age is the responsibility of the MCH services. Children from six years onwards are supposed to be looked after by the school health services. It is the children of ages between these two groups that seem to be nobody's responsibility. Their health care will be provided for if the MCH services take it on themselves to do it, as suggested above. MCH centers appropriately equipped to discharge the above functions and staffed with nurses and physicians should be able to do a great deal of good by reducing the incidence of malnutrition in infants and preschool children. An informed public health nutritionist supervising nutrition work in three or four MCH centers under the guidance of the physician and with nutrition aides could relieve the latter of much of the responsibility and at the same time ensure adequate nutritional service.

The idea of nutrition rehabilitation centers was developed originally in 1955 by Bengoa of the World Health Organization at a nutrition-training course for countries south of the Sahara organized by FAO, WHO, and the French government. Since then it has been discussed several times on formal and informal occasions and has been assuming a concrete shape. In 1967 several such centers were functioning in Algeria, Colombia, Costa Rica, Guatemala, Haiti, Uganda, and Venezuela. A detailed description of the day and residential types of rehabilitation centers, their organization, functions, and cost of operation will be found in an article by Bengoa (1967). This author rightly points out that the organization of the nutrition-rehabilitation service should not be considered in isolation but must form part of the basic health services of the country. Nutritional rehabilitation is but one plank in the program of prevention of malnutrition but at the same time is an extremely important one. It can be easily fitted in with the maternal- and child-health services we have proposed above. In our opinion, nutrition rehabilitation of infants and young children rightfully fits in with the objectives and scope of activities of MCH services.

INSTITUTIONAL AND GROUP FEEDING

Another specific measure of importance in the context of the prevention of malnutrition in a community is institutional feeding or feeding of sizable population groups. This includes provision of midday meals or breakfasts for day-school children, meals to industrial workers at canteens, and supervision of feeding in students' hostels, orphanages, prisons, messes of the armed forces, and hospitals. The feeding of the armed forces tends to be looked after fairly well for obvious reasons. On the other hand institutional feeding of other groups is generally a haphazard business in which the considerations of cost and convenience predominate to the neglect of the nutritional needs of those at the receiving end. Whereas each one of the categories needing group or institutional feeding is important, the most important group is that of school children because of their numbers and of the age at which they are more vulnerable to malnutrition than the adults in a population.

School Feeding

The purpose of providing school meals to the day scholars is to afford nourishment at a suitable hour during their long day at school. The school meal should also supplement the habitual diet which the child receives at home. In determining the composition of the school meal, an attempt should be made to correct the common nutritional deficiencies known to occur among school children of the locality. The meal itself could be a school breakfast or school lunch, depending upon the school hours. If the school meets early, many children are apt to leave home without breakfast.

In most cases, distance from the home precludes the children's return for a midday meal at home, and school children are usually averse to carrying pack meals with them. Often the parents are unable to provide such a meal for a variety of reasons. It is all the more imperative that the school children should receive a nutritious meal at school. The general idea about the nutritional content of a school meal is that it should provide approximately one third of the child's daily requirements. This has not always been possible, but it is a desirable target at which to aim.

School meal programs are thus beneficial from the nutritional point of view. They can also serve an educational purpose. With the nutritious meal that the child receives, he is in a position to be taught the elements of practical nutrition. School meal programs with or without the educational component have only slowly evolved in developing countries. An indication of the developments within the region is given below with reference to three countries,—Egypt, Iraq, and Libya.

Egypt. School feeding has been practiced in Egypt for a long time. Old records indicate that in A.D. 696 pupils in the two schools attached to the Amr-Ibn-El-As and Ahmed-Ibn-Touloon mosques had meals served to them. The theological university of Al-Azhar in Cairo has attracted since its foundation students from Islamic countries all over the world, and their feeding was attended to by the university authorities. In A.D. 1415, 750 Egyptian and foreign students at Al-Azhar were provided with hot meals. This is understandable, for the students were usually boarders receiving stipends and the responsibility for feeding them devolved on the university. A reference to the provision of school meals in the 19th century, when modern systems of education were being introduced in Egypt, can be found in an FAO publication (1953).

In 1942, the Egyptian government, satisfied with the results of a pilot trial conducted earlier in two villages near Cairo, enacted a law for free feeding at school of all elementary school children. The program of feeding included the distribution of snacks consisting of bread, local cheese, cooked beans, and a sweet (*halawa*) to more than 125,000 children. In 1951 another law brought under one feeding program all the kindergartens and the primary schools. About two million school children received free school meals. Soon after, however, the budget provision was drastically reduced, with the result that the amount of food given as well as the number of beneficiaries decreased. In 1951–52 the meal provided about 620 calories and 18 g protein, whereas in 1954–55 it contained only 420 calories and 14 g protein (Hegazi, 1959). Surplus wheat flour and skim milk powder imported from U.S.A. for a few years from 1954 onwards helped the school meal program. Eventually this source was depleted.

In 1958, 31% of all school age children were enrolled; of these, 0.52% were boarders who received all meals and 3.33% were day school children who were given hot or cold snacks; the majority of the remainder in primary and preparatory schools received bread only. When the U.S. surplus food stopped coming, the Egyptian government had to find food and additional funds for its purchase in order to ensure the continuation of the school feeding programs. Financial stringency and possibly priorities for other national activities resulted in the drying-up of funds for the school meal program, and the activity gradually diminished after 1960–61, so much so that during the last two years only the boarders have received free meals.

This is a sorry state of affairs, for Egypt had such fine tradition and the country did attempt to meet the modern concept of health care of school children by introducing the school meal program much earlier than had most other developing countries. Egypt had furthermore made rapid progress in expanding it, as the above account must show. It is all the more unfortunate, therefore, to have to record that school feeding in Egypt is now in the doldrums. One cannot predict when the program will get going again.

Iraq. The FAO publication of 1953 mentions only Egypt among the Arab countries which had a school meal program. In that year plans were set afoot in Iraq for initiating a school meal project with international assistance. UNICEF agreed to provide dry skim milk powder and vitamin A and D capsules; the government of Iraq had to find local foods, provide the organization, and make available some funds for the conduct of the project. The project envisaged the feeding of 40,000 school children in the first year, followed by a continuous increase in the number of beneficiaries in successive years. School feeding started in Baghdad in November 1953, and it was intended to cover 14 other provinces (Liwa) by the end of that year. The meal was to consist of locally produced foodstuffs such as eggs, cheese, chick-peas, beans, and citrus fruit, sugar (5 g), bread (100 g), dates and raisins, and reconstituted skim milk (equivalent to 40 g dry powder).

The program got off to a good start. The distribution of meals, however, was not uniform in all areas. Milk and vitamin capsules were given to school children in the urban areas, whereas in the village schools a meal composed from local foodstuffs was the general rule. In 1957, FAO conducted a survey of school feeding on request from the government of Iraq. According to this survey, school feeding was working reasonably well in most provinces visited by the survey team. There were difficulties, of course, mainly with regard to the uncertainty of funds promised by the local administration. Soon after this, other difficulties arose. Surplus skim milk powder was no longer available to UNICEF, and hence no supplies could be made for school feeding in Iraq. This was a great blow, for it meant that Iraq had to find a substitute and funds to buy it. In 1961, the government showed an inclination to curtail the allocation for school feeding, which it did in later years. As a result, the school feeding programs must have suffered a serious setback. In 1960, which was the peak year for the program, 400,000 children out of an estimated total of 1,000,000 primary school children received some kind of a school meal (DeMarchi and Hamandi, 1961). Of the beneficiaries, 140,000 children received mid-morning meals, and 260,000 received a glass of milk and vitamin A and D capsules each three times a week. The mid-morning meal provided 465 calories, 21 g protein, 330 mg calcium, 2 mg iron, 2,620 I.U. vitamin A activity, 0.2 mg thiamine, 0.65 mg riboflavin, 1.4 mg niacin, and 23 mg ascorbic acid. The nutritional value of the meal is considered reasonably good. DeMarchi and Hamandi (1961) found a significant difference in heights and weights between the children who received the school meal for 150 days a year and others who did not receive it at all. This was useful evidence for the beneficial effect of school meals. Greater is the pity therefore that other considerations interfered with the expansion of the program or even its continuation at the level which it had reached in 1960–61.

Libya. In marked contrast to the experience in Egypt and Iraq is the development and status of school feeding in Libya. The initiation of the project was facilitated by the preliminary consultations between the government of Libya, FAO, WHO, and UNICEF, which took place in 1953 and 1954. Skim milk powder, vitamin A and D capsules, distribution equipment, and transportation were supplied by UNICEF on a two-year basis to begin with. The school feeding program was started under the supervision of an expert nominated by FAO who was working in the Libyan Ministry of Education. Funds from the Libyan side were assured through the levy of a 5% supplementary tax on certain imported goods.

The school meal was in the form of a breakfast of milk reconstituted from 40 g dry skim milk powder, 100 g dates, and vitamin A and D capsules. The school breakfast began in the spring of 1955 with 3,500 school children, but within a year 60,000 children in 357 schools all over the country were benefiting from school meals. Certain changes in the meal were introduced. Bread became a regular constituent, and cheese donated by CARE was also included. This was later replaced by local cheese. Among other foods included as components of school meals were tuna fish, sardines, peanuts, and orange marmalade. The distribution of these foods varied in the three provinces of Libya. In 1959, Barakat surveyed the school feeding program on behalf of FAO. He found that 110,000 school children received meals at school. The distribution of various foods was uneven: in some schools meals were defective; in others no meals were served. Barakat made recommendations for eliminating the defects that he observed.

School feeding continued to expand in the 1960s, and its progress was twice reviewed by FAO,—once in 1962 and again in 1964. At some stage milk distribution had to be discontinued, probably because dry skim milk powder was no longer available as surplus. However, unlike other countries, the government of Libya has continued to press on with the program. In 1961–62 the school meal was estimated to provide 590 calories and 15 g protein with very small quantities of other essential nutrients. FAO made recommendations for improvement in the composition of the school meal. There is not much evidence, however, whether these are being put into practice. In 1963–64 the school meal allocations per child were tuna fish, 15 g; *halawa,* 20 g; orange marmalade, 20 g; cheese, 35 g. These were in addition to 100 g bread. Dates, 125 g, and peanuts, 50 g, were given twice a week beginning with that year. The school year extended over 180 days; the school meal was given for 130 days. In 1963–64, almost the total population of the elementary and primary school children numbering about 170,000 received benefit from the school meal program. By this time the government of Libya had agreed to place the program on a permanent basis. Funds for it were being derived from the supplementary import duty levied since 1955. Plans for expanding school feeding were being made to cover the preparatory and secondary schools, so as to include all children attending schools of one type or another.

It is unfortunate that at no stage was an attempt made to demonstrate the beneficial effects of school meals by surveys on the nutritional status of school children. Strictly speaking, such surveys ought not to be necessary, for in the long run, school meals must benefit the school children in terms of better health, reduced absenteeism, and improved scholastic performance.

One of the major difficulties in organizing and maintaining a school meal program is its cost. Reliable estimates which include the cost of food, its transport and storage; preparation and distribution of meals; space, furniture and eating utensils, and washing arrangements; and personnel involved in these operations and for supervision were not readily available from the sources we consulted. The reports from Egypt, Iraq, and Libya have given the cost of school meals to the governments as varying between 2.0 to 2.5 piastres (equivalent to about 6 U.S. cents) per child per day. This was exclusive of the food received free from such agencies as UNICEF, CARE, and U.S. AID. It also excluded the cost of the administration at the national level.

In the FAO report on the assessment of school feeding in Libya for 1963–64 it is stated that the budget allocation for school feeding in that year was approximately £ 1,400,000 Libyan, of which 80% was for the cost of food and 20% for administration. Taking into account the number of children (181,972) fed and the number of days (130) in a school year on which school meals were provided, one arrives at 4.7 piastres (11 U.S. cents) per child per day as being the cost of the meal. This seems to be a more realistic estimate than 2 to 2.5 piastres mentioned above. In countries with large child-populations, this would mean a substantial outlay on the part of the government, making considerable demand on their annual budgets. It is no wonder that the governments of Egypt and Iraq in recent years have drastically curtailed or nearly abolished the school meal programs.

The three examples of Egypt, Iraq, and Libya and their experiences in the domain of school feeding should indicate that, given the will and determination to care for the young generation, it should not be beyond the means of the national governments to make school feeding a permanent feature of government-sponsored health and educational activities. Libya has done this; let us hope that the present setbacks in Egypt and Iraq are only temporary and that better days for school feeding are ahead.

Feeding the boarders involves greater responsibility than feeding day scholars, for the boarders receive all their daily meals at the place of residence. It is essential therefore to ensure that the diets provided adequately meet their nutritional needs. One wonders whether proper thought is given to the composition of diets to satisfy the requirements. The same can probably be said of the feeding of the inmates of prisons and of patients in hospitals. A re-examination of the current schedules of institutional feeding with a view to improving them so as to ensure nutritional adequacy should be undertaken.

Industrial Feeding

Industrialization is proceeding apace in the Near East. New industries are being established, employing progressively larger numbers of people. Most of such industries will be located in and around large cities; their workers will come from the urban areas and from villages whose inhabitants will migrate to the cities in search of better living and find it difficult to adapt themselves to new eating habits. The collection of a large number of workers in one establishment and the long hours of work expected from them create a responsibility for feeding at work. However, the problem is not so simple. Eating out is not a habit which comes easily in Africa and Asia. The reasons may be partly tradition and partly economic. However, when a new way of life has to be adopted, as is inevitable under the conditions of industrialization, certain adjustments have to be made. Admittedly this will take time. Until such time, industrial feeding must be organized in such a way that, apart from being nutritious, the meals will appeal to the worker and be priced within the means of the lowest-paid employee. This is not possible unless the meals are subsidized. Probably even this will not attract all the workers to the canteen, for tradition and habits die hard. Education and experience alone will bring about changes in their outlook and behavior.

The Arab countries of the Near East now in the process of industrialization are apparently conscious of the benefits of industrial feeding so far as the health of the worker and its direct effect on productivity are concerned. Egypt entered the field of industrial feeding in 1959. Other countries are trying to introduce canteens to industries where they did not exist and to improve the existing ones. In 1963, FAO in consultation with WHO arranged for a survey of industrial feeding in the Near East. Among the countries visited by the consultant were Egypt and Jordan. A summary of his findings is given below.

Egypt. In 1959, a presidential decree made industrial feeding obligatory for workers in mining and quarrying industries. In 1961 another presidential decree brought under this law all factories employing 25 or more workers.

A committee consisting of representatives of workers and management in each factory is responsible for managing and directing the work of the canteen. The law relating to industrial canteens has laid down specifications concerning the provision of adequate space, seating arrangements, washing facilities, provision of potable drinking water, and maintenance of hygienic and sanitary standards including safe handling of foods.

The canteens are able to buy foodstuffs at controlled prices. This keeps the cost of meals low. The meals are, however, subsidized; the subsidy may be as high as 75%. According to law a worker is required to contribute not more than one third of the cost of the meal served at the canteen. At the time of the survey the workers paid approximately 2-1/2 piastres per meal.

Jordan. In Jordan, labor laws are permissive concerning the provision of meals at work in industrial establishments. The government may issue orders requiring provision of meals, when it considers them necessary. This has not often been done. As a result, at the time of the consultants' visit, about 90% of the industrial workers in Jordan were not provided with food during their working hours. In the opinion of the consultant, not much could be done at the time to improve the nutrition of industrial workers in Jordan unless the laws regulating their feeding at work obliged the establishments to organize canteens. As it was, a large proportion of workers brought food from their homes or bought it from small restaurants and peddlers and ate it in the dining area within the factory.

The FAO survey included four factories in Jordan and thirteen in Egypt, each employing more than 250 workers. The total number of workers covered in the survey was 1,696 in Jordan and 65,613 in Egypt. In Jordan three of the four factories visited had canteens operated voluntarily by the employers, and in the fourth factory a canteen was run by agreement with workers. In Egypt the employers operated all the industrial canteens so as to conform to the Egyptian labor laws. In both countries food was provided below its actual cost, the difference being made up by the factory. The proportion of workers who had meals exclusively in the canteen was 50% in Jordan and 75% in Egypt. The remainder brought their own food, some of them supplementing it with food from the canteens.

FAO and WHO jointly followed up the survey by organizing a seminar on industrial feeding in which the member governments of the region participated. It is hoped that the seminar will have provided sufficient stimulus for the improvement and expansion of the industrial feeding programs in the Arab countries. Egypt has set a good example, and the experience will be found useful by other countries launching on the expansion of their national programs of industrial canteens.

FEEDING OF REFUGEES

One cannot fail to take note of a large-scale group-feeding program which has been operating within the region for nearly twenty years. The circumstances under which it had to be organized were unfortunate but not unusual in the modern, politically disturbed world. That it has continued for twenty years and is likely to continue for some years to come is, however, unusual. The organization and the conduct of the program are subjects of sufficient interest and significance from the standpoint of the health of the Palestine refugees to warrant a short description here to supplement the brief reference to UNRWA activities made in Chapter 13.

The partition of Palestine in 1948 and the Arab-Israeli conflict which followed had the unfortunate consequence of rendering about a million Palestinian Arabs homeless. They migrated to the neighboring Arab countries and were forced to live as refugees. In order to meet the urgent situation, the United Nations created a new organization known as the United Nations Relief and Works Agency (UNRWA) for Palestine refugees. UNRWA had to take care of these refugees by providing them with shelter, food, and medical and health care. As the prospects of early settlement of the problem receded, UNRWA had to expand its activities and make long-term provision for the comprehensive care of refugees. The majority of refugees were settled in camps; some chose to stay in border villages, and others migrated to urban areas seeking employment. To the relief services already being provided by UNRWA were added educational and training services, and other methods of assisting refugees had to be developed over the years.

Feeding nearly a million refugees was a tremendous task for UNRWA, and continuation of the responsibility required the establishment within UNRWA of an organization capable of finding and distributing food. Whereas the procurement of food is the responsibility of the administrative branch of UNRWA, the supervision of services concerning distribution of dry rations, provision of supplements, and feeding of infants, children, and the sick is done by the UNRWA Directorate of Health.

All refugees registered with UNRWA are not eligible for rations. The proportion of recipients of rations to the total number of refugees has decreased from 97.5% in 1951 to 65.5% in 1966. There are several reasons for this decrease, the chief of which is lack of sufficient funds. The amount spent by UNRWA on procurement of food and its distribution to beneficiaries forms a substantial proportion of its budget. According to the report of the Commissioner General for 1966–67, this cost represented 37% of the total UNRWA budget in that year.

The food and nutrition service of UNRWA distributes food in three main categories—dry rations, milk, and supplementary feeding. UNRWA has sought advice and help from WHO and FAO in formulating rations and in developing the milk and supplementary feeding programs.

All refugees registered to receive full rations are issued foodstuffs

TABLE 1
UNRWA SCALE OF DRY RATIONS FOR PALESTINE REFUGEES

	Ration Scale g/Person/Day	
	Summer 7 Months	Winter 5 Months
Wheat flour	333	347
Pulses	20	30
Rice	20	20
Sugar	16.7	16.7
Oils and fats	12.5	12.5

according to a fixed scale. Summer and winter rations differ in quantity as shown in Table 1.

The rations provide 1,500 calories and 42 g protein per day per person in summer and 1,600 calories and 45 g protein in winter. These are subsistence rations midway between the relief rations and those designed to meet full nutritional needs. Realizing their inadequacy, UNRWA provides additional rations to pregnant and nursing women beginning with the fifth month of pregnancy and lasting until the end of twelfth month after delivery. This supplementary ration consists of wheat flour, 100 g; pulses, 27.5 g; and oils and fats, 6.7 g per day.

Special milk-distribution programs are organized for infants and children. All infants between 6 and 12 months in age and those below 6 months who are not breast fed are eligible to receive 480 ml each of milk reconstituted from a mixture of 30 g whole milk powder and 30 g dried skim milk. Children above one year and up to 15 years and pregnant and nursing women receive a supplement of milk reconstituted from 20 g dried skim milk on 26 days in each month. In addition, and depending upon the availability of milk supply, elementary school children are given milk reconstituted from 40 g of skim milk powder on 22 days per month. This service has varied in its incidence during any given year for financial reasons and has been practically abolished since November 1966.

Another commendable feature of the UNRWA feeding scheme is the provision daily of hot meals to children below 6 years of age at supplementary feeding centers. This meal is based on foodstuffs mentioned in the ration scale and includes skim milk as well. The meal is expected to provide 520 calories and 21 g protein per child per day. Older children on medical advice are entitled to receive the supplementary hot meals.

TABLE 2
BENEFICIARIES OF RATIONS AND OTHER UNRWA FEEDING PROGRAMS IN 1966

Particulars	No. of Beneficiaries per Day
1. Dry rations	851,166
2. Supplementary dry rations	
(a) pregnant and nursing women	33,034
(b) tuberculous outpatients	1,157
3. Supplementary cooked meal	38,421
4.[1] Milk (Jan.–Oct. 1966)	
(a) at milk-distribution centers	97,686
(b) in schools	89,916
(c) in orphanages and on medical prescription	683

1. Milk distribution program was curtailed from November 1966, so that in the remaining two months of the year only 51,986 beneficiaries received milk. No milk was distributed in schools.

An idea of the scale of the UNRWA feeding operation can be had from Table 2, prepared from figures contained in the report of the Director of Health, UNRWA, for the year 1966.

The feeding of refugees has been the best possible under the circumstances. A large majority of women of child-bearing age and infants and children have benefited most, as they should, since they represent the vulnerable groups in the population. Demands on UNRWA to raise the scale of rations have been made from time to time, and several complaints have been voiced in the lay, and even in the local medical, press about the inadequacy and unsuitability of UNRWA rations. Few people, however, make any constructive suggestions of how to meet the cost of this operation without increasing the burden on the contributing nations who expected that a permanent solution to the refugee problem would be found within a reasonable time. Recent happenings, unfortunately, do not hold out any promise of finding such a solution in the foreseeable future.

In fairness to UNRWA it must be said that the feeding programs and medical and health care provided by the agency have contributed to the maintenance of the health of refugees at a level which is not significantly different from that of the populations of the host countries in which the refugees have been living. The same applies to the nutritional status of infants, children, and adults among refugees.

TRAINING OF PERSONNEL

Preventive programs in nutrition cannot be implemented without trained personnel. It is not too much to ask that all those who have to do with food production and health should receive some training in nutrition appropriate to their respective specialties and functions. In this category could be included agriculture and veterinary science graduates and their auxiliaries, food technologists and food caterers on the one hand, and physicians, public health nurses, nurses in general, and dietitians on the other. The courses in human nutrition which the students of agriculture, veterinary science, and medicine receive as part of their undergraduate curricula are didactic and seem to have little relation to the problem of malnutrition in its various aspects, which these people in their professional life are likely to encounter. It is necessary therefore to reorient the nutrition-teaching in undergraduate years on a realistic basis. The universities need to be persuaded to appreciate this point of view in order to bring about the desired changes in the undergraduate curricula in the faculties of agriculture, veterinary science, food science, and medicine. The course in nursing schools also needs to be revised so as to improve nutrition-teaching with greater emphasis on the teaching of practical nutrition.

There are institutions in some of these countries which can assist in nutrition-teaching at the universities and in organizing special training courses for various categories of personnel. For example, institutes of food and nutrition exist in Egypt and Iraq. In Egypt the High Institute of Public Health, Alexandria, has a good department of nutrition engaged in teaching and research. In Lebanon, an active nutrition research laboratory in the Faculty of Medicine at the American University of Beirut functions under the Columbia University Nutrition Research Program. The Faculty of Agricultural Sciences of A.U.B. is also very much involved in nutritional investigations in Lebanon. It seems therefore that facilities exist within the region, not only for training national personnel, but also for training personnel from other countries of the region which do not have such facilities. It will be a pity if they are not put to good use.

REFERENCES

Abdou, I. A., H. E. Ali, and A. K. Lebshtein. 1965. A Study of the Nutritional Status of Mothers, Infants, and Young Children Attending Maternity and Child Health Centers in Cairo. Part I—The Nutritional Status of Infants and Young Children. *Bull. Nutr. Inst., U.A.R.* 1: 9.

Allcroft, R. 1965. Aspects of Aflatoxicosis in Farm Animals. In *Mycotoxins in Foodstuffs*. Ed. Gerald N. Wogan. Cambridge, Mass.: M.I.T. Press.

Badiali, L., M. H. Abou-Youssef, A. I. Radwan, F. M. Hamdy, and P. K. Hildebrandt. 1968. Moldy Corn Poisoning as the Major Cause of an

Encephalomalacia Syndrome in Egyptian Equidae. *Amer. J. Vet. Res.* 29: 2029.

Bengoa, J. M. 1967. Nutrition Rehabilitation Centers. *J. Trop. Pediatrics* 13: 169.

DeMarchi, M., and F. Hamandi. 1961. A Study on the Evaluation of the School Meal Supplement. *J. Fac. Med. Baghdad* 3: 12.

Elwood, P. C. 1963. A Clinical Trial of Iron-Fortified Bread. *Brit. Med. J.* i: 224.

Hegazi, L. M. A. 1959. Present Status of School Feeding in Egypt. Thesis (M.P.H.), High Institute of Public Health, Alexandria, Egypt, U.A.R.

World Health Organization. 1966. *Industrial Feeding in the Near East.* Report of the Joint FAO/WHO Seminar. Alexandria, Egypt, Regional Office for the Eastern Mediterranean.

Issawi, A., M. Khatib, and M. Pont-Flores. 1964. An Assessment of the School Feeding and Nutrition Education Program. Report to the Government of Libya. Rome, Italy: Food and Agriculture Organization of the United Nations.

Joint FAO/WHO Experiment Committee on Nutrition. 1967. Seventh Report. Technical Report Series No. 377. Geneva, Switzerland: World Health Organization.

Kotschevar, L. H. 1964. *The Feeding of Industrial Workers in the Near East.* Rome, Italy: Food and Agriculture Organization of the United Nations.

Lauersen, F. 1957. *Report to the Government of Libya on School Feeding.* Rome, Italy: Food and Agriculture Organization of the United Nations.

Scott, M. L. 1953. *School Feeding: Its Contribution to Child Nutrition.* Rome, Italy: Food and Agriculture Organization of the United Nations.

Wilson, B. J. 1966. Fungal Toxins. *In Toxicants Occurring Naturally in Foods.* National Research Council Publication 1354. Washington, D.C.: National Academy of Sciences.

United Nations. 1966, 1967. *Reports of the Commissioner General of the United Nations Relief and Works Agency for Palestine Refugees in the Near East.* General Assembly, Official Records: Supplement 13 (A/6313). 21st Session, 22nd Session, Supplement 13 (A/6713). New York.

United Nations Relief and Works Agency for Palestine Refugees. 1967. *Annual Report of the Director of Health 1966.* Beirut, Lebanon: UNRWA Headquarters.

INDEX

Adrenal glands: histopathological changes in protein-calorie deficiency disease, 156-157
Agricultural Marketing Bureau in Jordan, 286
Agriculture. *See* Food production
Aish shamy, 21
Amino acid deficiency in pellagra, 48
Anemia: and hookworm, 63-65; and parasitism in Egypt, 61-66; and protein-calorie deficiency disease, 70-71, 76-80; in Cairo infants, 242; in Cairo school children, 243; in Egypt, 57-66; in Iraq, 275-277; in Libya, Lebanon, Jordan, 73-80; iron-deficiency, 65, 76-80; iron deficiency, and kwashiorkor, 70-72, 76-80; iron deficiency, and pregnancy, 67-70, 75
Animals, domestic: consumption of contaminated food, 283
Anklostomiasis: and Pellagra, 37-38, 50; and malnutrition and anemia in Egypt, 57; in Arab countries, 17; in Egypt, 62, 66; in oases, 66
Antibiotics, 159, 177
Ascorbic acid: absorption in pellagra, 54; deficiency, in scurvy, 116-119

Balady bread, 20
Barley, 20
Bedouins, 8-9
Bétau, 22
Bilharziasis: and malnutrition and anemia in Egypt, 57; in Arab countries, 17; in Egypt, 65; in oases, 66
Birth rates, 15
Birth weights and lengths: of Egyptian infants, 192-194; of Jordanian infants, 195-199; of Lebanese infants, 195-199
Bitot's spot, 101, 102, 244
Blood transfusion, 159, 180
Bread, 20-22. *See also* Maize, and names of bread
Breast-feeding: in Arab countries, 182-184; in Egypt, 184-186; in Jordan, 186-187; in Lebanon, 187-190
Burghul, 21, 189

Calorie supply, 26
Cereals, 20
Chromium, 164-165
Codex Alimentarius Commission, 287
Communicable diseases: in Arab countries, 16-17. *See also* names of specific diseases, e.g., Malaria
Cornea, xerosis, 101, 102
Crops. *See* Food production

Dairy husbandry, 24
Dietary habits: in Egypt, 214-226, 237-238; in Iraq, 269-273; in Jordan, 234-238; in Lebanon, 230-234; in Libya, 226-230, 237-238; in the Near East, 213
Doctors, ratio to population, 17
Dwarfism, *See* Growth retardation

305

Economic situation, 13–14
Education: in Arab countries, 12–13; role in nutritional status, 265; trained nutrition personnel needed, 302–303
Eggs, 23
Eye: manifestations of vitamin A deficiency, 101, 108–111, 256. See also names of diseases, e.g., Trachoma

FAFA, 169–170
Feeding: industrial, 297–298; industrial, in Egypt, 298; industrial, in Jordan, 299; institutional, 292; refugees, 299–302; school meals, 292–293; school meals in Egypt, 293–294; school meals in Iraq, 294–295; school meals in Libya, 295–297; unhygienic practices, 146. See also Breast-feeding
Fish, 23–24
Follicular hyperkeratosis, 101, 257
Food: adulteration, 283; composition, 32–33; consumption patterns. See Dietary habits; Food Balance Sheets, 25–26; imports, 25; need for enrichment, 285; processing, 284–285; production, 6–7, 13, 14, 19–33; production in Iraq, 267; production improvement needed, 282
Food standards and laws: in Egypt, 286–287; in Jordan, 286; in Lebanon, 286; need, 285–287
Fruits, 25, 119, 267

GNP, 14
Gastroenteritis, 175, 177
Goiter: in Egypt, 86–91; in Jordan, 96–97; in Lebanon, 91–95; in Libya, 91; in oases, 86
Goiter, endemic: definition, 85; 4 categories, 85; in Iraq, 277–279; iodization of salt not adopted, 288
Growth rate: school-age children and adolescents, 200–211; of children 2–6 years, 199–200; of Egyptian infants, 194–195, 197; of Iraqi infants and children, 273–275; of Jordanian infants, 197–199; of Lebanese infants, 196–199
Growth retardation: and hookworm, 122; and zinc deficiency, 123–125; of Egyptian infants and children, 194–195, 241; hemoglobin values, 61; in marasmus, 144; in protein-calorie-deficiency disease, 146, 147

Health situation, 14–17

Height of children, 200–211
Hemoglobin: levels in Egyptian population, 58–61, 66–67; levels in the oases, 66; values for Egyptian population, 58; values in growth retardation, 61
Hookworm: and anemia, 63–65; and growth retardation, 122; and pellagra, 38, 50, 51
Hyperkeratosis follicularis. See Follicular hyperkeratosis
Hypoglycemia, 180

Illiteracy, 265
Immunization programs, 17
INCAPARINA, 169
Indicative World Plan for Agricultural Development, 32
Industry: in Arab countries, 13–14; feeding, 297–299; nutritional status of workers in Egypt, 241–242
Infants: birth weights and lengths, 192–199; in Iraq, nutritional status, 273–275; infantile pellagra, 145n; mortality, 15
Infections, 177–179
Iodine: deficiency in Lebanon, 94; in Egyptian water, 89; requirement, 84
Iodization of salt, 287–288
Iron: deficiency in Libya, Lebanon, Jordan, 73–80; deficiency, and pellagra, 50; treatment of marasmus, 179

Keratinization, 101
Keratomalacia, 101–103 passim
Khubz balady, 21
Kishk, 21
Kuwait, 208
Kwashiorkor: and anemia, 70–72, 76–79; and xerophthalmia, 110; associated infections, 157–158, 177–179; biochemical investigations in Egypt, 150–155; clinical features, 144, 142–144, 147–149; dietary management, 178–179; enlarged liver, 155–156; global importance, 142; prevalence in Egypt, 145–146; rehydration programs, 175–177

Lactation. See Pregnancy
Land: geography, 3–7, 19; reforms, 11
Language, 10
Legumes, 23
Liver, 148, 155–156

Maize: and pellagra, 41–44, 50; bread, 22; crop, 20; fortification of flour with nicotinic acid, 289; mold infected, 283; treated with lime water, 49

Index

Malaria, 16
Marasmus: and growth retardation, 144; and protein-calorie malnutrition, 76, 79; and xeropthalmia, 110; associated conditions, 157–158, 177–179; biochemical investigations, 150–155; dietary management, 178–179; in Egypt, 149–150; rehydration programs, 175–177; treatment, 178–181
Maternal and Child-health (MCH) services, 290–291
Meat, 23–24
Mental disease, 35, 53
Milk and milk products, 24–25, 77, 158, 178
Milk substitutes, 160–161, 164, 166–167, 189, 190
Mineral resources, 13

Najjar's solution, 176
National Institute of Nutrition of Iraq, 268
Net Protein Utilization (NPU), 29
Niacin deficiency, 49
Nicotinic acid: fortification of maize flour, 289; role in causation of pellagra, 35, 49
Night blindness. *See* Xerophthalmia
Nutrition Committee of Egypt, 240
Nutrition Institute of Egypt, 240
Nutrition recovery syndrome, 180
Nutrition surveys: in Egypt, 240–245, 262–265; in Iraq, 268, 270; in Jordan, 246–247, 254–265; in Lebanon, 246–247, 251–254, 262–265; in Libya, 247–251, 262–265
Nutritional rehabilitation centers, 291–292
Nuts, 25. *See also* Peanuts

Oases: dietary habits, 218; growth pattern of children, 205–207; hemoglobin levels of populations, 66; nutritional deficiency in school children, 244; parasitic infections, 66. *See also* under names of diseases, e.g., Ankylostomiasis
Oil, 13
Oil seeds, 25
Osteomalacia, 113

PCM. *See* Protein-calorie malnutrition
Parasitism: and anemia in Egypt, 61–66; and protein-calorie malnutrition, 158; in Iraq, 275–277; in oases, 66. *See also* names of diseases, e.g., Bilharziasis
Pasta, 21–22

Peanut preparation: treatment of protein-calorie malnutrition, 160
Peanuts, 25, 283–284
Pellagra: and ankylostomiasis, 37–38; and schizophrenia, 53; and zinc deficiency, 123; caused by maize diets, 50; effect of solar radiation, 52–53; etiology in Egypt, 41–51; first recorded account in Egypt, 36; gastrointestinal absorption function, 54; in Arab countries, 36; in prisoners of war, 49; in refugees, 45; infantile, 145n; mental aspects, 35, 53; neurological symptoms, 54; prevalence in Egypt, 36–41, 49–51; prevention by fortification of maize flour with nicotinic acid, 289; rare in Central America, 49; seasonal variations, 51; symptoms, 34–35; 1954 survey in Egypt, 57
People (racial stock), 7–9
Personnel: need for trained personnel, 302–303; shortage, 17
Pests, 282–284
Plasma transfusion, 159, 180
Population, 10–12
Pregnancy: and anemia, 67–70, 75; and zinc deficiency, 133; diets in, 221–226; need for nutrition-rehabilitation services, 290–291; nutritional deficiencies, 252; plasma ascorbic acid levels, 117
Prisoners of war and pellagra, 49
Protein: and pellagra, 44–48; food production, 29
Protein-calorie malnutrition: and anemia, 70–71, 76–80; and zinc deficiency, 123, 131–133; associated infections, 157–158, 177–179; biochemical investigations, 150–155; deaths, 161–162; etiology and course, 146–147; first use of term, 142; histopathological changes, 156–157; in Egypt, 144–145; in infants in Middle East, 131–133; in Iraqi infants and children, 273–275; in Jordan, 163–165, 254–256; in Lebanon, 165–167; in Libya, 162; in Sudan, 162–163; milk substitutes in treatment, 160–161; treatment, 158–161, 164, 166–167, 178–181

Racial stock, 7–9
Refugees: feeding, 299–302; pellagra, 45
Rehydration, 175–177
Religion, 9–10
Rice, 20, 22

Rickets: and marasmus, 179; classical studies, 111; in Egypt, 112–115; in Egyptian infants, 242; in Lebanese refugee infants, 254

Salt, iodization, 287–288
Schistosomiasis: and pellagra, 50, 51; in Egypt, 62, 65
Schizophrenia and pellagra, 53
School meals. *See under* feeding
Scurvy, 116–119
Skin: in protein-calorie deficiency disease, 156–157; keratinization, 101; signs of nutritional deficiencies, 243, 244, 245, 251, 257
Solar radiation, 52–53
Sorghum: and pellagra, 50; cereal, 22; crop, 20
Sudan, protein-calorie malnutrition, 162–163
Sugar, 25

Thyroid gland: 4 categories of enlargement, 85; function, 84. *See also* Goiter, and Goiter, endemic
Trachoma, 17, 157
Tryptophan, 48, 49
Tuberculosis, 157, 177, 179

UNRWA, 246, 300–302

Vegetables, 23, 119, 267
Vitamin A: deficiency, effects, 101–102; deficiency in Jordan, 106–111, 256; deficiency in Lebanon, 106; deficiency in Libya, 106; deficiency, ocular manifestations, 101, 108–110; fortification of foods needed, 288–289; intake, 100; sources, 99; treatment of protein-calorie malnutrition, 179
Vitamin B: deficiency, and pellagra, 53, 54; treatment of protein-calorie malnutrition, 179
Vitamin B_{12}, 77
Vitamin C. *See* Ascorbic acid
Vitamin D: deficiency, 111–115; treatment of protein-calorie malnutrition, 179
Vitamin E, 77, 78, 79, 80

Weaning:foods, 167–170; practices, 184–190
Weight of children, 200–211. *See also* Birth weights and lengths
Wheat, 20, 21, flour, fortification needed, 288

Xerophthalmia: in Egypt, 102–104; in Jordan, 106–111; in Lebanon, 106; symptom of vitamin A deficiency, 101, 179

Zinc: biochemistry, 134–136; deficiency, and protein-calorie malnutrition, 123, 131–133; deficiency, clinical features, 123–125; deficiency, history, 122–123; deficiency, in pregnancy, 133; deficiency, laboratory examination, 125–129; deficiency, public health significance, 136–137; deficiency, treatment, 130–133; physiology, 133–134